An Integrated Approach on Cerebral Venous Sinus Thrombosis (CVST)

An Integrated Approach on Cerebral Venous Sinus Thrombosis (CVST)

Guest Editors

Dragos Catalin Jianu
Jean Claude Sadik
Dafin Fior Mureşanu

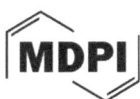

Basel • Beijing • Wuhan • Barcelona • Belgrade • Novi Sad • Cluj • Manchester

Guest Editors

Dragos Catalin Jianu
Department of Neurosciences
"Victor Babes" University of
Medicine and Pharmacy
Timisoara
Romania

Jean Claude Sadik
Department of
Radiology-Imaging
Foundation Ophtalmologique
"Adolphe de Rothschild"
Hospital
Paris
France

Dafin Fior Mureşanu
Department of Neurosciences
"Iuliu Hatieganu" University
of Medicine and Pharmacy
Cluj-Napoca
Romania

Editorial Office
MDPI AG
Grosspeteranlage 5
4052 Basel, Switzerland

This is a reprint of the Special Issue, published open access by the journal *Life* (ISSN 2075-1729), freely accessible at: www.mdpi.com/journal/life/special_issues/cvst.

For citation purposes, cite each article independently as indicated on the article page online and using the guide below:

Lastname, A.A.; Lastname, B.B. Article Title. *Journal Name* **Year**, *Volume Number*, Page Range.

ISBN 978-3-7258-3744-1 (Hbk)
ISBN 978-3-7258-3743-4 (PDF)
https://doi.org/10.3390/books978-3-7258-3743-4

© 2025 by the authors. Articles in this book are Open Access and distributed under the Creative Commons Attribution (CC BY) license. The book as a whole is distributed by MDPI under the terms and conditions of the Creative Commons Attribution-NonCommercial-NoDerivs (CC BY-NC-ND) license (https://creativecommons.org/licenses/by-nc-nd/4.0/).

Contents

About the Editors vii

Preface ix

Dragos Catalin Jianu, Silviana Nina Jianu, Traian Flavius Dan, Georgiana Munteanu, Alexandra Copil and Claudiu Dumitru Birdac et al.
An Integrated Approach on the Diagnosis of Cerebral Veins and Dural Sinuses Thrombosis (a Narrative Review)
Reprinted from: *Life* **2022**, *12*, 717, https://doi.org/10.3390/life12050717 1

Jean-Claude Sadik, Dragos Catalin Jianu, Raphaël Sadik, Yvonne Purcell, Natalia Novaes and Edouard Saragoussi et al.
Imaging of Cerebral Venous Thrombosis
Reprinted from: *Life* **2022**, *12*, 1215, https://doi.org/10.3390/life12081215 25

Natalia Novaes, Raphaël Sadik, Jean-Claude Sadik and Michaël Obadia
Epidemiology and Management of Cerebral Venous Thrombosis during the COVID-19 Pandemic
Reprinted from: *Life* **2022**, *12*, 1105, https://doi.org/10.3390/life12081105 45

Dragos Catalin Jianu, Silviana Nina Jianu, Nicoleta Iacob, Traian Flavius Dan, Georgiana Munteanu and Anca Elena Gogu et al.
Diagnosis and Management of Cerebral Venous Thrombosis Due to Polycythemia Vera and Genetic Thrombophilia: Case Report and Literature Review
Reprinted from: *Life* **2023**, *13*, 1074, https://doi.org/10.3390/life13051074 57

Adina Stan, Silvina Ilut, Hanna Maria Dragos, Claudia Bota, Patricia Nicoleta Hanghicel and Alexander Cristian et al.
The Burden of Cerebral Venous Thrombosis in a Romanian Population across a 5-Year Period
Reprinted from: *Life* **2022**, *12*, 1825, https://doi.org/10.3390/life12111825 70

Georgiana Munteanu, Andrei Gheorghe Marius Motoc, Traian Flavius Dan, Anca Elena Gogu and Dragos Catalin Jianu
Aphasic Syndromes in Cerebral Venous and Dural Sinuses Thrombosis—A Review of the Literature
Reprinted from: *Life* **2022**, *12*, 1684, https://doi.org/10.3390/life12111684 82

Sorin Tuță
Cerebral Venous Outflow Implications in Idiopathic Intracranial Hypertension—From Physiopathology to Treatment
Reprinted from: *Life* **2022**, *12*, 854, https://doi.org/10.3390/life12060854 93

Any Docu Axelerad, Lavinia Alexandra Zlotea, Carmen Adella Sirbu, Alina Zorina Stroe, Silviu Docu Axelerad and Simona Claudia Cambrea et al.
Case Reports of Pregnancy-Related Cerebral Venous Thrombosis in the Neurology Department of the Emergency Clinical Hospital in Constanta
Reprinted from: *Life* **2022**, *12*, 90, https://doi.org/10.3390/life12010090 115

Timothy C. Frommeyer, Tongfan Wu, Michael M. Gilbert, Garrett V. Brittain and Stephen P. Fuqua
Cerebral Venous Sinus Thrombosis Following an mRNA COVID-19 Vaccination and Recent Oral Contraceptive Use
Reprinted from: *Life* **2023**, *13*, 464, https://doi.org/10.3390/life13020464 129

Florentina Cristina Pleșa, Alina Jijie, Gabriela Simona Toma, Aurelian Emilian Ranetti, Aida Mihaela Manole and Ruxandra Rotaru et al.
Challenges in Cerebral Venous Thrombosis Management—Case Reports and Short Literature Review
Reprinted from: *Life* **2023**, *13*, 334, https://doi.org/10.3390/life13020334 . . . . **137**

About the Editors

Dragos Catalin Jianu

Dragoş Cătălin Jianu is a professor of neurology, MD, Ph.D., Dr. Habil., Ph.D., coordinator, head of the Advanced Centre for Cognitive Research in Neuropsychiatric Pathology, and head of the first division of neurology, Department of Neurosciences, "Victor Babes" University of Medicine and Pharmacy, Timişoara, Romania. He is a senior consultant neurologist, certified in neurosonology, and head of the first department of neurology at the "Pius Branzeu" Clinical Emergency County Hospital, Timisoara, Romania.

His research topics include the following: 1) Ischemic stroke: a) large-artery diseases/extra and transcranial Doppler sonography (TIPIC syndrome, carotid body paragangliomas, congenital anomalies of supra-aortic arteries, giant cell arteritis with large artery involvement, and extracranial and intracranial arterial stenoses); b) small-artery diseases (cerebral vessel endothelial dysfunction in patients with type 2 diabetes mellitus and chronic kidney disease); c) cerebral veins and dural sinuses thrombosis (inherited thrombophilia, emissary veins, cavernous sinus thrombosis, and lateral sinus thrombosis); and d) cardio-embolic stroke. 2) Neuro-ophthalmology/color Doppler imaging of orbital vessels: anterior ischemic optic neuropathies, central retinal artery occlusion, and giant cell arteritis with eye involvement. 3) Vascular aphasias, including aphasias in cerebral venous thrombosis, examination procedures (Western Aphasia Battery, Romanian version), and rehabilitation. 4) Vascular cognitive impairment: mild cognitive impairment and cognitive dysfunction in young subjects with periodontal disease. 5) Parkinson's disease: management of the patients with advanced Parkinson's disease.

Jean Claude Sadik

Jean-Claude Sadik, M.D., Ph.D., is a senior consultant radiologist, and head of the Department of Radiology Imaging, Foundation Ophtalmologique "Adolphe de Rothschild" Hospital, Paris, Île-de-France, France.

His interests include the following: stroke; noninvasive explorations of large-artery diseases/extra- and transcranial Doppler sonography; cerebral venous thrombosis; neuro-ophthalmology; and color Doppler imaging of orbital vessels.

Dafin Fior Mureşanu

Fior-Dafin Muresanu is a professor of Neurology, M.D., Ph.D., MBA, and senior consultant neurologist. He is the president of the European Federation of NeuroRehabilitation Societies (EFNR); co-chair at the EAN Scientific Panel Neurorehabilitation; past president of the Romanian Society of Neurology; chairman at the "Iuliu Hatieganu" University of Medicine and Pharmacy, Cluj-Napoca, Romania; chairman at the "RoNeuro" Institute for Neurological Research and Diagnostic, Cluj-Napoca, Romania; and president of the Society for the Study of Neuroprotection and Neuroplasticity (SSNN).

His interests include the following: cerebrovascular diseases, neurodegenerative diseases, traumatic brain injury, brain protection and Recovery, neurorehabilitation, and neuroimmunology.

Preface

Cerebral vein and intracranial dural sinus thrombosis (CVT) is a relatively uncommon disease in the general population. At least one risk factor can be identified in 85% of CVT cases. Searching for a thrombophilic state should be realized for patients with CVT who present a high pretest probability of severe thrombophilia. Two pathophysiological mechanisms determine their highly variable clinical spectrum, i.e., the augmentation of venular and capillary pressure and the diminution of cerebrospinal fluid absorption. The clinical spectrum of CVT is usually non-specific. The following four major syndromes have been observed: isolated intracranial hypertension, seizures, focal neurological signs, and encephalopathy. Cavernous sinus thrombosis represents the only CVT that produces a characteristic clinical syndrome.

Non-enhanced computer tomography (NECT) of the head is the most frequently performed imaging technique in the emergency department. CVT diagnosis is confirmed with CT venography (CTV), directly detecting the venous clot as a filling defect, or magnetic resonance imaging (MRI)/MR venography (MR-V), which also realizes a better description of parenchymal abnormalities.

Acute-phase therapy for CVT focuses on anticoagulation, the management of seizures and increased intracranial pressure, and the prevention of cerebral herniation. The majority of patients have a complete or partial recovery; however, they have an increased incidence of venous thromboembolism. Clinical and imaging follow-ups 3–6 months after diagnosis are recommended to assess for recanalization.

Dragos Catalin Jianu, Jean Claude Sadik, and Dafin Fior Mureşanu
Guest Editors

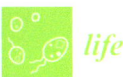

Review

An Integrated Approach on the Diagnosis of Cerebral Veins and Dural Sinuses Thrombosis (a Narrative Review)

Dragos Catalin Jianu [1,2,3,4], **Silviana Nina Jianu** [5], **Traian Flavius Dan** [1,2,3,*], **Georgiana Munteanu** [1,2,3], **Alexandra Copil** [2,3], **Claudiu Dumitru Birdac** [2,3], **Andrei Gheorghe Marius Motoc** [2,6], **Any Docu Axelerad** [2,7], **Ligia Petrica** [2,4,8], **Sergiu Florin Arnautu** [2,3,9], **Raphael Sadik** [10], **Nicoleta Iacob** [11] and **Anca Elena Gogu** [1,2,3]

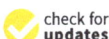

Citation: Jianu, D.C.; Jianu, S.N.; Dan, T.F.; Munteanu, G.; Copil, A.; Birdac, C.D.; Motoc, A.G.M.; Docu Axelerad, A.; Petrica, L.; Arnautu, S.F.; et al. An Integrated Approach on the Diagnosis of Cerebral Veins and Dural Sinuses Thrombosis (a Narrative Review). *Life* **2022**, *12*, 717. https://doi.org/10.3390/life12050717

Academic Editor: Nicola Smania

Received: 10 March 2022
Accepted: 9 May 2022
Published: 11 May 2022

Publisher's Note: MDPI stays neutral with regard to jurisdictional claims in published maps and institutional affiliations.

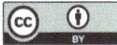

Copyright: © 2022 by the authors. Licensee MDPI, Basel, Switzerland. This article is an open access article distributed under the terms and conditions of the Creative Commons Attribution (CC BY) license (https://creativecommons.org/licenses/by/4.0/).

1. Department of Neurosciences-Division of Neurology, Victor Babes University of Medicine and Pharmacy, E. Murgu Sq., no.2, 300041 Timisoara, Romania; jianu.dragos@umft.ro (D.C.J.); georgiana.munteanu@umft.ro (G.M.); anca.gogu@umft.ro (A.E.G.)
2. Centre for Cognitive Research in Neuropsychiatric Pathology (NeuroPsy-Cog), Department of Neurosciences, Victor Babes University of Medicine and Pharmacy, 156 L. Rebreanu Ave., 300736 Timisoara, Romania; alexandra.copil@yahoo.com (A.C.); claudiubirdac8@gmail.com (C.D.B.); amotoc@umft.ro (A.G.M.M.); axelerad.docu@365.univ-ovidius.ro (A.D.A.); petrica.ligia@umft.ro (L.P.); arnautu.sergiu@umft.ro (S.F.A.)
3. First Department of Neurology, Pius Branzeu Clinical Emergency County Hospital, 156 L. Rebreanu Ave., 300736 Timisoara, Romania
4. Centre for Molecular Research in Nephrology and Vascular Pathology, Department of Internal Medicine II, Victor Babes University of Medicine and Pharmacy, 156 L. Rebreanu Ave., 300736 Timisoara, Romania
5. Department of Ophthalmology, Dr. Victor Popescu Military Emergency Hospital, 7 G. Lazar Ave, 300080 Timisoara, Romania; silvianajianu@yahoo.com
6. Department of Anatomy and Embryology, Victor Babeș University of Medicine and Pharmacy, E. Murgu Sq., no.2, 300041 Timisoara, Romania
7. Department of Neurology, General Medicine Faculty, Ovidius University, 900527 Constanța, Romania
8. Department of Internal Medicine II-Division of Nephrology, Victor Babeș University of Medicine and Pharmacy, E. Murgu Sq., no.2, 300041 Timișoara, Romania
9. Department of Internal Medicine I, Victor Babeș University of Medicine and Pharmacy, E. Murgu Sq., no.2, 300041 Timișoara, Romania
10. Department of Geriatrics-Rehabilitation, Riviera-Chablais Hospital, 3 Prairie Av, 1800 Vevey, Switzerland; raphaelsadik@hopitalrivierachablais.ch
11. Department of Multidetector Computed Tomography and Magnetic Resonance Imaging, Neuromed Diagnostic Imaging Centre, 300218 Timișoara, Romania; nicoiacob@yahoo.co.uk
* Correspondence: traian.dan@umft.ro; Tel.: +40-745035178

Abstract: (1) Objective: This review paper aims to discuss multiple aspects of cerebral venous thrombosis (CVT), including epidemiology, etiology, pathophysiology, and clinical presentation. Different neuroimaging methods for diagnosis of CVT, such as computer tomography CT/CT Venography (CTV), and Magnetic Resonance Imaging (MRI)/MR Venography (MRV) will be presented. (2) Methods: A literature analysis using PubMed and the MEDLINE sub-engine was done using the terms: cerebral venous thrombosis, thrombophilia, and imaging. Different studies concerning risk factors, clinical picture, and imaging signs of patients with CVT were examined. (3) Results: At least one risk factor can be identified in 85% of CVT cases. Searching for a thrombophilic state should be realized for patients with CVT who present a high pretest probability of severe thrombophilia. Two pathophysiological mechanisms contribute to their highly variable clinical presentation: augmentation of venular and capillary pressure, and diminution of cerebrospinal fluid absorption. The clinical spectrum of CVT is frequently non-specific and presents a high level of clinical suspicion. Four major syndromes have been described: isolated intracranial hypertension, seizures, focal neurological abnormalities, and encephalopathy. Cavernous sinus thrombosis is the single CVT that presents a characteristic clinical syndrome. Non-enhanced CT (NECT) of the Head is the most frequently performed imaging study in the emergency department. Features of CVT on NECT can be divided into direct signs (demonstration of dense venous clot within a cerebral vein or a cerebral venous sinus), and more frequently indirect signs (such as cerebral edema, or cerebral venous infarct). CVT diagnosis is confirmed with CTV, directly detecting the venous clot as a filling defect, or MRI/MRV, which also realizes a better description of parenchymal abnormalities. (4) Conclusions: CVT is a relatively rare disorder in the general population and is frequently misdiagnosed upon initial examination. The knowledge of wide clinical aspects and imaging signs will be essential in providing a timely diagnosis.

Keywords: cerebral veins and dural sinuses thrombosis (CVT); thrombophilia; headache; native and contrast-enhanced Head Computed Tomography (CT); Magnetic Resonance Imaging (MRI) of the Head; Magnetic Resonance (MR) Venography

1. Introduction
1.1. Background

While rare in the adult population, but far more common than previously known, cerebral venous thrombosis (CVT) presents a higher frequency among young adults, children, patients with thrombophilia, pregnant women, puerperium, or women with oral contraceptives therapy [1–3].

The clinical spectrum of CVT can be highly variable and usually not specific [4–6]. CVT cases rarely present as an arterial stroke syndrome, which is an acute onset of focal neurological deficits associated with classic vascular risk factors [1–3].

Because CVT can be produced by multiple predisposing causes and precipitants, it may be encountered not only by neurologists, and neurosurgeons, but also by ear, nose, and throat specialists, ophthalmologists, obstetricians, oncologists, hematologists, rheumatologists, emergency clinicians, family practitioners, and pediatricians [5–7]. Different imaging techniques are essential in accurately diagnosing patients with clinically suspected CVT. These are represented by native and contrast-enhanced Head Computed Tomography (CT), CT Venography (CTV), Magnetic Resonance Imaging (MRI) of the Head combined with MR Venography (MRV), and, in peculiar cases, cerebral intra-arterial angiography with venous phase imaging, direct cerebral venography, or ultrasound (US) [3–5].

This paper will review the cerebral veins and dural sinuses anatomy, the epidemiology, etiology, pathophysiology, and clinical and imagistic aspects of CVT. The advantages and disadvantages of each imaging method will be analyzed to help the neurologists and radiologists in the selection of the most adequate method/methods to establish a faster and more accurate diagnosis in each peculiar CVT case [5–7].

1.2. Cerebral Veins and Dural Sinuses Anatomy

Familiarity with the anatomic variants of cerebral veins and dural sinuses is essential to accurately detect CVT.

1.2.1. Cerebral Veins

The cerebral veins are represented by three groups: the superficial cerebral venous system, the deep cerebral venous system, and the posterior fossa veins. (Figure 1) [1,8].

In contrast with other veins, including the internal jugular veins (IJV), the cerebral veins develop certain peculiarities that can explain some of the clinical aspects of CVT. On one hand, the cortical veins, and the posterior fossa veins present wide anatomic variability (in number, location, and anastomoses), thus explaining why the angiographic diagnosis of their isolated occlusion is very difficult. On the other hand, the occlusion of the deep cerebral veins is easy to detect, because these veins (with the exception of the anatomic variations of the basal veins) are constant and are always detected at angiography [1,8].

Cerebral veins have thin walls, without a muscular tunic, possess no valves, and are linked by different anastomoses, which enable both their dilatation and the inversion of venous flow toward the brain if there is an occlusion of the sinus into which they empty. Thus, the presence of anastomoses allows the development of collateral venous circulation in the situation of vessel occlusion, explaining the good prognosis in such patients [1,8].

1.2.2. Intracranial Dural Sinuses

They are divided into two groups: the posterior-superior, and the antero-inferior. (Figure 1) The former group includes the Superior Sagittal Sinus (SSS), Inferior Sagittal Sinus (ISS), Lateral Sinus (LS), consisting of transverse sinus and sigmoid sinus, Straight Sinus (SS), and occipital sinus; the torcular Herophili represents the junction of SSS, SS, transverse sinus, and occipital sinus and is frequently asymmetrical [1,8,9]. The latter group comprises the cavernous sinus, and the superior and inferior petrosal sinuses. The great majority of the cerebral venous blood collects posteriorly, from the SSS or the SS into the LSs, and only a smaller part flows to the cavernous sinuses [1,8].

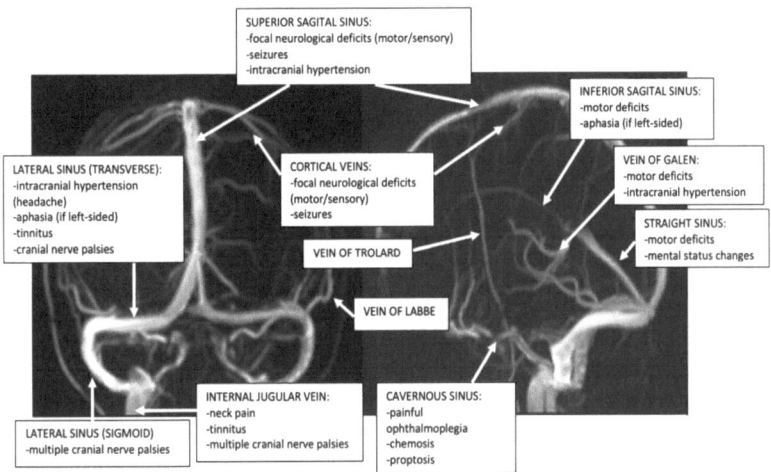

Figure 1. Dural sinuses and cerebral veins anatomy and major clinical syndromes according to the topography of CVT (archive of the First Department of Neurology, Clinical Emergency County Hospital, Timisoara, Romania).

The intracranial dural sinuses drain in adults into the two IJV, for the supine position, and into the vertebral venous system for the upright position [10].

2. Material and Methods

A literature search using PubMed and the MEDLINE sub-engine was completed using the terms: cerebral venous thrombosis, thrombophilia, and imaging. Different studies concerning epidemiology, etiology-risk factors, pathophysiology, clinical diagnosis, laboratory data, and imaging signs of patients with CVT were included.

3. Results

3.1. Epidemiology

No epidemiologic studies of CVT own the needed criteria for a good quality epidemiologic stroke study, due to multiple factors, including the wide clinical spectrum of CVT, frequently with subacute onset [6,11,12].

CVT represents only less than 1% of all strokes [12], its prevalence is higher than previously noted, due to an increased awareness of this type of disease among clinicians, and to improved and more accessible imaging methods, including MRI/MRV, for the examination of patients with unclear neurological clinical aspects, such as headache and seizures [6,11–14].

Annual incidence is noted to be between 0.22 to 1.57 per 100,000 citizens [11] and is sex-independent in children and the elderly [6,7]. CVT is more frequent in children (especially in neonates) than in adults [6,7]. In adults, CVT is observed in patients who are younger on average than those with arterial types of stroke [6]. Thus, in the International

Study on Cerebral Vein and Dural Sinus Thrombosis (ISCVT) cohort, the median age was 37 years [7], and only 8% of the patients were older than 65 [15]. Compared with men, women were significantly younger (median age of 34 years, vs. 42 years for men) [13]. In adult cases of the ISCVT cohort, CVT presented a female predominance (3:1) [9], which was higher between 31 to 50 years because of augmented risk attributed to a prothrombotic condition [6,7].

3.2. Etiology-Risk Factors

The most frequent risk factors detected in elder people with CVT are thrombophilia, neoplasms, and hematologic disorders [15,16].

In the Canadian pediatric ischemic stroke registry, a risk factor was detected in 98% of the children. Thrombophilia was found in 41% of all cases. In infants older than four weeks of age and children head and neck diseases, especially infections and chronic systemic diseases (e.g., connective tissue diseases, hematologic disorders, or malignancy) were frequent [17].

Different factors can determine or predispose adults to develop CVT (in 85% of cases at least one risk factor can be found), and in about half of CVT cases, they present multiple risk factors. For this reason, the detection of a cause or a risk factor should not stop a search for others [7]. The most common risk factors are represented by: genetic thrombophilia, oral contraceptives (OC), pregnancy, puerperium, malignancy, and infections [7,12]. Thus, a prothrombotic condition was detected in one-third of all cases of the ISCVT cohort, and a genetic thrombophilia was reported in 22% of all cases [7].

3.2.1. Genetic Thrombophilia

According to Marjot et al., the risk for CVT depends on the individual's genetic background [18]. If different prothrombotic aspects are noted, patients present an increased risk of CVT when they are exposed to a precipitant factor such as head trauma, pregnancy, infection, etc. [6].

The major genetic trombophilias as prothrombotic conditions include the following: factor V Leiden (FVL) pathologic variant; [17,19,20] G20210 A prothrombin gene pathologic variant; [17,20–22]; hyperhomocysteinemia; [23] antithrombin deficiency; [24] and protein C or protein S deficiencies [16,25].

In a meta-analysis of case-control studies, with more than 200 neonates and children with CVT, and 1200 control subjects, the prevalence of FVL variant among patients with CVT and controls was 12.8% and 3.6%, respectively, and carriers of the FVL variant were significantly more likely to present CVT (odds ratio [OR] 3.1, 95% CI 1.8–5.5) [26]. In the same meta-analysis, the prevalence of the G20210 A prothrombin gene pathologic variant among all patients and controls was 5.2% and 2.5%, respectively, and carriers were significantly more likely to develop CVT (OR 3.1, 95% CI 1.4–6.8) [26].

The association of hyperhomocysteinemia due to different genetic variants in methylene tetrahydrofolate reductase (MTHFR) with CVT is controversial [18,21,26]. On one hand, in a meta-analysis of case-control studies, Gouveia and Canhão reported that the frequency of the *MTHFR 677C > T* polymorphism in adults was similar for 382 cases with CVT compared with 1217 controls (15.7% vs. 14.6%; OR 1.12, 95% CI 0.8–1.58), thus indicating that the *MTHFR 677C > T* polymorphism is not a risk factor for CVT [27]. On the other hand, Marjot et al., asserted in a meta-analysis, after controlling for heterogeneity among studies, that the *MTHFR 677C > T* polymorphism was associated with CVT [OR 2.30, 95% CI 1.20–4.42) [18,28].

There is no association of CVT with PAI-1 or protein Z polymorphisms [6,29].

Acquired Thrombophilia

According to different studies, the most frequent acquired thrombophilia are due to pregnancy, puerperium, OC, and malignancy [30,31].

3.2.2. Pregnancy and Puerperium

In high-income countries, between 5–20% of all CVT patients present risk factors for pregnancy and puerperium; for example, in the ISCVT cohort, these risk factors appeared in 15% of all CVT patients [7]. In low-income countries, puerperium is the most frequent risk factor for CVT, with 31% of patients [32–35]. There are multiple favorable conditions, including the absence of antenatal care, home delivery, and depletion of vitamin and protein stores [32–35]. Usually, CVT appears in the third trimester or, more frequently, in the first three weeks after delivery. In the majority of cases, CVT could be associated with pulmonary embolism and/or lower extremity or pelvic phlebothrombosis, due to the hypercoagulability and the venous stasis that appear during pregnancy [32–35]. At this stage a significant increase of fibrinogen and different coagulation factors and a notable diminution of antithrombin III and plasminogen occurs. This state of hypercoagulability is accentuated during early puerperium due to multiple causes, including trauma-induced by instrumental delivery or cesarean section, volume depletion, and infections favored by precarious hygienic conditions at home. Pelvic phlebothrombosis may produce CVT via the venous plexuses of the vertebral channel, and the basilar venous plexus [32–35].

3.2.3. Therapy with Estrogens, such as Hormonal OC or Replacement Therapy

The most common risk factor for CVT in younger women is the use of OC [36,37]. In 10% of such cases, OC represents the only identifiable risk factor [1,7]. In the remaining cases, there are other risk factors for CVT, associated with the OC, such as different vasculitis (systemic lupus erythematous-SLE, Behçet's disease), obesity, [38] or genetic thrombophilia; in this last situation, the risk of intra-, or extracerebral thrombosis is 6 times higher than that of non-users [7,39].

Different case reports noted the association between tamoxifen (which is an estrogen receptor modulator) and CVT [40].

In contrast to inherited thrombophilia, pregnancy and OC therapy represent transient risk factors for CVT and they are not linked with a higher risk for recurrence [32–35].

3.2.4. Malignancy Disorders

In the ISCVT cohort, cancers represented 7.4% of all CVT cases [7]. The most frequent malignancy disorders associated with CVT are solid tumors outside the Central Nervous System (CNS) (breast tumors, medullary carcinoma of the thyroid, nephroblastoma, Ewings tumor, gallbladder carcinoma), hematologic malignancies, and CNS malignancies (medulloblastoma) [12]. The main mechanisms are direct tumor compression or invasion of dural sinuses, leukostasis, the hypercoagulable state produced by augmentation in acute-phase reactants, or modified coagulation factors from chemotherapy (L-asparaginase, cisplatin), or hormonal drugs [6,12].

3.2.5. Hematologic Disorders

Different Philadelphia-negative myeloproliferative disorders (MPDs), such as polycythemia vera (PV) or essential thrombocythemia, present an augmented risk of venous thrombosis, including CVT. The acquired Janus kinase 2 V617F mutation (JAK2 V617F), which appears in more than 90% of patients with PV, produces an augmented incidence of severe CVT with a poor prognosis [41]. Other hematological disorders that can produce CVT are represented by paroxysmal nocturnal hemoglobinuria, heparin-induced thrombocytopenia, thrombotic thrombocytopenic purpura, essential thrombocytosis, different gammapathies, iron deficiency anemia, and myelofibrosis [12].

3.2.6. COVID-19 Infection and COVID-19 Vaccine-Associated CVT

COVID-19 Infection-Associated CVT

Some cases of CVT have been noted in the setting of SARS-CoV-2 infection, usually without other associated predisposing risk factors [42]. According to the European Medicines Agency safety committee report concerning a review of 34,331 patients hospitalized with SARS-CoV-2 infection, the frequency of CVT was 0.08% (95% CI 0.01–0.5). The in-hospital mortality was 40% [43].

COVID-19 Vaccination-Associated CVT

Vaccine-induced immune-mediated thrombocytopenia (VITT) represents an infrequent process of thrombosis associated with thrombocytopenia, frequently producing CVT, and splanchnic veins thrombosis, that has been observed after adenovirus vector vaccines against COVID-19: ChAdOx1 nCOV-19 (AstraZeneca) and Ad26.COV2·S Johnson and Johnson (Janssen/J&J) [44]. Although there have been a few reports of CVT after mRNA vaccines, these did not have the features of VITT and could have been incidental [45].

Perry et al. [45] observed in their study that when they are compared with those without VITT, patients with VITT-associated CVT were younger, presented fewer venous thrombosis risk factors, and were more likely to have been administrated the ChAdOx1 vaccine. They presented more extensive CVT with more cerebral veins or dural sinuses thrombosed, and multiple intracerebral hemorrhages (ICH) were more frequent. They were more likely to have concomitant extracranial venous (especially splanchnic veins) or arterial thromboses. Their outcomes at the end of hospital admission were worse, with higher rates of death and disability, ranging from 22% to 47% in studies, compared with 3% to 5% among those with other causes of CVT [45,46].

The diagnostic criteria for definite VITT-associated CVT are post-vaccine CVT (between 4 and 28 days after COVID-19 vaccination), thrombocytopenia (lowest recorded platelet count <150 $\times$ 10^9 per L or documented platelet count), anti-platelet factor four (PF4) antibodies (detected on ELISA or functional assay) [45–47].

Other laboratory data are represented by high levels of D-dimer (>4000 mcg/L) and disseminated intravascular coagulation-like coagulopathy with a tendency to hemorrhage [44].

3.2.7. Infections

In the past, loco-regional or systemic infections represented the main cause of CVT. Nowadays, in developed countries (especially due to higher accessibility to antibiotics) septic thrombosis of cerebral veins and dural sinuses in adults has become a rare (6% to 12% of cases), but sometimes severe disease [7,30].

In developing countries, different infections remain an important cause (18% of cases) [34]. Localized acute pyogenic infections of the middle third of the face (especially with Staphylococcus aureus), of the paranasal sinuses, mouth with multiple dental abscesses, ears (otitis media), mastoid air cells (mastoiditis), throat, or scalp can produce septic CVT, especially for the cavernous and lateral sinuses. In chronic CVT, the main identified germs are gram-negative or fungi (especially Aspergillus). Cerebral thrombophlebitis may also appear as a complication of meningitis, epidural, or brain abscesses, or after an open traumatic injury of the head, pelvic phlebothrombosis, or after systemic infectious diseases (trichinosis, human immunodeficiency virus or cytomegalovirus) [1].

3.2.8. Systemic Autoimmune Disorders

The most frequent are SLE, with or without the nephrotic syndrome, Behçet disease, Sjögren's syndrome, Wegener's granulomatosis, sarcoidosis, and inflammatory bowel disease [6,12].

3.2.9. Head Injury and Mechanical Precipitants

These are less common causes of CVT. Cerebral veins and dural sinuses could be occluded by different local factors, including head trauma (with local injury to cerebral sinuses or veins), brain tumors, arachnoid cysts, arterio-venous malformations, and by mechanical causes, such as neurosurgical procedures or systemic surgery, epidural blood patch, jugular venous cannulation, spontaneous intracranial hypotension, lumbar puncture [1,48].

3.2.10. No Identified Cause

There is still an important number of idiopathic CVT patients. According to ISCVT cohort data, in 13% of adult CVT cases, no risk factors could be identified [7]. The percentage of idiopathic CVT was higher for older patients (37%) [7,15]. No identified etiology or risk factor for CVT was noted in a minority of children ($\leq$10%) [17].

3.3. Pathophysiology

The main two pathophysiological mechanisms implied in CVT are diminution of CSF absorption, and increase of venular and capillary pressure [3,49–51] (Figure 2).

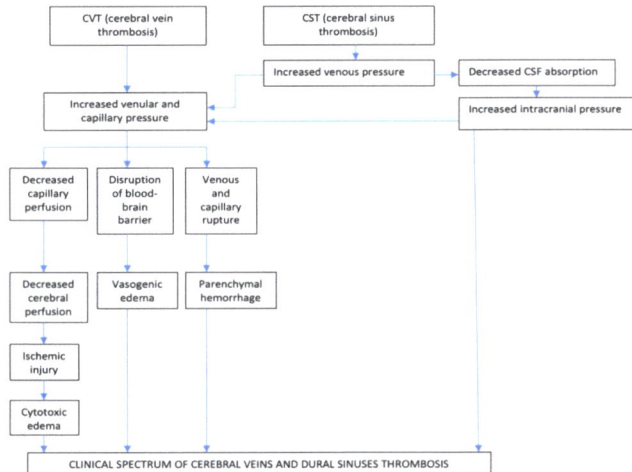

Figure 2. Pathophysiology of cerebral veins and dural sinuses thrombosis.

The Occlusion of the Intracranial Dural Sinuses May Determine a Diminution of CSF Absorption

The normal absorption of CSF is produced through arachnoid granulations, especially at the level of the SSS and LS. In the particular situation of dural sinuses occlusion, especially of the SSS and LS, appears a raise of the cerebral venous pressure, with subsequent diminution of CSF absorption which, consecutively, increases the intracranial pressure. This pathologic process produces a rise in venular and capillary hypertension and generates vasogenic and cytotoxic edema and cerebral hemorrhage [3,49–51].

The second mechanism is represented by the progressive increase of venular and capillary pressure.

This mechanism is the result of the thrombosis of dural sinuses and cerebral veins [3,49–51].

In the initial stages of venous obstruction, a diminished but still efficient perfusion of the correspondent brain tissue might be possible, due to the collateral venous circulation, which produces a significant degree of compensation, with consecutive neutralization of the pathological pressure modifications. For this reason, the corresponding areas of the brain can be functionally and metabolically affected, but not irreversibly injured [3,49–51]. As loco-regional venous pressure continues to increase, in the context of an ineffective collateral venous circulation, a rise of the thrombosis within cortical venous tributaries will reduce the cerebral perfusion pressure even more. Consequently, it will appear damage to the blood-brain barrier producing vasogenic edema, local ischemic lesions, cytotoxic edema, and venous and capillary lesions with consecutively parenchymal hemorrhage and, rarely, subarachnoid hemorrhages [3,49–51].

The diminution of the venous drainage consecutive to CVT determines raised venous pressure, with the backup of the fluid into the brain, producing vasogenic edema. This type of edema is situated within the extracellular compartment of the encephalic white matter/inside the glial cells, under the control of the hydrostatic pressure (augmented blood pressure and local blood flow) and osmotic gradients. Usually, the vasogenic edema does not produce neuronal lesions, because the fluid in excess in the extracellular space can, frequently, be removed [3,49–51].

Cytotoxic edema is produced by energy failure with a displacement of ions and water across the cell membranes into neurons. The intracellular edema, caused by ischemia, determines a great volume of dead or dying brain neurons with a bad prognosis [3,49–51].

In cerebral venous infarcts, the vasogenic edema represents the majority in comparison with the cytotoxic edema; these pathological aspects identified by diffusion-weighted imaging (DWI) confirm that the venous infarcts differ from arterial ones and present a significantly better recovery [1,49–51].

Brain edema and associated augmented intracranial pressure produce headache, vomiting, and diminished consciousness, but the most severe complications are represented by the pressure differences and the potential risk for brain herniation, which can determine death due to probable pressure-related lesions to neighboring areas [1].

The growth of the venous and capillary pressures produces vessel lesions and erythrocytes diapedesis due to disruptions of the blood-brain barrier both resulting in cerebral hemorrhage. The neuronal lesions determined by the cerebral hemorrhage induced by CVT are often milder than the damages induced by arterial infarcts [3,49–51].

Histological exam in CVT cases notes dilated cerebral veins, brain edema with flattened gyri, diminished sulci, compressed small ventricles, and ischemic neuronal lesions. The thrombus inside the cerebral veins is similar to other venous thrombi (when it is fresh, it presents a rich content in red blood cells and fibrin and a poor content in platelets; and, when it is chronic, it is replaced by fibrous tissue, frequently with recanalization) [1].

3.4. Clinical Diagnosis

The clinical spectrum and outcome of CVT are related to different factors: location and number of thrombosed sinuses and cerebral veins, as well as the presence of functional collateral pathways, absence or presence of parenchymal lesions (cytotoxic or vasogenic edema, hemorrhage), gender, age, etiology, and interval from onset to admission to hospital [4,6].

The clinical presentation of CVT can be polymorphous, and misleading. In the majority of cases (50–80% of patients), the onset is subacute [1,52].

3.4.1. Clinical Syndromes

In the majority of adult CVT cases, four major clinical syndromes have been noted in combination or isolation: Isolated intracranial hypertension, focal neurological deficits, seizures, and encephalopathy [1,2].

A minority of adult CVT patients develop a cavernous sinus thrombosis with a distinctive clinical picture: painful ophthalmoplegia. Collet-Siquard syndrome (consisting of multiple low cranial nerves palsies) represents a clinical syndrome of IJVs, posterior fossa veins, or LS thrombosis [1,2].

Rare adult CVT cases with unusual clinical aspects were also reported: subarachnoid hemorrhage, transient ischemic attacks, or psychiatric symptoms, mimicking a postpartum psychosis [1,2].

In neonates, CVT has a nonspecific clinical presentation with seizures, tetraparesis, and encephalopathy [17]. In older children, the clinical spectrum is more similar to the adult clinical aspects, with headache and paresis [53]. In elderly patients, symptoms of encephalopathy are more common than in adults, whereas isolated intracranial hypertension is less common [1,2].

Isolated Intracranial Hypertension

It is the most frequent clinical syndrome observed in CVT (40% of cases) [6]. It consists of headaches, associated with vomiting, papilledema, visual complaints, and sixth nerve palsy [54]. It is more common in patients with a chronic onset than in those cases that present acutely [55].

Headache is the most common symptom of CVT (about 90% of cases in the ISCVT cohort). It is usually the initial one, and can develop isolated, or can precede other symptoms or signs. Headache is more frequent in women and younger patients than in men or older patients [7,13,52,53]. The characteristics of headaches are polymorphic. It may be localized or diffused [54]. Frequently, headache is severe augmenting during the night and may worsen with Valsalva maneuvers or position changes (when the patient is lying down) [2,32].

However, its characteristics can be misleading, sometimes being initially diagnosed as a migraine with aura [56]. In a few cases, it occurs like a thunderclap headache (mimicking a subarachnoid hemorrhage) [57]. Some of the risk factors associated with CVT (such as meningitis, epidural or brain abscesses, meningiomas, dural arteriovenous fistulas, and different vasculitis) also clinically manifest as a headache. CVT must be suspected as a possible explanation of persisting headache after lumbar puncture because this maneuver can rarely precipitate a CVT [1]. Headache is noted more frequently in patients with CVT than in cases with cerebral arterial infarcts [1,6].

Papilledema is observed on funduscopy in 25–40% of CVT cases, especially in those with chronic onset or delayed clinical presentation. It can produce transient loss of vision (associated with intense headache), and if prolonged, optic atrophy and consecutive peripheral blindness [6,12].

Focal Neurological Deficits

They are noted in 37–50% of CVT patients and appear at onset in 15% of cases [1,7].

Paresis, sometimes bilateral, is the most frequent focal neurological deficit associated with CVT (in the ISCVT cohort was noted in 37% of cases) [1,7].

Other signs are less common: fluent aphasia (which is observed in left transverse sinus thrombosis associated with a posterior left temporal lesion), central sensory deficits, hemianopia, and ataxia (usually observed in posterior dural sinuses occlusion) [7]. Mixed transcortical aphasia is noted in left thalamus lesions due to deep cerebral vein thrombosis [58].

Seizures

Focal or generalized seizures, even status epilepticus, are more frequently noted during the evolution of CVT (in the ICSVT cohort in 40% of cases) [7] than in arterial strokes [59–61]. Seizures appear during the onset of CVT in about 12–15% of cases [59,60]. A higher incidence has been observed in peripartum (76%) [60] and neonates (44%) [61].

Early seizures are noted more frequently in cases with supratentorial parenchymal brain lesions (especially disposed anterior to the sulcus of Rolando), thrombosis of the SSS and cortical veins and in those patients who present motor deficits [59–61].

Encephalopathy

Subacute/chronic encephalopathy, presenting altered mental status with cognitive dysfunction (including delirium, apathy, and dysexecutive syndrome), and diminished level of consciousness (between drowsiness and deep coma) is frequently associated with multifocal neurological deficits and is observed especially in elderly patients or neonates with CVT [15,62]. Usually, the diminution of the level of consciousness is reversible; however, coma at onset represents the main predictor of a poor outcome [1,2].

3.4.2. Topographic Clinical Diagnosis

Due to frequent concomitant multiple cerebral veins and dural sinuses thrombosis (more than two-thirds of cases), the existence of multiple anatomic variants of some cerebral veins and dural sinuses, and action of venous collateral circulation, the topographic clinical diagnosis of CVT is not so well-defined like in arterial occlusion and frequent is misleading [1,7,63].

However, isolated thrombosis of the different dural sinuses and cerebral veins produces the following clinical aspects (Figure 1).

Superior Sagittal Sinus (SSS) Thrombosis

It represents the most frequent dural sinuses occlusion, especially during the puerperium (62–80% in association, and 30% in isolated thrombosis) [1,6,12]. The common clinical presentation is that of an isolated intracranial hypertension syndrome. The clinical aspects may vary depending on the concomitant occlusion of other dural sinuses, especially LSs cerebral, or tributaries cerebral veins. Bilateral motor/sensory signs (especially in the legs) and psychiatric symptoms (prefrontal syndrome) may also appear due to bilateral frontoparietal hemispheric lesions produced by the progression of the SSS thrombosis to tributaries bilateral cortical veins [1,6,12].

Lateral Sinus (LS) Thrombosis

LS thrombosis may present different clinical aspects. Cases with isolated LS thrombosis develop an isolated headache or frequently intracranial hypertension (pseudotumor) syndrome. Less often, these patients may also present with focal neurological deficits due to hemispheric lesions produced by the progression of the LS thrombosis to tributaries cortical veins.

In contrast to SSS thrombosis, the infectious etiology is much more common in LS thrombosis. Different localized pyogenic infections of the ears (otitis), mastoid air cells (mastoiditis), and the paranasal sinuses (sinusitis) can determine septic LS thrombosis: "otitic hydrocephalus" [1,63]. The clinical signs are relatively characteristic: fever, headache, neck pain, neck tenderness, nausea and vomiting, vertigo, diplopia produced by sixth nerve palsy, and temporal and retro-orbital pain due to symptomatic trigeminal neuralgia [1,12,63].

Since the left LS is often hypoplasic, the pseudotumor syndrome appears especially after right LS thrombosis. In such cases, a bilateral venous drainage impairment may be noted, affecting the inferior portions of both temporal lobes and cerebellum, with subsequent temporal lobe and cerebellar signs [1,2,63]. Fluent Wernicke aphasia is usually observed in left transverse sinus thrombosis associated with adjacent cerebral veins occlusion (40%) and can be associated with right hemianopia or superior quadrantanopia. Right temporal lobe lesions produce left hemianopia. Nystagmus and gait ataxia represent the markers of cerebellar affection [1,7,63].

Unusually, an isolated left LS thrombosis presents a misleading isolated headache (migraine-like). In such cases, the thrombosis is not due to an otitis, but a thrombophilia [3,63,64]. This is why screening for LS thrombosis (and other CVT) has to be done in young women with a recent headache even if this symptom is isolated and is not associated with otitis or mastoiditis [63,64]. LS thrombosis may present also as isolated pulsating tinnitus [65].

Cavernous Sinus Thrombosis

It is rare and usually has an infection etiology (pyogenic infections of the face, or the paranasal sinuses) [66,67].

In patients with classic acute unilateral septic cavernous sinus thrombosis, they present a typical clinical picture, with painful complete or partial ophthalmoplegia associated with chemosis, proptosis, and conjunctival edema. Frequently, a papilledema associated with hemorrhages of the retina can be observed. In the absence of an immediate diagnosis and treatment, it becomes bilateral via inter-cavernous sinuses. When the thrombosis progresses to other dural sinuses and cortical veins, seizures and paresis may associate [66,67].

In a minority of cases (head trauma, surgery on intracranial or facial structures, thrombophilia, and thrombosis of dural arteriovenous fistulas) an aseptic cavernous sinus thrombosis may be observed with an isolated abducens nerve palsy and mild proptosis [66].

Thrombosis of the Superior and Inferior Petrosal Sinuses

In the majority of cases, it represents a sequela of cavernous or sigmoid occlusion. The thrombosis of the superior petrosal sinus clinically manifests as a trigeminal palsy, while the occlusion of the inferior one occurs as an abducens palsy [1,2].

Cortical Veins Thrombosis

Isolated thrombosis of cortical veins without associated dural sinus thrombosis is considered a rare disease (2%), but it is probably underdiagnosed, due to difficulties to detect it using the traditional MRI sequences and MRV [68]. Occlusion appears especially at the levels of the superior cortical veins, producing seizures associated with motor/sensory deficits [68].

Thrombosis of the Deep Cerebral Venous System

Frequently associated with the thrombosis of the SS, it is a rare disease that occurs more often during childhood (especially in neonates). The clinical presentation is severe, with encephalopathy, and bilateral motor deficits [69,70].

In adults, a more limited thrombosis of the deep cerebral veins, without associated SS thrombosis, can produce relatively mild clinical aspects, such as headache, nausea and vomiting, gait ataxia, hemiparesis (that may be bilateral or alternating), neuropsychological symptoms, and mild disturbances of consciousness [69,70]. In rare situations, benign cases of thrombosis of the deep cerebral veins were noted with mixed transcortical aphasia [58].

Thrombosis of the Posterior Fossa Veins

Isolated venous infarctions in the posterior fossa are rare because the posterior fossa owns an efficient collateral venous circulation. However, this disease represents the main differential diagnosis in cases with concomitant risk factors for CVT, associated with some clinical aspects (intracranial hypertension syndrome, cerebellar-vestibular syndrome), and atypical aspects on brain CT (bilateral hemispheric and vermian cerebellar infarcts, irregular cerebellar hemorrhages) [71,72].

Internal Jugular Vein (IJV) Thrombosis

IJV thrombosis represents especially a progression of the sigmoid sinus thrombosis or may be produced by cannulation for long-term IJV access. It can be asymptomatic or its clinical picture consists of symptoms and signs of local infection (such as pain and swelling of the mastoid area, a painful and tender thrombosed IJV). The thrombophlebitis of the IJV can be a consequence of the syndrome of tonsillopharyngitis (Lemierre's syndrome). A jugular foramen syndrome (consisting of unilateral pulsatile tinnitus [65] or multiple cranial nerve palsies VIII-XII) occurs if the infection affects the skull base [73].

Emissary Veins (EV) Thrombosis

The EVs (e.g., petrosquamosal sinus (PSS)), are vestigial valve-less veins, which connect the intracranial dural venous sinuses and the extracranial venous system. Posterior fossa EVs pass through corresponding cranial apertures and ensure (together with the IJV) an additional extracranial venous drainage of the veins of the posterior fossa. In healthy people, EVs are small and have no clinical significance. In pathological cases (associated with high-flow arteriovenous malformations, IJV aplasia or IJV thrombosis, or even LS thrombosis) they are large with clinical significance (different craniofacial syndromes and pulsatile tinnitus) [65,72].

3.5. Laboratory Data

Unfortunately, there is no simple confirmatory laboratory test that can rule out an acute CVT.

3.5.1. Blood Assay

Guidelines from the American Heart Association/American Stroke Association (AHA/ASA) recommend obtaining a complete blood count, chemistry panel, prothrombin time and activated partial thromboplastin time for cases with clinically suspected CVT [12]. These data may reveal conditions that contribute to the appearance of CVT such as a hypercoagulable state, infective, or inflammatory, diseases.

Anti-platelet factor four (PF4) antibodies are searched for COVID 19-vaccination-associated CVT [45]. An assessment for paroxysmal nocturnal hemoglobinuria should be done if the complete blood count indicates hemolytic anemia, iron deficiency, or pancytopenia [6].

The guidelines recommend screening for use of oral contraceptives, at the initial clinical presentation of young women, and for an occult neoplasm or hematologic disorder in patients older than 40 years with suspected CVT [12,74].

3.5.2. D-Dimer

An elevated plasma D-dimer level suggests the diagnosis of CVT, but a normal D-dimer level does not exclude the CVT diagnosis, especially in those cases with predisposing factors and a compatible clinical presentation for CVT, such as isolated headache or in those patients with a subacute or chronic clinical presentation before the D-dimer test [75,76].

3.5.3. Lumbar Puncture and Cerebrospinal Fluid (CSF) Examination

They may be useful to exclude meningitis in cases with CVT who clinically present with isolated intracranial hypertension, and in cases with sepsis, or with fever and no obvious cause of infection [7,12,77]. Increased opening pressure during the exam of CSF pressure represents a frequent feature in CVT cases presenting isolated intracranial hypertension. Other significant data are nonspecific and may be represented by a mild lymphocytosis, hyperproteinorahia, and numerous red blood cell count; these abnormalities are noted in 30% to 50% of cases with CVT [77].

Lumbar puncture is contraindicated in cases with CVT and with large brain lesions because they present an augmented risk of herniation [6,77].

3.5.4. Evaluation for Thrombophilic State

Searching for a thrombophilia should be realized for cases with CVT who present an elevated pretest probability of severe thrombophilia (patients with a personal and/or family history of venous thrombosis, CVT in young people, or CVT in the absence of a transient or permanent risk factor) [6].

When indicated, screening should contain factor V Leiden, prothrombin G20210A pathologic variant, antithrombin, protein C, protein S, lupus anticoagulant, anticardiolipin, and anti-beta2 glycoprotein-I antibodies [6,7,74].

3.6. Imaging

Neuroimaging data are essential for the diagnosis of CVT [74,78].

3.6.1. Head Computed Tomography (CT)

Head CT is usually the first technique to be performed in the emergency department in cases with acute/subacute clinical suspicion for CVT [12]. It should be done initially native (NCECT), and then (if hemorrhagic infarcts, cerebral hemorrhage, subdural hematoma, or subarachnoid hemorrhage are absent) with contrast enhancement (CECT) [12,74,78] (Table 1).

Table 1. CT and MRI features in CVT.

Direct Signs	Indirect Signs
-Dense triangle sign (acute clot in dural sinus on NCECT) -Replacement of normal dark flow void with a clot on MRI -Cord sign (acute thrombosed cerebral vein on NCECT) -MRI equivalent: acute thrombosed cerebral vein on T2* GRE images or T2*SW images. -Empty delta sign (chronic clot in dural sinus) on CTV/ Contrast Enhancement-MRV	-Cerebral edema (on CT or MRI-T1 WI/T2WI) with elevated or mixed diffusion characteristics (on DWI) -Hemorrhagic infarction -Subarachnoid hemorrhage -Subdural hemorrhage

Head CT presents the following advantages:

First, it may identify alternative diagnoses that CVT can clinically resemble, such as subdural hematoma, abscess, or different tumors. Second, sometimes, CT diagnoses diseases that can themselves produce CVT, such as sinusitis, mastoiditis, abscesses, or meningiomas. Third, Head CT can detect direct and indirect signs of CVT [1,74,78].

Direct Signs of CVT on Head CT

They represent the direct visualization of the venous clot inside the occluded cerebral vein, or dural sinus, and can be observed in about one-third of all CVT patients. They are the "cord sign", the "dense triangle sign," and the "empty delta sign" [6,74,79,80]. (Figure 3) [58].

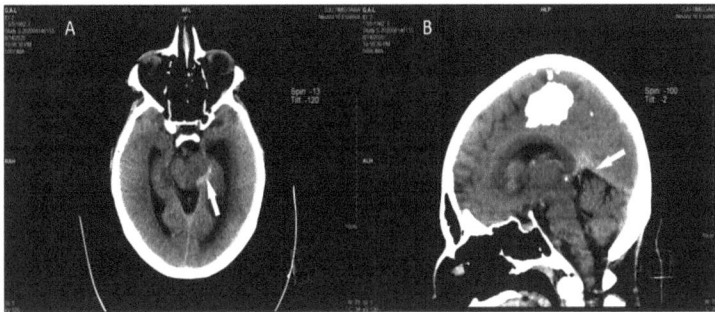

Figure 3. A, B. Axial (**A**) and MPR sagittal (**B**) non-contrast head computed tomography performed in the acute phase shows hyperdense appearance (acute thrombosis) of the left lateral mesencephalic [58].

The "cord sign" represents an acute thrombosed cerebral vein on NCECT and is reported in a quarter of CVT cases. It appears as a curvilinear or linear hyperdensity representing a fresh clot in-side an occluded cerebral vein and it is best visualized within the first 7 days of CVT clinical onset [8]. After 1 to 2 weeks, the thrombus appears isodense and then hypodense. Mimicking appears in slow flow cases; thus, its specificity is considered to be rather low [1,74,78].

The "dense triangle sign" (acute thrombus in dural sinus on NCECT) is identified in less than 2% of CVT patients [78]. It appears as a hyperdensity with a triangular or round shape in the posterior part of the SSS caused by the fresh clot inside the sinus [6]. It can be detected during the first 2 weeks of the disease. Because cases with increased hematocrit or dehydration can also produce this sign, its specificity is considered to be rather low, especially in other sinuses than SSS [79–81]. Measurement of the venous sinus density and Hounsfield unit-to-hematocrit (H:H) ratio has been noted to raise the sensitivity in detecting CVT, as attenuation of 62HU and higher is suggestive of thrombosis [82]. If a hyperdense sinus is detected, consecutive investigation with CTV and/or MRI/MRV should be realized [1,2].

The "empty delta sign" is detected on CECT scans in 10–20% of CVT cases. It appears as a triangular hyperdensity of contrast enhancement of the walls of the dural sinus surrounding a hypodense central region lacking contrast enhancement inside the posterior part of the SSS [6,83,84]. This sign occurs between day 5 to 2 months after onset. The sensitivity and specificity of the "empty delta sign" are augmented to 30% of all CVT cases with CT scans with orthogonal sectioning, different window and level settings, and multi-planar reformations. Furthermore, an early division of the SSS can mimic a false "empty delta sign", so this sign is not pathognomonic [83,84].

Indirect Signs of CVT on Head CT

They are more frequent than direct signs and can include intense contrast enhancement of falx and tentorium, dilated cerebral veins, small or enlarged ventricles, and cerebral parenchyma abnormalities [7,12].

Intense contrast enhancement of falx and tentorium represents venous stasis or hyperemia of the cranial dura mater and is detected in 20% of cases. The former can be difficult to examine, especially in older patients, but the latter is more easily identified, denoting especially SS and, sometimes, SSS thrombosis [1,7,83].

The cortical veins may appear dilated on the CECT exam due to collaterally veins development [83].

Diffuse brain edema (20–50% of CVT cases) can secondarily produce effacement of cerebral sulci and small ventricles (diminution of the ventricular dimensions); this imaging sign may be difficult to differentiate from normal aspects with small ventricles in young adults [7,83].

The identification of the opposite sign (enlarged ventricles) cannot remove the diagnosis of CVT, because it may be produced by the hydrocephalus appearing from raised CSF production and diminished resorption from augmented venous pressure; usually, it can be associated with posterior fossa veins occlusion. In both cases (small, vs. enlarged ventricles), a comparison with precedent CT exams may be necessary [7,83].

Cerebral parenchyma abnormalities may be nonhemorrhagic or hemorrhagic and may be detected in 60–80% of CVT cases [83].

The first type includes focal areas of hypodensity produced by edema or venous infarction, usually not respecting the arterial boundaries, as well as diffuse brain edema. With serial imaging, some of them may disappear ("vanishing infarcts"), and new lesions may be detected. The latter type includes hemorrhagic infarcts, intracerebral hemorrhage, or rarely (<1%) subarachnoid hemorrhage usually limited to convexity [6,83].

Peculiar forms of CVT may present on CT different aspects. First, many irregular filling defects with enlarged cavernous sinuses and orbital veins show up on CECT of cavernous sinus thrombosis; in septic cavernous sinus thrombosis, air can be detected inside the sinus on coronal sections [12,74]. Second, bilateral parasagittal hemispheric lesions are highly suggestive of thrombosis of the SSS [12,74]. Third, temporo-occipital lesions indicate LS thrombosis or occlusion of the vein of Labbe [12,74]. Forth, in cases of deep cerebral veins thrombosis, the main features are represented by: bilateral hypodensities, denoting infarcts at the level of the thalami, basal ganglia, and internal capsule; bilateral hyperdensities (hemorrhages or hemorrhagic infarcts) with the same topography; severe edema with compression of the third ventricle and consecutive hydrocephalus, and hyperdense appearance (fresh clot) at the level of the occluded sinuses. Thus, the appearance of hemorrhage or edema near a main dural sinus or deep cerebral vein should suggest CVT [12,74]. Last, cerebellar venous infarctions can determine hydrocephalus and compression of the fourth ventricle [12,74].

Unfortunately, head CT diagnosis of CVT is insensitive, findings being pathologic only in one-third of real CVT cases, and different CT signs are mostly nonspecific in the rest of detected CVT cases [12]. Furthermore, several normal anatomic variants may mimic sinus thrombosis, including sinus atresia, sinus hypoplasia, asymmetric sinus drainage, and normal sinus filling defects associated with arachnoid granulations or intrasinus septa [7,12]. For this reason, normal Head CT results will not exclude a diagnosis of CVT; therefore, in clinically suspected cases, a CT Venography or MRI Venography is essential for CVT positive diagnosis [79,80].

3.6.2. CT Venography-CTV (Multi-Detector CT Angiography-MDCTA) with Bolus Injection of Contrast Material

When associated with head CT, it adds important information in suspected clinical cases of CVT [6]. The combined accuracy of head CT and CTV is 90–100%, depending on the occlusion site [85–88]. According to AHA/ASA guidelines published in 2011, CTV is considered equivalent to MRV in the diagnosis of CVT [12]. Compared with digital subtraction intra-arterial angiography, the combination of head CT and CTV presents sensitivity and specificity of 95 and 91% [12] (Table 2).

Table 2. Comparison of CTV and MRV in CVT.

Imaging Method	Advantages	Disadvantages
CTV	-More widely accessible than MRV -Generally costs less than MRV -Faster image acquisition than MRV -More suitable for unstable patients -Less prone to motion artifact -Better detection of cerebral small vessels	-Radiation risk -Higher rate of adverse reactions to Iodinated contrasts, including the risk of contrast-induced nephropathy -Potentially reduced visualization of skull base structures in 3D display -Acute thrombus, which is hyperdense, may mimic opacified sinus resulting in false-negative results
MRV	-No radiation risk -Low rate of adverse reactions to Gadolinium -Indicated in cases with severe renal failure if done without contrast enhancement contrast technique) -Higher sensitivity for small parenchymal lesions	-Contraindicated in cases with ferromagnetic devices and most pacemakers -More prone to motion artifact -TOF-MRV may present false-positive results from a flow that has a parallel direction with the acquisition plane. -For this reason, phase contrast MRV has to be used to identify the thrombus. -Stenotic, hypoplastic, or aplastic dural sinuses may be misdiagnosed as CVT.
CTV and MRV	Noninvasive imaging methods with indirect signs possible to detect	-Inferior resolution to detect the patency of the posterior part or entire SSS, both LSs of the deep cerebral veins to DSA

This method is used especially in acute cases, in the emergency department, when it can be performed immediately after NCECT. It ensures an excellent visualization of the cerebral venous system and can detect filling defects in the thrombosed sinuses or cerebral veins, sinus wall enhancement, and augmented collateral venous circulation. In addition, in subacute or chronic CVT phases, it can identify a heterogeneous clot [6,83].

It presents some advantages compared to intra-arterial angiography: it is less expensive and less invasive, and faster (rapid image acquisition); it detects better the inferior sagittal and cavernous sinuses, and the basal vein of Rosenthal (with multiplanar reformatted images) than conventional intra-arterial angiography [85–88].

The main advantages of CTV vs. MRV are: it is much more accessible and less expensive, faster, has no contraindications to ferromagnetic devices, augmented imaging resolution for the major dural sinuses, much easier to interpret, with fewer artifacts than MRV. MDCTA has been demonstrated to be as accurate as time-of-flight (TOF) MRV in the identification of the dural sinuses, with superior capability vs. MRV to visualize: the ISS and the non-dominant transverse sinus thrombosis; the cortical vein thrombosis (especially for single cortical vein occlusion); and cerebral veins or dural sinuses with low flow [85–88].

Unfortunately, CTV is less sensitive in the assessment of the deep venous system and cortical veins. This disadvantage can be ameliorated by realizing multiplanar reformations, which increases the sensitivity of CTV beyond angiography [85,86]. Maximum intensity projection (MIP) image generation occasionally presents diminished detection of skull base components in three-dimensional display, with inadvertent sinus exclusion from bone subtracting algorithms; however, this can be improved with specific software for mask bone elimination [88]. CTV also presents different concerns (contrast allergy, contrast nephropathy due to contrast material, and radiation exposure), which may contraindicate its use during pregnancy, childhood, or renal failure [88].

3.6.3. Magnetic Resonance Imaging (MRI) of the Head

MRI pathological features in CVT cases are represented by direct signs (visualizing the clot itself inside the cerebral veins and dural sinuses) and indirect signs (detected especially at the level of the brain parenchyma) [12,89,90] (Table 1).

The MRI direct signs:

The main characteristic of thrombosis is the absence of a flow void or a flow signal with altered intensity in the dural sinus or cerebral vein. The signal intensity of the thrombus on T1-, and T2-weighted MR images is similar to a hematoma, and it is evolving depending on clot age. The successive intensity modifications noted in the clot are the results of the paramagnetic features of the hemoglobin molecule and its secondary products [12,89–94].

Acutely (0–5 days after the onset of the clinical aspects), flow void is missing and the thrombosed dural sinus or cerebral vein is isointense with brain tissue on T1-WI and hypointense on T2-WI, due to the abundance of deoxyhemoglobin in red cells within the clot. The detection of CVT in this phase is practically very difficult on MRI alone because the MRI aspect is similar to normal flow. For this reason, other MRI sequences, MRV, CTV, or cerebral intra-arterial angiography are needed to certify the absence of flow in the occluded venous channel [12,89,90] (Figure 4) [58].

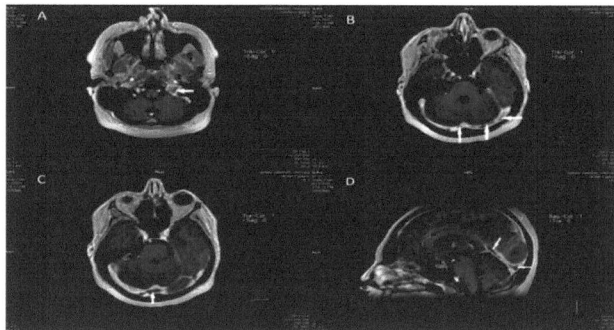

Figure 4. A, B, C, D. Axial and sagittal T1 post-contrast magnetic resonance demonstrate extensive filling defects throughout the dural sinuses (arrows-left sigmoid and jugular bulb (**A**), left and right transverse sinuses (**B**), sinus confluence (**C**), straight sinus (**D**)) [58].

In the subacute phase (between days 6 and 15 after the onset), the venous clot becomes more apparent because the signal is hyperintense in both T1-, and T2-WI, due to the accumulation of methemoglobin inside the venous thrombus. This imaging pattern certifies the aging of the clot, rather than its progression. Practically, these intermediate imaging aspects (increased signals on both T1-, and T2-WI) are specific for CVT and are the most common imagistic sign [89,90].

In the chronic stage (between two and four weeks after onset), the beginning of recanalization of the anteriorly occluded cerebral vein or dural sinus determines the recommencing of the flow void. In this phase, the clot, which is heterogeneous, is isointense on T1-WI, with variable intensity (iso-, or hyperintense) on T2-WI, due to the deoxygenated hemoglobin and methemoglobin components. In consequence, in this phase, the diagnosis of CVT can be overlooked [89,90].

After 4–6 months, no signal abnormality is seen on T1-WI or DWI; however, subtle changes (heterogeneous topic signal abnormalities) can be noted in T2-WI or FLAIR, which can remain for years, and should not be confused for a recurrent acute CVT [89,90].

Unfortunately, in a significant number of situations, we can detect false-negative or false-positive appearances. The former situations are relatively rare and represent a supra-acute or very late phase of CVT, or an isolated cortical vein thrombosis, which will be diagnosed especially by angiography. The later situations are the result of slowly flowing venous blood. To reduce these artifacts, we have to reposition the patient, repeat the sequence in a different plane, using at least two sequences, and using special acquisitions, such as [74,83].

Gradient echo T2*-weighted (T2*GRE) MRI sequences identify CVT, as deposited blood breakdown products (i.e., hemosiderin, methemoglobin, deoxyhemoglobin), which can produce increased signal drop-out, detecting intravessel clots in stages where the thrombus can be unapparent in other sequences [91]. Thus, on T2*GRE MRI sequences, the acute clot can be directly detected as an area of hypointensity in the affected cortical vein and/or dural sinus. However, a chronically thrombosed sinus may still have a low signal on these sequences [92].

Echo-planar T2 susceptibility-weighted imaging (T2* SWI) MRI sequences represent a complementary T2* GRE sequence to evaluate CVT. SWI identifies the isolated cortical vein thrombosis during the first days of acute CVT when T1 and T2 are less sensitive. This imagistic method detects the intraluminal clot as a hypointense area. The exaggeration of magnetic susceptibility effect (MSE) helps detection of discrete thrombosis (as it is noted in more than 90% of cases), and it also detects venous stasis, presence of collateral venous pathways, and possible associated intracranial hemorrhage [93]. Supplementary, SWI indicates a blooming artifact better observed than regular T2* GRE sequences, realizing a better location of the thrombus or hemorrhage. Isolated cortical vein thrombosis may be easier to observe on the maximum-intensity projections (MIPs) of SWI compared to dedicate venous imaging [80,93].

The MRI indirect signs:

A variety of parenchymal brain lesions secondary to venous occlusion (brain edema, cerebral infarct, and/or cerebral hemorrhage) noted in CVT cases are better detected by MRI, than by CT [79].

Cerebral edema consists of an increased signal on T2-WI and an isointense or hypointense signal on T1-WI. Isolated cerebral edema, without cerebral infarcts or hemorrhages, may appear in 50% of CVT patients, and may be associated with cortical sulcal effacement and small ventricles. When these MRI signs are detected, CTV or MRV should be done to confirm the CVT diagnosis [89,90].

An augmented signal in both T1- and T2-WI is a hallmark of cerebral hemorrhage (one-third of the CVT patients). Usually, in the case of an SSS occlusion, we can note flame-shaped, irregular, and heterogeneous areas of lobar hemorrhages in the parasagittal areas of both frontal and parietal lobes. Frequently, LS thrombosis is associated with both temporal and occipital lobes abnormalities. Deep brain lesions, especially bilateral thalamic hemorrhages, extensive brain edema, or intraventricular hemorrhage indicate an occlusion of the vein of Galen or SS [12,89,90].

All the MRI indirect signs are nonspecific, but their interpretation is clear because of the associated MRI direct signs of dural sinus thrombosis [89,90].

After contrast (gadolinium) injection, intense contrast enhancement and flow voids may be noted within the occluded sinuses, diminished flow in sinuses and intra-clot collateral channels, or recanalization of the thrombus [1,7].

Diffusion-Weighted Imaging (DWI) Techniques

DWI directly identifies the clot as a high signal intensity within the occluded vessel, with decreased apparent diffusion coefficient (ADC). Cases with restrictions on DWI present longer recovery time and a lower probability of total thrombus recanalization (DWI-prognostic factor) [12,94].

DWI also detects cerebral edema, which can be differentiated in:

- Vasogenic edema, which is represented by different signal abnormalities in the affected region, and augmented ADC values, practically without significantly lower ADC values than in unaffected areas [1,94].
- Cytotoxic edema, which is represented by high signal intensity, and low ADC values [1,94].

On perfusion-weighted (PWI) MRI, relative cerebral blood volume (rCBV), and mean transit time (MTT) are increased in affected regions, with preserved relative cerebral blood flow (rCBF) [1,94].

Due to the prominence of vasogenic edema vs. cytotoxic edema in CVT cases, corresponding regions of the brain may be functionally and metabolically affected, but not irreversibly. The reversibility of different cerebral venous lesions is characteristic of CVT cases and is manifested in both a better recovery in venous infarcts than in arterial strokes and vanishing lesions on MRI [89,90,94].

The main MRI advantages vs. CT in CVT diagnosis are represented by sensitivity to venous flow, better capacity to identify the clot itself, and easily repeatable and noninvasive. However, conventional MRI presents limitations, such in comatose patients or in cases of isolated cortical vein thrombosis, (when intra-arterial angiography is mandatory to confirm the diagnosis of CVT) [90]. (Table 1).

3.6.4. Magnetic Resonance Venography (MRV)

MRV can detect the thrombus and can assess the spontaneous recanalization or recanalization following therapy. Total recanalization is not mandatory for symptomatic recovery, and the presence of collateral pathways may also be identified in MRV [95,96]. (Table 2) (Figure 5) [81].

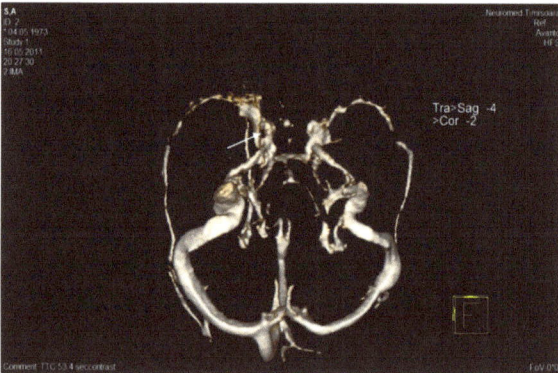

Figure 5. CE–MRA, venous time—VRT reconstruction in the axial plane: lacunar image in right cavernous sinus (arrow). CE–MRA: Contrast-enhanced–magnetic resonance angiography; VRT: Volume rendering technique [81].

MRV may be done without contrast enhancement (using the TOF technique or phase contrast technique) or with a contrast-enhanced technique [95,96].

The two-dimensional (2D-TOF) method (with 1.5, and 3-mm thick slices in the coronal and axial planes) represents the most frequent technique and is essential in pregnant or breastfeeding women, as well as in case of severe renal failure, where contrast enhancement is prohibited. It detects the absence of flow signal (absence of opacification) of dural sinuses in the case of an occlusion of the vessel, though interpretation can be confounded by normal anatomic variants such as sinus hypoplasia and asymmetric flow [12,95,96].

The indirect signs of CVT include delayed emptying, collateral venous circulation, dilated veins, and tortuous collateral cortical veins (corkscrew veins) [2]. The 2D-TOF technique is superior to its 3D counterpart due to a relative lack of saturation effects and superior sensitivity in the setting of slow venous flow but has a low sensitivity to small vessels with a slow flow [95,96].

Other MR techniques may be useful to differentiate sinus hypoplasia from venous thrombosis. Contrast-enhanced MRV can ensure better detection of cerebral venous vessels, and T2*GRE or T2*SWI MRI sequences will detect normal signals in a hypoplastic sinus and abnormally low signals in the presence of a clot [91–93]. A chronically thrombosed hypoplastic sinus will indicate the absence of flow on 2D-TOF MRV and enhancement on contrast-enhanced MRI and MRV [6]. MRV with gadolinium realizes a direct examination of cerebral veins and dural sinuses filling similar to that of CTV, with comparable sensitivity and specificity. Supplementary, both CTV and contrast-enhanced MRV are superior to the TOF and phase-contrast methods, due to different artifacts in these sequences [83].

Unfortunately, conventional MRV presents some limitations: it has a reduced role in detecting: cortical veins and cavernous sinus occlusions, partial thrombosis of other cerebral veins and dural sinuses, or net differentiation between hypoplasia and occluded sinus [6]. A major disadvantage of MRV compared to CTV is that acquisition times are long, and motion artifacts may appear in comatose patients (Table 2) [83,95,96].

Contrast-enhanced MRV with elliptic centric ordering is a newer method, which realizes better examination of smaller cerebral veins and dural sinuses, in which the paramagnetic effect of gadolinium shorts T1 and determines positive intravascular contrast enhancement [83,96]. 3D phase-contrast (PC) MRV presents a better capacity to identify slow flow and may better differentiate between slow flow and thrombus [95,96]. Static contrast-enhanced 3D MRV detects better the intracranial venous system; unfortunately, it may present some limitations in chronic dural sinus thrombosis as the thrombus may be enhanced, miming a patent dural sinus [95,96]. This problem is solved with time-resolved 3D MRV (4D MRV), which produces images with different delays for better detection of the venous thrombus [95]. 4D MRV presents better sensitivity to diagnose CVT than T2-WI, T2*GRE, and TOF-MRV; supplementary, it has better specificity than TOF- MRV, and it identifies chronic CVT [95].

MRI using gradient-echo T2* SW sequences in combination with MRV is the most sensitive imaging technique for detecting the clot and the occluded dural sinus or cerebral vein [92,95,96].

Unfortunately, the interobserver agreement on CVT MRI diagnostic imaging is not perfect, percentages vary depending on which sinuses or veins are occluded: it is good or very good for most of the occluded sinus and veins; moderate to very good for the left LS and SS; and poor to good for the cortical veins [6,89].

3.6.5. Cerebral Intra-Arterial Angiography with Venous Phase Imaging and Direct Cerebral Venography

These are invasive diagnostic methods that are used for the peculiar cases when: The clinical suspicion of CVT is high, but MR or CT Venography data are ambiguous (such as in cases of isolated cortical vein thrombosis), or when required to exclude a dural arteriovenous fistula or distal aneurysm, like in subarachnoid hemorrhage cases [12,97].

Cerebral Intra-Arterial Angiography with Venous Phase Imaging

It requires a four-vessel angiography (conventional or digitized intra-arterial) with detection of the whole venous phase on at least two projections (frontal and lateral) and three oblique views for the detection of the whole SSS [12,97].

Characteristic imagistic signs of CVT on angiography are: partial lack of opacification or absence of filling of dural sinuses or cerebral veins delayed emptying, dilatation of cortical, scalp, or facial veins, dilatation of collateral veins, reversal of venous flow, and the sudden stopping of cortical veins surrounded by tortuous and dilated collateral "corkscrew" veins [12,97]. CVT is easy to detect on angiography when it occludes the posterior part of the entire SSS, both LSs of the deep cerebral veins, but it can be misdiagnosed with hypoplasia or aplasia when the anterior third of the SSS or the left LS are thrombosed [1,12,97]. In such situations, it is mandatory to detect other imagistic signs: thrombosis of another venous channel or delayed emptying and dilatation of collateral veins in occlusion of the anterior part of the SSS and total lack of opacification of the whole sinus or its sigmoid portion in LS thrombosis. The detection of different collateral veins usually is a hallmark of SSS occlusion and is noted in nearly half of CVT patients [1]. This technique has some limitations: it does not indicate the clot itself, it is invasive, the associated risk of surgery complications, radiation exposure, needs homogeneous teams of experts who act in dedicated hospital departments, and some subjects are allergic to the iodine contrast material [1,12,97].

Direct Cerebral Venography

This technique is done during endovascular therapeutic techniques, detecting the clot within the lumen either as an intraluminal filling defect (no occlusive thrombosis) or as a complete no filling (occlusive thrombosis); complete thrombosis may also indicate a "cupping appearance" within the sinus [12,97].

While the inter-observer agreement for a diagnosis of CVT is not perfect, the association of conventional contrast angiography plus brain MRI has a higher inter-observer agreement than angiography alone (94% vs. 62%) [6,97].

3.6.6. Transcranial Doppler Ultrasonography (TCD) and Transcranial Color-Coded Duplex Sonography (TCCDS), or Transcranial Power Imaging, with or without the Use of a Contrast Agent

They represent the initial method used when CVT is clinically suspected in neonates and infants with opened fontanelles, identifying different aspects, depending on the size of the fontanelle: echogenic clot, intracranial hemorrhage, cerebral edema, or hydrocephalus [98].

4. Conclusions

CVT adult patients are younger, usually female, and present diminished frequencies of classical vascular risk factors when compared with patients with the arterial occlusive disease.

The major risk factors for CVT in adults are prothrombotic conditions, either genetic or acquired, oral contraceptives, pregnancy and the puerperium, malignancy (including myeloproliferative diseases) infection, and adenovirus-based COVID-19 vaccine-induced thrombocytopenia and thrombosis.

The pathophysiology of CVT determines the clinical spectrum and the abnormal imaging aspects. The wide clinical spectrum of CVT, often with a misleading presentation, may cause delays in diagnosis, and it is frequently represented by headache or intracranial hypertension, seizures, focal neurological deficits, and/or encephalopathy.

Both CT-CTV and MRI-MRV are excellent techniques to diagnose CVT and detect different complications. They may be combined for efficient assessment in complex or equivocal cases and must be associated with ultrasound in neonates.

Author Contributions: Conceptualization, D.C.J.; methodology, D.C.J., T.F.D., G.M., A.C., C.D.B. and A.E.G.; software, T.F.D., G.M., S.F.A. and R.S.; validation, D.C.J., S.N.J., T.F.D., G.M., A.C., C.D.B., A.G.M.M., A.D.A., L.P., S.F.A., R.S., N.I. and A.E.G.; formal analysis, D.C.J., T.F.D. and N.I.; investigation, D.C.J., S.N.J., T.F.D., N.I. and G.M.; resources, D.C.J.; data curation, D.C.J.; writing—original draft preparation, D.C.J.; writing—review and editing, D.C.J. and T.F.D.; visualization, D.C.J., S.N.J., T.F.D., G.M., A.C., C.D.B., A.G.M.M., A.D.A., L.P., S.F.A., R.S., N.I. and A.E.G.; supervision, D.C.J.; project administration, D.C.J.; funding acquisition, D.C.J. All authors have read and agreed to the published version of the manuscript.

Funding: This research received no external funding.

Institutional Review Board Statement: The study was conducted according to the guidelines of the Declaration of Helsinki and approved by the Institutional Review Board (or Ethics Committee) of Pius Brînzeu Emergency County Hospital, Timisoara, Romania, Protocol code 247/23 April 2021.

Informed Consent Statement: Informed consent was obtained from all subjects involved in the study.

Data Availability Statement: First Department of Neurology, Pius Brînzeu Emergency County Hospital, Timisoara, Romania; Department of Multidetector Computed Tomography and Magnetic Resonance Imaging, Neuromed Diagnostic Imaging Centre, Timisoara, Romania.

Conflicts of Interest: The authors declare no competing interest.

References

1. Bousser, M.G.; Barnett, H.J.M. Chapter Twelve: Cerebral Venous Thrombosis. In *Stroke (Pathophysiology, Diagnosis, and Management)*, 4th ed.; Mohr, J.P., Choi, D.W., Grotta, J.C., Weir, B., Wolf, P.A., Eds.; Churchill Livingstone: London, UK, 2004; pp. 301–325.
2. Stam, J. Thrombosis of the cerebral veins and sinuses. *N. Engl. J. Med.* **2005**, *352*, 1791–1798. [CrossRef] [PubMed]
3. Piazza, G. Cerebral Venous Thrombosis. *Circulation* **2012**, *125*, 1704–1709. [CrossRef] [PubMed]
4. Dmytriw, A.A.; Song, J.S.A.; Yu, E.; Poon, C.S. Cerebral venous thrombosis: State of the art diagnosis and management. *Neuroradiology* **2018**, *60*, 669–685. [CrossRef] [PubMed]
5. Ferro, J.M.; Canhão, P. Chapter 45: Cerebral Venous Thrombosis. In *Stroke (Pathophysiology, Diagnosis, and Management)*, 6th ed.; Grotta, J.C., Albers, G.W., Broderick, J.P., Kasner, S.E., Lo, E.H., Mendelow, A.D., Sacco, R.L., Wong, L.K.S., Eds.; Elsevier: Amsterdam, The Netherlands, 2016; pp. 716–730.
6. Ferro, J.M.; Canhão, P. Cerebral Venous Thrombosis: Etiology, Clinical Features, and Diagnosis. Available online: https://www.uptodate.com/contents/cerebral-venous-thrombosis-etiology-clinical-features-and-diagnosis (accessed on 15 October 2021).
7. Ferro, J.M.; Canhao, P.; Stam, J.; Bousser, M.G.; Barinagarrementeria, F. Prognosis of cerebral vein and dural sinus thrombosis: Results of the International Study on Cerebral Vein and Dural Sinus Thrombosis (ISCVT). *Stroke* **2004**, *35*, 664–670. [CrossRef]
8. Egemen, E.; Solaroglu, I. Chapter 5: Anatomy of Cerebral Veins and Dural Sinuses. In *Primer on Cerebrovascular Diseases*, 2nd ed.; Caplan, L.R., José Biller, J., Leary, M.C., Eng, H., Lo, E.H., Thomas, A.J., Yenari, M., Zhang, J.H., Eds.; Gulf Professional Publishing: Oxford, UK, 2017; pp. 32–36. [CrossRef]
9. Satyarthee, G.D.; Moscote-Salazar, L.R.; Agrawal, A. Persistent enlarged occipital sinus with absent unilateral transverse sinus. *J. Neurosci. Rural. Pract.* **2019**, *10*, 519–521. [CrossRef]
10. Valdueza, J.M.; von Münster, T.; Hoffman, O.; Schreiber, S.; Einhäupl, K.M. Postural dependency of the cerebral venous outflow. *Lancet* **2000**, *355*, 200–201. [CrossRef]
11. Coutinho, J.M.; Zurbier, S.M.; Aramideh, M.; Stam, J. The Incidence of Cerebral Venous Thrombosis A Cross-Sectional Study. *Stroke* **2012**, *43*, 3375–3377. [CrossRef]
12. Saposnik, G.; Barinagarrementeria, F.; Brown, R.D.; Bushnell, C.D.; Cucchiara, B.; Cushman, M.; de Veber, G.; Ferro, J.M.; Tsai, F.Y.; on behalf of the American Heart Association Stroke Council and the Council on Epidemiology and Prevention. Diagnosis and management of cerebral venous thrombosis: A statement for healthcare professionals from the American Heart Association/American Stroke Association. *Stroke* **2011**, *42*, 1158–1192. [CrossRef]
13. Coutinho, J.M.; Ferro, J.M.; Canhão, P.; Barinagarrementeria, F.; Bousser, M.G.; Stam, J. Cerebral Venous and Sinus Thrombosis in Women. *Stroke* **2009**, *40*, 2356–2361. [CrossRef]
14. Devasagayam, S.; Wyatt, B.; Leyden, J.; Kleinig, T. Cerebral Venous Sinus Thrombosis Incidence Is Higher Than Previously Thought: A Retrospective Population-Based Study. *Stroke* **2016**, *47*, 2180. [CrossRef]
15. Ferro, J.M.; Canhão, P.; Bousser, M.-G.; Stam, J.; Barinagarrementeria, F. Cerebral vein and dural sinus thrombosis in elderly patients. *Stroke* **2005**, *36*, 1927. [CrossRef]
16. Zuurbier, S.M.; Hiltunen, S.; Lindgren, E.; Silvis, S.M.; Jood, K.; Devasagayam, S.; Kleinig, T.; Silver, F.; Mandell, D.M.; Putaala, J.; et al. Cerebral Venous Thrombosis in Older Patients. *Stroke* **2018**, *49*, 197. [CrossRef]
17. DeVeber, G.; Andrew, M.; Adams, C.; Bjornson, B.; Booth, F.; Buckley, D.J.; Camfield, C.S.; David, M.; Humphreys, P.; Langevin, P.; et al. Cerebral sinovenous thrombosis in children. *N. Engl. J. Med.* **2001**, *345*, 417. [CrossRef]
18. Marjot, T.; Yadav, S.; Hasan, N.; Bentley, P.; Sharma, P. Genes associated with adult cerebral venous thrombosis. *Stroke* **2011**, *42*, 913. [CrossRef]
19. Lüdemann, P.; Nabavi, D.G.; Junker, R.; Wolff, E.; Papke, K.; Buchner, H.; Assmann, G.; Ringelstein, E.B.; Factor, V. Leiden mutation is a risk factor for cerebral venous thrombosis: A case-control study of 55 patients. *Stroke* **1998**, *29*, 2507. [CrossRef]
20. Weih, M.; Junge-Hülsing, J.; Mehraein, S.; Ziemer, S.; Einhäupl, K.M. Hereditary thrombophilia with ischemiC stroke and sinus thrombosis. Diagnosis, therapy and meta-analysis. *Nervenarzt* **2000**, *71*, 936. [CrossRef]
21. Biousse, V.; Conard, J.; Brouzes, C.; Horellou, M.H.; Ameri, A.; Bousser, M.G. Frequency of the 20210 G→A mutation in the 3′-untranslated region of the prothrombin gene in 35 cases of cerebral venous thrombosis. *Stroke* **1998**, *29*, 1398. [CrossRef]
22. Reuner, K.H.; Ruf, A.; Grau, A.; Rickmann, H.; Stolz, E.; Jüttler, E.; Druschky, K.F.; Patscheke, H. Prothrombin gene G20210→A transition is a risk factor for cerebral venous thrombosis. *Stroke* **1998**, *29*, 1765. [CrossRef]

23. Lauw, M.N.; Barco, S.; Coutinho, J.M.; Middeldorp, S. Cerebral venous thrombosis and thrombophilia: A systematic review and meta-analysis. *Semin. Thromb. Hemost.* **2013**, *39*, 913–927.
24. Lee, M.K.; Ng, S.C. Cerebral venous thrombosis associated with antithrombin III deficiency. *Aust. N. Z. J. Med.* **1991**, *21*, 772. [CrossRef]
25. Deschiens, M.A.; Conard, J.; Horellou, M.H.; Ameri, A.; Preter, M.; Chedru, F.; Samama, M.M.; Bousser, M.G. Coagulation studies, factor V Leiden, and anticardiolipin antibodies in 40 cases of cerebral venous thrombosis. *Stroke* **1996**, *27*, 1724. [CrossRef]
26. Hillier, C.E.; Collins, P.W.; Bowen, D.J.; Bowley, S.; Wiles, C.M. Inherited prothrombotic risk factors and cerebral venous thrombosis. *QJM* **1998**, *91*, 677. [CrossRef]
27. Gouveia, L.O.; Canhão, P. MTHFR and the risk for cerebral venous thrombosis–a meta-analysis. *Thromb. Res.* **2010**, *125*, e153. [CrossRef]
28. Gogu, A.E.; Jianu, D.C.; Dumitrascu, V.; Ples, H.; Stroe, A.Z.; Docu Axelerad, D.; Docu Axelerad, A. MTHFR Gene Polymorphisms and Cardiovascular Risk Factors, Clinical-Imagistic Features and Outcome in Cerebral Venous Sinus Thrombosis. *Brain Sci.* **2021**, *11*, 23. [CrossRef]
29. Gogu, A.E.; Motoc, A.G.; Stroe, A.Z.; Docu Axelerad, A.; Docu Axelerad, D.; Petrica, L.; Jianu, D.C. Plasminogen Activator Inhibitor-1 (PAI-1) Gene Polymorphisms Associated with Cardio-vascular Risk Factors Involved in Cerebral Venous Sinus Thrombosis. *Metabolites* **2021**, *11*, 266. [CrossRef]
30. Duman, T.; Uluduz, D.; Midi, I.; Bektas, H.; Kablan, Y.; Goksel, B.K.; Milanlioglu, A.; Necioglu Orken, D.; Aluclu, U.; VENOST Study Group. A Multicenter Study of 1144 Patients with Cerebral Venous Thrombosis: The VENOST Study. *J. Stroke Cerebrovasc. Dis.* **2017**, *26*, 1848. [CrossRef]
31. Ferro, J.M.; Canhão, P. Cerebral venous sinus thrombosis: Update on diagnosis and management. *Curr. Cardiol. Rep.* **2014**, *16*, 523. [CrossRef] [PubMed]
32. Bousser, M.G.; Crassard, I. Cerebral venous thrombosis, pregnancy and oral contraceptives. *Thromb. Res.* **2012**, *130*, S19–S22. [CrossRef]
33. Cantu, C.; Barinagarrementeria, F. Cerebral venous thrombosis associated with pregnancy and puerperium. Review of 67 Cases. *Stroke* **1993**, *24*, 1880–1884. [CrossRef]
34. Lanska, D.J.; Kryscio, R.J. Stroke and intracranial venous thrombosis during pregnancy and puerperium. *Neurology* **1998**, *51*, 1622–1628. [CrossRef]
35. Kashkoush, A.I.; Maa, H.; Agarwal, N.; Panczykowski, D.; Tonetti, D.; Weiner, G.M.; Ares, W.; Kenmuir, C.; Jadhav, A.; Jovin, T.; et al. Cerebral venous sinus thrombosis in pregnancy and puerperium: A pooled, systematic review. *J. Clin. Neurosci.* **2017**, *39*, 9–15. [CrossRef] [PubMed]
36. Martinelli, I.; Sacchi, E.; Landi, G.; Taioli, E.; Duca, F.; Mannucci, P.M. High risk of cerebral-vein thrombosis in carriers of a prothrombin-gene mutation and in users of oral contraceptives. *N. Engl. J. Med.* **1998**, *338*, 1793–1797. [CrossRef] [PubMed]
37. de Bruijn, S.F.; Stam, J.; Koopman, M.M.; Vandenbroucke, J.P. Case-control study of risk of cerebral sinus thrombosis in oral contraceptive users and in [correction of who are] carriers of hereditary prothrombotic conditions. *Cereb. Venous Sinus Thromb. Study Group. BMJ* **1998**, *316*, 589.
38. Zuurbier, S.M.; Arnold, M.; Middeldorp, S.; Broeg-Morvay, A.; Silvis, S.M.; Heldner, M.R.; Meisterernst, J.; Nemeth, B.; Meulendijks, E.R.; Stam, J.; et al. Risk of Cerebral Venous Thrombosis in Obese Women. *JAMA Neurol.* **2016**, *73*, 579. [CrossRef]
39. Dentali, F.; Crowther, M.; Ageno, W. Thrombophilic abnormalities, oral contraceptives, and risk of cerebral vein thrombosis: A meta-analysis. *Blood* **2006**, *107*, 2766–2773. [CrossRef]
40. Knox, A.M.; Brophy, B.P.; Sage, M.R. Cerebral venous thrombosis in association with hormonal supplement therapy. *Clin. Radiol.* **1990**, *41*, 355. [CrossRef]
41. Godeneche, G.; Gaillard, N.; Roy, L.; Mania, A.; Tondeur, S.; Chomel, J.; Lavabre, T.; Arquizan, C.; Neau, J. JAK2 V617F Mutation Associated with Cerebral Venous Thrombosis: A Report of Five Cases. *Cerebrovasc. Dis.* **2010**, *29*, 206–209. [CrossRef]
42. Baldini, T.; Asioli, G.M.; Romoli, M.; Carvalho Dias, M.; Schulte, E.C.; Hauer, L.; Aguiar De Sousa, D.; Sellner, J.; Zini, A. Cerebral venous thrombosis and severe acute respiratory syndrome coronavirus-2 infection: A systematic review and meta-analysis. *Eur. J. Neurol.* **2021**, *28*, 3478. [CrossRef]
43. European Medicines Agency Safety Committee Report. Available online: https://www.ema.europa.eu/en/news/astrazenecas-covid-19-vaccine-ema-finds-possible-link-very-rare-cases-unusual-blood-clots-low-blood (accessed on 14 April 2021).
44. Thakur, K.T.; Tamborska, A.; Wood, G.K.; McNeill, E.; David Roh, D.; Akpan, I.J.; Miller, E.C.; Bautista, A.; Claassen, J.; Kim, C.Y.; et al. Clinical review of cerebral venous thrombosis in the context of COVID-19 vaccinations: Evaluation, management, and scientific questions. *J. Neurol. Sci.* **2021**, *427*, 117532. [CrossRef]
45. Perry, R.J.; Tamborska, A.; Singh, B.; Craven, B.; Marigold, R.; Arthur-Farraj, P.; Yeo, J.M.; Zhang, L.; Hassan-Smith, G.; Jones, M.; et al. Cerebral venous thrombosis after vaccination against COVID-19 in the UK: A multicenter cohort study. *Lancet* **2021**, *398*, 1147–1156. [CrossRef]
46. Pavord, S.; Scully, M.; Hunt, B.J.; Lester, W.; Bagot, C.; Craven, B.; Rampotas, A.; Ambler, G.; Makris, M. Clinical Features of Vaccine-Induced Immune Thrombocytopenia and Thrombosis. *N. Engl. J. Med.* **2021**, *385*, 1680. [CrossRef]
47. Greinacher, A.; Thiele, T.; Warkentin, T.E.; Weisser, K.; Kyrle, P.A.; Eichinger, S. Thrombotic thrombocytopenia after ChAdOx1 nCov-19 vaccination. *N. Engl. J. Med.* **2021**, *384*, 2092–2101. [CrossRef]

48. Dobbs, T.D.; Barber, Z.E.; Squier, W.L.; Green, A.L. Cerebral venous sinus thrombosis complicating traumatic head injury. *J. Clin. Neurosci.* **2012**, *19*, 1058. [CrossRef]
49. Schaller, B.; Graf, R. Cerebral Venous Infarction-The Pathophysiological Concept. *Cerebrovasc. Dis.* **2004**, *18*, 179–188. [CrossRef]
50. Gotoh, M.; Ohmoto, T.; Kuyama, H. Experimental study of venous circulatory disturbance by dural sinus occlusion. *Acta Neurochir.* **1993**, *124*, 120. [CrossRef]
51. Lövblad, K.O.; Bassetti, C.; Schneider, J.; Guzman, R.; El-Koussy, M.; Remonda, L.; Schroth, G.S.O. Diffusion-weighted mr in cerebral venous thrombosis. *Cereb. Dis.* **2001**, *11*, 169. [CrossRef]
52. Bousser, M.G.; Chiras, J.; Bories, J.; Castaigne, P. Cerebral venous thrombosis-a review of 38 cases. *Stroke* **1985**, *16*, 199. [CrossRef]
53. Ichord, R.N.; Benedict, S.L.; Chan, A.K.C.; Kirkham, F.; Nowakgottl, U. Paediatric cerebral sinovenous thrombosis: Findings of the International Paediatric Stroke Study. *Arch. Dis. Child.* **2015**, *100*, 174. [CrossRef]
54. Biousse, V.; Ameri, A.; Bousser, M.G. Isolated intracranial hypertension as the only sign of cerebral venous thrombosis. *Neurology* **1999**, *53*, 1537. [CrossRef]
55. Lopes, M.G.; Ferro, J.; Pontes, C. Henriques I for the Venoport Investigators. Headache and cerebral venous thrombosis. *Cephalalgia* **2000**, *20*, 292.
56. Cumurciuc, R.; Crassard, I.; Sarov, M.; Valade, D.; Bousser, M.G. Headache as the only neurological sign of cerebral venous thrombosis: A series of 17 cases. *J. Neurol. Neurosurg. Psychiatry* **2005**, *76*, 1084. [CrossRef]
57. de Bruijn, S.F.; Stam, J.; Kappelle, L.J. Thunderclap headache as first symptom of cerebral venous sinus thrombosis. CVST Study Group. *Lancet* **1996**, *348*, 1623. [CrossRef]
58. Jianu, D.C.; Jianu, S.N.; Dan, T.F.; Iacob, N.; Munteanu, G.; Motoc, A.G.M.; Baloi, A.; Hodorogea, D.; Axelerad, A.D.; Ples, H.; et al. Diagnosis and Management of Mixed Transcortical Aphasia Due to Multiple Predisposing Factors, including Postpartum and Severe Inherited Thrombophilia, Affecting Multiple Cerebral Venous and Dural Sinus Thrombosis: Case Report and Literature Review. *Diagnostics* **2021**, *11*, 1425. [CrossRef]
59. Ferro, J.M.; Canhão, P.; Bousser, M.G.; Stam, J.; Barinagarrementeria, F. Early Seizures in Cerebral Vein and Dural Sinus Thrombosis Risk Factors and Role of Antiepileptics. *Stroke* **2008**, *39*, 1152–1158. [CrossRef]
60. Ferro, J.M.; Correia, M.; Rosas, M.J.; Pinto, A.N.; Neves, G.; The Cerebral Venous Thrombosis Portuguese Collaborative Study Group [VENOPORT]. Seizures in cerebral vein and dural sinus thrombosis. *Cereb. Dis.* **2003**, *15*, 78–83. [CrossRef]
61. Lancon, J.; Killough, K.; Tibbs, R.; Lewis, A.; Parent, A. Spontaneous dural sinus thrombosis in children. *Pediatr. Neurosurg.* **1999**, *3*, 23. [CrossRef]
62. Ferro, J.M.; Correia, M.; Pontes, C.; Baptista, M.V.; Pita, F. Cerebral vein and dural sinus thrombosis in Portugal: 1980–1998. *Cerebrovasc. Dis.* **2001**, *11*, 177. [CrossRef]
63. Damak, M.; Crassard, I.; Wolff, V.; Bousser, M.G. Isolated Lateral Sinus Thrombosis A Series of 62 Patients. *Stroke* **2009**, *40*, 476–481. [CrossRef] [PubMed]
64. Jianu, D.C.; Jianu, S.N.; Motoc, A.G.M.; Poenaru, M.; Petrica, L.; Vlad, A.; Ursoniu, S.; Gogu, A.E.; Dan, T.F. Diagnosis and management of a young woman with acute isolated lateral sinus thrombosis. *Rom. J. Morphol. Embryol.* **2017**, *58*, 1515–1518. [PubMed]
65. Waldvogel, D.; Mattle, H.P.; Sturzenegger, M.; Schroth, G. Pulsatile tinnitus—A review of 84 patients. *J. Neurol.* **1998**, *245*, 137. [CrossRef] [PubMed]
66. Sakaida, H.; Kobayashi, M.; Ito, A.; Takeuchi, K. Cavernous sinus thrombosis: Linking a swollen red eye and headache. *Lancet* **2014**, *384*, 928. [CrossRef]
67. Ebright, J.R.; Pace, M.T.; Niazi, A.F. Septic thrombosis of the cavernous sinuses. *Arch. Intern. Med.* **2001**, *161*, 2671. [CrossRef]
68. Jacobs, K.; Moulin, T.; Bogousslavsky, J.; Woimant, F.; Dehaene, I.; Tatu, L.; Besson, G.; Assouline, E.; Casselman, J. The stroke syndrome of cortical vein thrombosis. *Neurology* **1996**, *47*, 376. [CrossRef]
69. Lacour, J.C.; Ducrocq, X.; Anxionnat, R.; Taillandier, L.; Auque, J.; Weber, M. Thrombosis of deep cerebral veins in form adults: Clinical features and diagnostic approach. *Rev. Neurol.* **2000**, *156*, 851.
70. van den Bergh, W.M.; van der Schaaf, I.; van Gijn, J. The spectrum of presentations of venous infarction caused by deep cerebral vein thrombosis. *Neurology* **2005**, *65*, 192. [CrossRef]
71. Pekçevik, Y.; Pekçevik, R. Why should we report posterior fossa emissary veins? *Diagn. Interv. Radiol.* **2014**, *20*, 78–81. [CrossRef]
72. Jianu, D.C.; Jianu, S.N.; Dan, T.F.; Motoc, A.G.M.; Poenaru, M. Pulsatile tinnitus caused by a dilated left petrosquamosal sinus. *Rom. J. Morphol. Embryol.* **2016**, *57*, 319–322. Available online: www.rjme.ro (accessed on 16 May 2021).
73. Kuehnen, J.; Schwartz, A.; Neff, W.; Hennerici, M. Cranial nerve syndrome in thrombosis of the transverse/sigmoid sinuses. *Brain* **1998**, *121*, 381. [CrossRef]
74. Ferro, J.M.; Bousser, M.-G.; Canhãoa, P.; Coutinho, J.M.; Crassard, I.; Dentali, F.; di Minnof, M.; Mainoh, A.; Martinelli, I.; Masuhr, F.; et al. European Stroke Organization guideline for the diagnosis and treatment of cerebral venous thrombosis—Endorsed by the European Academy of Neurology. *Eur. J. Neurol.* **2017**, *24*, 1203–1213. [CrossRef]
75. Dentali, F.; Squizzato, A.; Marchesi, C.; Bonzini, M.; Ferro, J.; Ageno, W. D-dimer testing in the diagnosis of cerebral vein thrombosis: A systematic review and a meta-analysis of the literature. *J. Thromb. Haemost.* **2012**, *10*, 582. [CrossRef]
76. Meng, R.; Wang, X.; Hussain, M.; Dornbos, D.; Meng, L.; Liu, Y.; Wu, Y.; Ning, M.; Buonanno, F.S.; Lo, E.H.; et al. Evaluation of plasma D-dimer plus fibrinogen in predicting acute CVST. *Int. J. Stroke* **2014**, *9*, 166. [CrossRef]

77. Canhão, P.; Abreu, L.F.; Ferro, J.M.; Stam, J.; Bousser, M.G.; Barinagarrementeria, F.; Fukujima, M.M.; for the ISCVT Investigators. Safety of lumbar puncture in patients with cerebral venous thrombosis. *Eur. J. Neurol.* **2013**, *20*, 1075. [CrossRef]
78. Rizzo, L.; Crasto, S.G.; Rudà, R.; Gallo, G.; Tola, E.; Garabello, D.; De Lucchi, R. Cerebral venous thrombosis: Role of CT, MRI and MRA in the emergency setting. *Radiol. Med.* **2010**, *115*, 313. [CrossRef]
79. Qu, H.; Yang, M. Early imaging characteristics of 62 cases of cerebral venous sinus thrombosis. *Exp. Med.* **2013**, *5*, 233–236. [CrossRef]
80. Boukobza, M.; Crassard, I.; Bousser, M.G.; Chabriat, H. MR Imaging Features of Isolated Cortical Vein Thrombosis: Diagnosis and Follow-Up. *Am. J. Neuroradiol.* **2009**, *30*, 344–348. [CrossRef]
81. Dan, T.F.; Jianu, S.N.; Iacob, N.; Motoc, A.G.M.; Munteanu, G.; Baloi, A.; Albulescu, N.; Jianu, D.C. Management of an old woman with cavernous sinus thrombosis with two different mechanisms: Case report and review of the literature. *Rom. J. Morphol. Embryol.* **2020**, *61*, 1329–1334. [CrossRef]
82. Buyck, P.-J.; De Keyzer, F.; Vanneste, D.; Wilms, G.; Thijs, V.; Demaerel, P. CT density measurement and H:H ratio are useful in diagnosing acute cerebral venous sinus thrombosis. *Am. J. Neuroradiol.* **2013**, *34*, 1568–1572. [CrossRef]
83. Poon, C.S.; Chang, J.-K.; Swarnkar, A.; Johnson, M.H.; Wasenko, J. Radiologic diagnosis of cerebral venous thrombosis: Pictorial review. *Am. J. Roentgenol.* **2007**, *189*, S64–S75. [CrossRef]
84. Virapongse, C.; Cazenave, C.; Quisling, R.; Sarwar, M.; Hunter, S. The empty delta sign: Frequency and significance in 76 cases of dural sinus thrombosis. *Radiology* **1987**, *162*, 779. [CrossRef]
85. Majoie, C.B.; van Straten, M.; Venema, H.W.; den Heeten, G.J.; Multisection, C.T. Venography of the dural sinuses and cerebral veins by using matched mask bone elimination. *AJNR Am. J. Neuroradiol.* **2004**, *25*, 787.
86. Khandelwal, N.; Agarwal, A.; Kochhar, R.; Bapuraj, J.R.; Singh, P.; Prabhakar, S.; Suri, S. Comparison of CT Venography with MR Venography in cerebral sinovenous thrombosis. *AJR Am. J. Roentgenol.* **2006**, *187*, 1637. [CrossRef] [PubMed]
87. Leach, J.L.; Fortuna, R.B.; Jones, B.V.; Gaskill-Shipley, M.F. Imaging of cerebral venous thrombosis: Current techniques, spectrum of findings, and diagnostic pitfalls. *Radiographics* **2006**, *26* (Suppl. 1), S19. [CrossRef]
88. Rodallec, M.H.; Krainik, A.; Feydy, A.; Hélias, A.; Colombani, J.-M.; Jullès, M.-C.; Marteau, V.; Zins, M. Cerebral venous thrombosis and multidetector CT angiography: Tips and tricks. *Radiographics* **2006**, *26* (Suppl. 1), S5. [CrossRef] [PubMed]
89. Dormont, D.; Anxionnat, R.; Evrard, S.; Louaille, C.; Chiras, J.; Marsault, C. MRI in cerebral venous thrombosis. *J. Neuroradiol.* **1994**, *21*, 81. [PubMed]
90. Isensee, C.; Reul, J.; Thron, A. Magnetic resonance imaging of thrombosed dural sinuses. *Stroke* **1994**, *25*, 29. [CrossRef] [PubMed]
91. Fellner, F.A.; Fellner, C.; Aichner, F.T.; Mölzer, G. Importance of T2*-weighted gradient-echo MRI for diagnosis of cortical vein thrombosis. *Eur. J. Radiol.* **2005**, *56*, 235. [CrossRef] [PubMed]
92. Selim, M.; Fink, J.; Linfante, I.; Kumar, S.; Schlaug, G.; Caplan, L.R. Diagnosis of cerebral venous thrombosis with echo-planar T2*-weighted magnetic resonance imaging. *Arch. Neurol.* **2002**, *59*, 1021. [CrossRef] [PubMed]
93. Mittal, S.; Wu, Z.; Neelavalli, J.; Haacke, E.M. Susceptibility weighted imaging: Technical aspects and clinical applications. Part 2. *AJNR Am. J. Neuroradiol.* **2009**, *30*, 232–252. [CrossRef]
94. Favrole, P.; Guichard, J.-P.; Crassard, I.; Bousser, M.-G.; Chabriat, H. Diffusion-weighted imaging of intravascular clots in cerebral venous thrombosis. *Stroke* **2004**, *35*, 99. [CrossRef]
95. Meckel, S.; Reisinger, C.; Bremerich, J.; Damm, D.; Wolbers, M.; Engelter, S.; Scheffler, K.; Wetzel, S.G. Cerebral venous thrombosis: Diagnostic accuracy of combined, dynamic and static, contrast-enhanced 4D MR venography. *AJNR Am. J. Neuroradiol.* **2010**, *31*, 527–535. [CrossRef]
96. Pallewatte, A.S.; Tharmalingam, T.; Liyanage, N. Anatomic variants and artefacts in non enhanced MRV—Potential pitfalls in diagnosing cerebral venous sinus thrombosis (CVST). *SLJR* **2016**, *1*, 40–46. [CrossRef]
97. Wetzel, S.G.; Kirsch, E.; Stock, K.W.; Kolbe, M.; Kaim, A.; Radue, E.W. Cerebral veins: Comparative study of CT venography with intraarterial digital subtraction angiography. *AJNR Am. J. Neuroradiol.* **1999**, *20*, 249.
98. Yang, J.Y.K.; Chan, A.K.C.; Callen, D.J.A.; Paes, B.A. Neonatal cerebral sinovenous thrombosis: Sifting the evidence for a diagnostic plan and treatment strategy. *Pediatrics* **2010**, *126*, e693–e700. [CrossRef]

Review

Imaging of Cerebral Venous Thrombosis

Jean-Claude Sadik [1,*], Dragos Catalin Jianu [2], Raphaël Sadik [3], Yvonne Purcell [1], Natalia Novaes [4], Edouard Saragoussi [1], Michaël Obadia [4], Augustin Lecler [1] and Julien Savatovsky [1]

1. Department of Diagnostic Neuroradiology, Hôpital Fondation A. de Rothschild, 75019 Paris, France
2. First Department of Neurology, "Victor Babes" University of Medecine and Pharmacy, 300041 Timisoara, Romania
3. Geriatrics Rehabilitation, Hospital Riviera Chablais—la Providence, 1800 Vevey, Switzerland
4. Department of Neurology, Stroke Unit, Hôpital Fondation A. de Rothschild, 75019 Paris, France
* Correspondence: jcsadik@for.paris

Abstract: Cerebral venous thrombosis is a rare cause of stroke. Imaging is essential for diagnosis. Although digital subtraction angiography is still considered by many to be the gold standard, it no longer plays a significant role in the diagnosis of cerebral venous thrombosis. MRI, which allows for imaging the parenchyma, vessels and clots, and CT are the reference techniques. CT is useful in case of contraindication to MRI. After presenting the radio-anatomy for MRI, we present the different MRI and CT acquisitions, their pitfalls and their limitations in the diagnosis of cerebral venous thrombosis.

Keywords: cerebral vein; cerebral venous thrombosis; venous stroke; dural sinus thrombosis; intracranial hypertension; MR venography; MRI; CT venography

1. Introduction

Cerebral venous thrombosis is a rare but potentially serious disease. It accounts for 0.5% to 1% of all strokes in adult populations. It can occur at any age but more frequently affects young people, particularly pregnant women and women on estrogen–progestin contraceptives.

Cerebral imaging is fundamental for detecting cerebral venous thrombosis and the parenchymal complications. Cerebral venous thrombosis is not diagnosed without imaging. Noninvasive cerebral imaging (CT and MRI) has completely replaced digital subtraction angiography (DSA), which is now used to guide exceptional endovascular treatments of the most severe forms that worsen despite effective anticoagulation.

Imaging cerebral venous thrombosis has a poor reputation because in the absence of good knowledge of the anatomy and the different results of CT and MRI, it is exposed to pitfalls that can be easily avoided [1].

This review are to illustrate the anatomy of the cerebral venous system and the accuracy of CT and MRI for cerebral venous thrombosis diagnosis. We present the main findings and pitfalls of these two imaging modes.

2. Pathophysiology

Cerebral venous thrombosis is secondary to a local or general imbalance of the coagulation system that leads to a thrombus developing in the dural sinuses or cerebral veins. Thrombosis of the dural sinuses leads to a delay in venous emptying and a decrease in the reabsorption of cerebral spinal fluid. Because of the obstruction, there is an increase in venous and capillary pressure.

If the collaterals are of good quality, the only symptoms are those related to intracranial hypertension. However, if the collaterals are insufficient or with extension to the cortical veins, the intracranial pressure may increase until it exceeds the cerebral perfusion pressure, thus increasing the ischemic risk.

Cerebral venous thrombosis leads to the formation of areas of focal edema related to increased retrograde pressure, characterized by venous dilatation, petechiae that are sometimes confluent and lead to hematomas, and focal non-systematized ischemic damage. Parenchymal lesions occur in 60% of patients with cerebral venous thrombosis and differ significantly from those in arterial stroke because they cross arterial boundaries, have a hemorrhagic component in nearly two-thirds of cases, and often feature a combination of vasogenic and cytotoxic edema.

3. Clinical Presentations

A wide range of symptoms should cause suspicion of cerebral venous thrombosis. These symptoms, which progressively worsen and fluctuate, are mostly nonspecific. The condition is diagnosed by imaging at 7 days on average after the onset of clinical symptoms.

The most common symptoms are headache that indicates intracranial hypertension, diplopia related to a sixth nerve palsy, papilledema [2], and an altered mental status. If symptoms appear suddenly, they can also reveal a subarachnoid hemorrhage [3–5] without arterial cause [Figure 1].

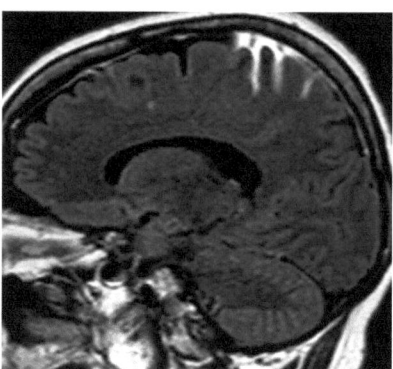

Figure 1. Sagittal fluid attenuated inversion recovery (FLAIR) image. Spontaneous subarachnoid hemorrhage in the precentral, central, and postcentral sulci in the context of cerebral venous thrombosis. Some cortical veins are visible, but their thrombosis cannot be verified because they are drowned in the spontaneous FLAIR signal of the subarachnoid hemorrhage.

Focal neurological motor or sensory deficits, aphasia, or hemianopsia are most often the result of a hematoma or parenchymal ischemia easily diagnosed on MRI and CT. Focal or generalized seizures are more common in cerebral venous thrombosis than in other causes of stroke.

Cerebral venous thrombosis occurs most often in populations with predisposing risk factors such as pro-thrombotic factors (genetic or acquired), autoimmune diseases, use of hormones for contraception or hormone replacement therapy, pregnancy, being in the postpartum period, heart failure, brain tumors (especially hematological diseases), and infections; however, in about 30% of cases, no cause is found.

4. Cerebral Venous Anatomy

The clinical presentation depends on the location and extension of the thrombus as well as parenchymal abnormalities [2]. Cerebral veins do not have valves [6] and are largely anastomosed to each other, which allows for the development of collateral circulation in case of occlusion.

Anatomical description is difficult due to the great variability of the cortical veins. However, the large deep veins and the dural sinuses can be easily identified. The walls of dural sinuses are formed by the dural mater.

The venous blood of the brain is drained by three networks of cerebral veins: the superficial veins (cortical), the deep veins, and the veins of the posterior fossa. These veins terminate in the dural venous sinuses, which are themselves collected by the jugular veins [7]. The superior sagittal sinus, the straight sinus, and the occipital sinus converge toward the posterior confluence of the sinuses (torcular Herophili), located at the level of the internal occipital protuberance [8] [Figure 2]. From the torcular Herophili, venous blood flows into the jugular veins after travelling through the transverse and sigmoid sinuses. The dural sinuses contain the Pacchionian arachnoidian granulations that are used for the resorption of cerebrospinal fluid. The superficial system begins with the subcortical veins that drain the outer surfaces of the cortex; these subcortical veins drain into the pial veins located on the surface of the cortex. The pial veins drain into the cerebral veins, which are located on the surface of the brain.

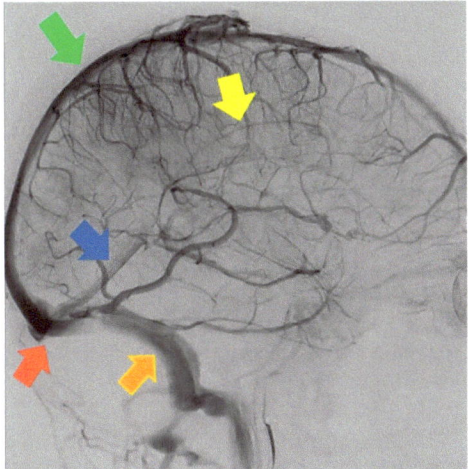

Figure 2. Digital subtraction angiography, sagittal plane. Green arrow: superior sagittal sinus. Yellow arrow: inferior sagittal sinus. Blue arrow: straight sinus. Orange arrow: lateral sinus. Red arrow: torcular Herophili.

There are many cerebral veins, but the three most important are the superficial middle cerebral veins; Trolard's vein (also known as the superior anastomotic vein), which connects the superior sagittal sinus to the middle cerebral vein; and Labbé's vein (also known as inferior anastomotic vein), which connects the middle cerebral vein to the lateral sinus [Figure 3].

The superficial cerebral veins can be divided into three collecting systems: a mediodorsal group draining into the superior sagittal sinus and straight sinus, a lateroventral group draining into the lateral sinus, and an anterior group draining into the cavernous sinus. These veins are connected by the superior anastomotic vein (Trolard's vein), which connects the superior sagittal sinus to the middle cerebral veins. The inferior anastomotic vein (Labbé's vein) connects the superior sagittal sinus and middle cerebral veins to the lateral sinus.

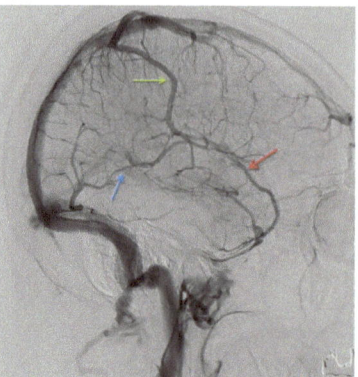

Figure 3. Digital subtraction angiography, sagittal plane. Red arrow: superficial middle cerebral vein. Green arrow: superior anastomotic vein (Trolard's vein). Blue arrow: inferior anastomotic vein (Labbé's vein).

MR Anatomy of the Superior Sagittal, Straight, Lateral and Torcular Sinuses

The superior sagittal single sinus drains most of the cortex. Its size increases from front to back. The anterior part may be absent and then replaced by two superior cerebral veins. It joins the straight sinus at the level of the torcular Herophili [Figure 2].

The inferior sagittal sinus, which is also single, drains the inner side of the middle part of the hemispheres and the corpus callosum.

The straight sinus, which is single, is the confluence of the vein of Galen and the inferior longitudinal sinus [Figure 4]. It drains into a transverse sinus (most often the left one) or into the torcular Herophili.

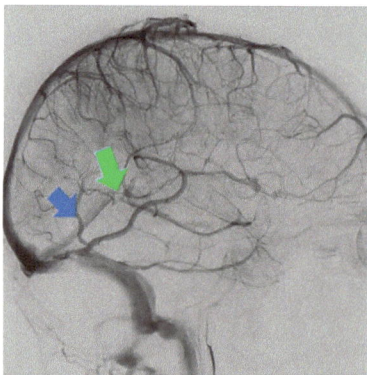

Figure 4. Digital subtraction angiography, sagittal plane. Anatomy of Galen's ampulla and straight sinus. The straight sinus receives blood from the inferior sagittal sinus and the vein of Galen. It flows into the torcular Herophili, where it joins the superior sagittal sinus. Green arrow: Galen's ampulla. Blue arrow: straight sinus.

The lateral sinuses are divided into the transverse sinus and sigmoid sinus. They are usually asymmetrical, with the right lateral sinus frequently larger than the left. This asymmetry and the frequent hypoplasia of the left lateral sinus are important to be aware of so as to not interpret poor filling as a thrombosis of the left lateral sinus.

Thus, the torcular Herophili receives blood from the superficial veins through the superior sagittal sinus and blood from the deep veins through the straight sinus [Figures 5 and 6].

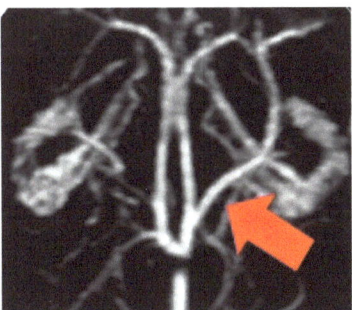

Figure 5. CE-MRV, axial and sagittal planes. MR anatomy of the basal veins. Red arrow: basal veins (former basal veins of Rosenthal).

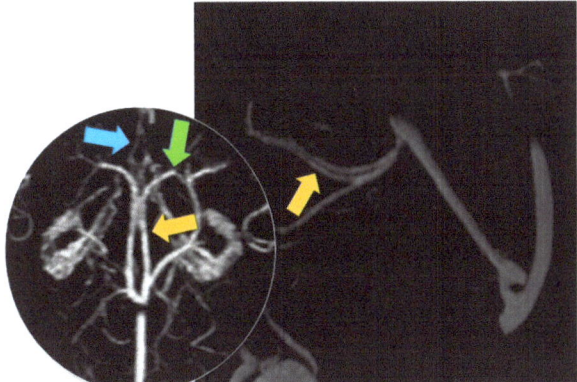

Figure 6. CE-MRV, axial and sagittal planes. MR anatomy of the septal, thalamostriate, and internal cerebral veins. Blue arrow: septal veins. Green arrow: thalamostriate veins. Yellow arrow: internal cerebral veins.

With symptoms suggesting cerebral venous thrombosis and knowledge of anatomy, what imaging techniques should be used?

5. Brain Imaging

DSA has long been considered the gold standard for the diagnosis of CVT. Today, it is used almost exclusively to guide interventional radiology procedures. The diagnosis is based on CT, CT venography, MRI, and MR venography. DSA is still superior to MR venography and CT venography in terms of dynamic information and can yield important additional information, particularly in collateral venous drainage.

Noninvasive neuroimaging with CT and MRI allows for the rapid diagnosis of cerebral venous thrombosis and thus affects the prognosis by improving the speed of management and monitoring. It provides two types of findings: direct signs corresponding to the visualization of the thrombus or venous thrombosis and indirect signs such as the presence of cerebral ischemia or hemorrhage.

Direct signs include "positive" visualization of the thrombus on nonenhanced CT and MRI and "negative" visualization of the thrombotic material as a filling defect on CT venography and MR venography.

Indirect signs refer to brain changes in the brain parenchyma that occurred after the thrombosis and include venous edema, venous infarction, subarachnoid hemorrhage, and parenchymal hemorrhage. Unlike arterial infarcts, venous infarcts do not respect arterial territories or cross territory boundaries.

The different imaging techniques are mainly noninjected or postinjection CT with venous time acquisition and MRI with MR venography. CT provides less information on the clot, the vessels, and the parenchyma and few clues favoring intracranial hypertension [9]. CT venography was found accurate for diagnosing cerebral sinus thrombosis [10,11]. MRI provides information on the clot, the vessels, the parenchyma, and possible signs of intracranial hypertension [5,9,12,13].

Although less efficient than MRI for the detection of parenchymal abnormalities, CT is the first-line examination because of its greater availability [1]. It is used for examining patients with contraindications to MRI.

Both CT and MRI should look for local causes that may have contributed to the cerebral venous thrombosis, especially staphylococcal infection on the face, mastoiditis, or sphenoidal or ethmoidal sinusitis.

6. MRI

From a clinical point of view, in a patient presenting headache, the question that every radiologist asks is: Should I look for a ruptured brain aneurysm or cerebral venous thrombosis? If an aneurysm is clearly suspected, arterial 3D time of flight (TOF) imaging should be systematically performed, covering the posterior inferior cerebellar arteries to the callosal marginal arteries.

In case of any unusual headache with neurological or visual signs or confusion, even if the onset is sudden, MR venography should be performed [4], with 2D or 3D phase contrast and 2D TOF or 3D T1 elliptical post-gadolinium enhancement [Figure 7].

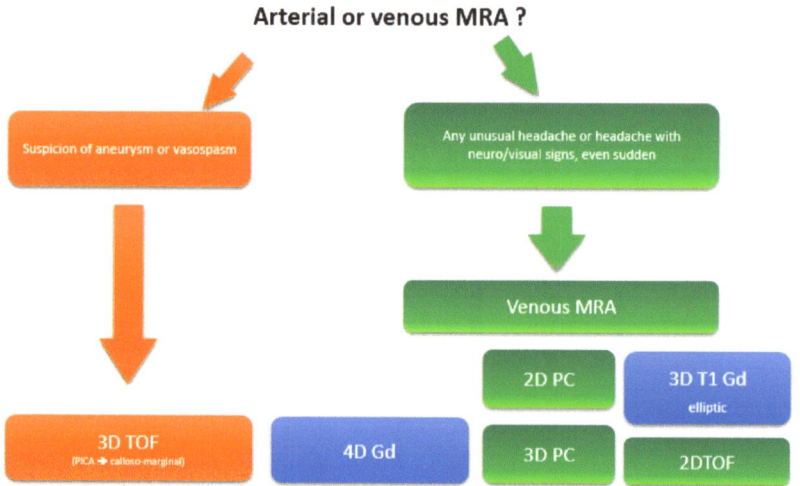

Figure 7. Decisional algorithm for choosing arterial or venous MR angiography. PC: phase contrast, Gd, gadolinium, TOF, time of flight.

Performed in the venous phase, 3D elliptical T1 post-gadolinium enhancement requires a bolus injection of gadolinium (0.1 mmol/kg with an injection flow rate of 2 to 3 mL/s) starting when the cerebral veins and/or the jugular veins are visible on the dynamic imaging detection of contrast arrival. Compared with 2D TOF and 2D phase contrast sequences, this sequence seems more efficient for visualizing the cortical veins, the deep system, and the sinuses of the base of the skull (petrous, cavernous, and basilar plexus). It also provides very good visualization of the lateral sinuses, even in cases of hypoplasia [12,14]. It also overcomes the limitations of other MR techniques, in particular signal losses in the event of slow or turbulent flows (2D TOF, 2D, and 3D phase contrast), not perpendicular to the acquisition plane (TOF) and in the event of inappropriate selection of encoding speed (2D and 3D phase contrast).

7. MRI Sequences and Semiology

Distinctions should be made between vascular semiology, the thrombus signal, and any parenchymal or meningeal repercussions [Figure 8 and Table 1].

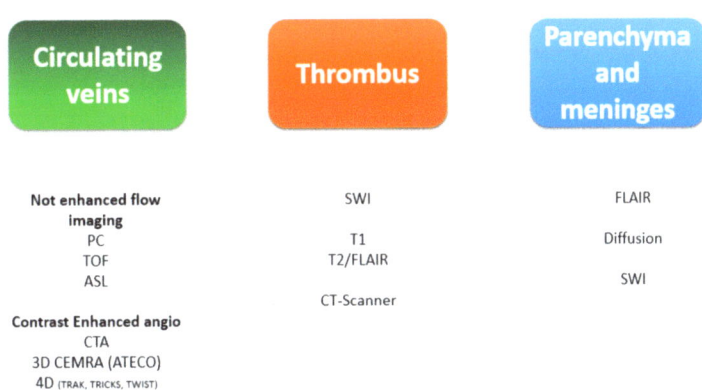

Figure 8. MRI sequences for imaging the veins, the thrombus, the parenchyma, and the meninges [15]. PC: phase contrast, TOF: time of flight, ASL: arterial spin labeling, CTA: CT angiography. 3D CE-MRA (ATECO): 3D contrast-enhanced MR angiography (auto-triggered elliptic centric ordered), 4D (TRAK, TRICKS, TWIST): dynamic contrast-enhanced MR angiography, FLAIR: fluid-attenuated inversion recovery, Diffusion: diffusion-weighted imaging, SWI: susceptibility-weighted imaging.

Table 1. MRI results according to sequences.

	Thrombus-Veins	Parenchyma	Optic Nerves	Sella
T1	Loss of flow hyposignal Thrombus in iso/hypersignal	Hypo/isosignal edema Hemorrhages-Petechiae		
T2	Thrombus in hypo/iso signal at the acute stage then hypersignal	High signal edema Sometimes: Small ventricles and ptosis of the cerebellar tonsils. Parenchymal hematoma	Intracranial hypertension: dilation of the optic nerve sheaths. Papilledema	intracranial hypertension: "Empty" sella turcica.
Axial T2* or SWI	Frank hyposignal. High sensitivity for cortical veins.	Hemorrhages-Petechiae.		
Axial DWI.	Thrombus in hypersignal	Hypersignal B1000 and decreased ADC in ischemic lesions.		
Enhanced 3DT1EG	Intraluminal defect			
Non-enhanced Venous MRA	Specifies the location of the occlusion.			
CE-MRA	Defect in the vein. Not very sensitive to slow flows. Good filling of the cortical veins.			
3D Flair	Thrombus in hypersignal.	Edema. Intra parenchymal hematoma. Subarachnoid hemorrhage.		

SWI: susceptibility-weighted imaging. DWI: diffusion-weighted imaging, CE-MRA: contrast-enhanced magnetic resonance angiography, ADC: apparent diffusion coefficient, FLAIR: fluid-attenuated inversion recovery.

Parenchymal abnormalities are found in only 40% [8] of patients with cerebral venous thrombosis. They are edema and ischemic and/or hemorrhagic softening [4]. The edema presents a hyposignal on T1 sequences and a hypersignal on T2 sequences, whereas the hemorrhage is globally hypersignal on T1 and T2 sequences and hyposignal on T2 gradient-echo sequences. Ischemia and hemorrhage areas [4] cross arterial boundaries, readily bilateral and asymmetrical.

Thrombosis of the superior sagittal sinus is often accompanied by frontal or parietal lobar hematomas, whereas thrombosis of the lateral sinus is accompanied by temporal or occipital lesions. Deep parenchymal abnormalities involving the thalami suggest thrombosis of the vein of Galen or the straight sinus.

The thrombus signal evolves in the same way as a hematoma. The progressive changes in clot signal are related to the paramagnetic properties of hemoglobin. The acute thrombus generally presents a hyposignal on T2* sequences and susceptibility-weighted imaging (SWI) and a hypersignal on spin-echo T1, T2, diffusion-weighted imaging (DWI) and fluid-attenuated inversion recovery (FLAIR) sequences. SWI and T2 gradient-echo sequences are useful because they are sensitive to hemoglobin breakdown products that cause an exaggerated signal drop-out [Figures 9 and 10]. However, the hyperintense signal on DWI has a lower sensitivity, but higher specificity, than the hyperintense on T2WI for the diagnosis of cerebral venous thrombosis [16,17].

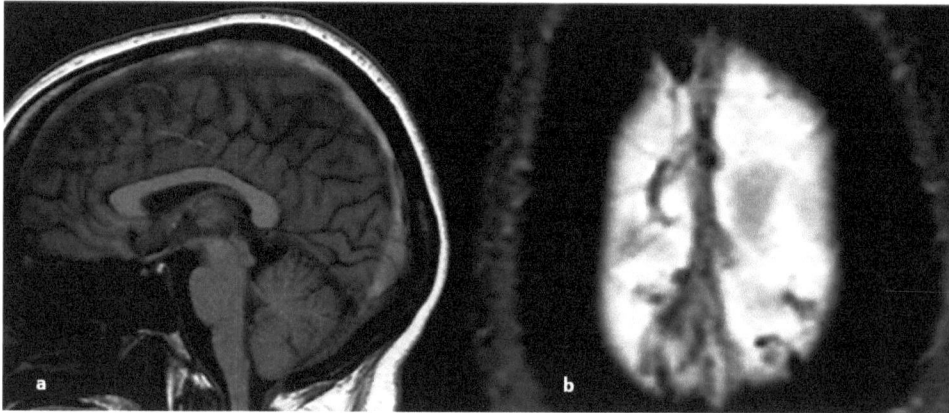

Figure 9. (a) Nonenhanced T1-weighted images, sagittal plane. Spontaneous hypersignal of the superior sagittal sinus suggests thrombosis. (b) T2* images, axial plane. Spontaneous hyposignal of the cortical veins of the vertex suggests cortical vein thrombi.

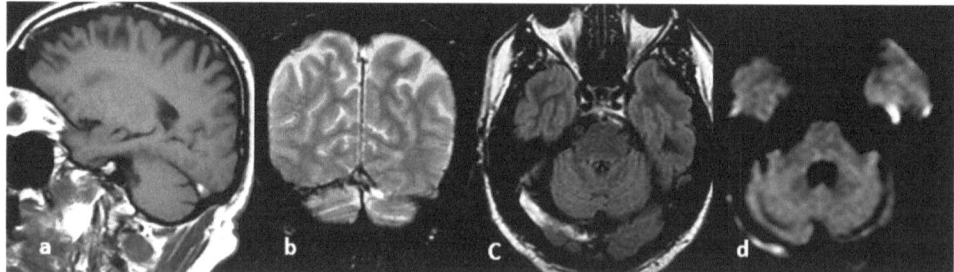

Figure 10. From left to right, spontaneous signal of the right lateral sinus suggesting thrombosis: (a) T1 hypersignal, (b) T2* hyposignal, (c) FLAIR hypersignal, (d) diffusion-weighted imaging hypersignal.

On enhanced morphological sequences after the injection of gadolinium, such as 3D T1 gadolinium enhancement, we look for a sign of "empty delta," revealing venous enhancement around the thrombus [6,13], which is not particularly enhanced. To be positive, the empty delta sign must be visualized on several sections [Figure 11].

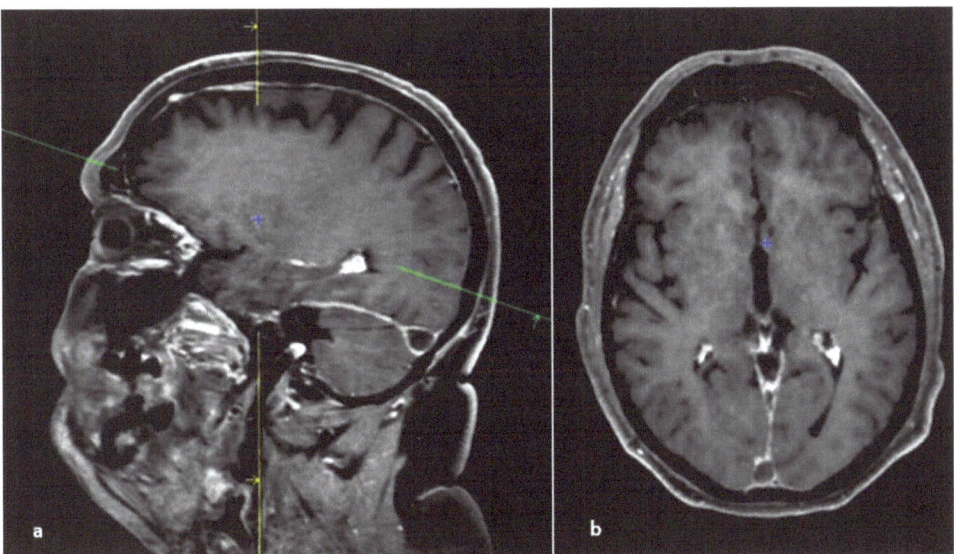

Figure 11. 3D contrast-enhanced T1-weighted gradient-echo images. (**a**) Sagittal plane; "empty delta" sign in the lateral sinus. (**b**) Axial plane; empty delta sign in the superior sagittal sinus. The enhancement related to the injection occurs around the thrombus, which appears in relative hyposignal.

Beyond 15 days, the diagnosis of cerebral venous thrombosis can be delicate because of the possible partial recanalization.

On 3D contrast-enhanced MR venography (CE-MRV) auto-triggered elliptic centric ordered (ATECO), we can observe the filling defect of the vein [8] linked to the presence of the thrombus [Figure 12]. The ATECO technique allows the bolus to be synchronized with the acquisition.

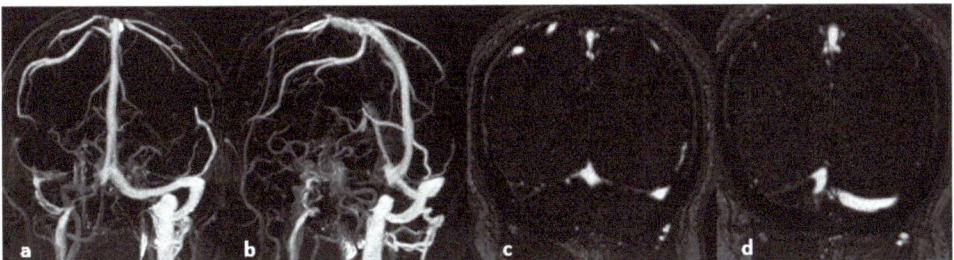

Figure 12. CE-MRV. From left to right: (**a,b**) maximum intensity projection (MIP) reconstructions; interruption of the proximal portion of the right lateral sinus; (**c,d**) native slices; defect in the lateral sinus suggests a thrombus.

Time-resolved MRA techniques: 4D-TRAK—Philips (4D Time Resolved Angiography using Keyhole), TRICKS—GE (Time Resolved Imaging of Contrast KineticS), TWIST—Siemens (time-resolved angiography with stochastic trajectories) allow for obtaining a sequential visualization of the arteries and then the veins and for answering the various questions when the symptomatology is too uncertain to engage directly in the search for cerebral venous thrombosis. A typical-time resolved MRA study might contain 20 images obtained at rates as rapid as 1–2 frames per second. An inherent trade-off exists between spatial and temporal resolution [18].

In case of intracranial hypertension, there will also be a dilation of the optic nerve sheaths and an empty sella turcica [Figure 13].

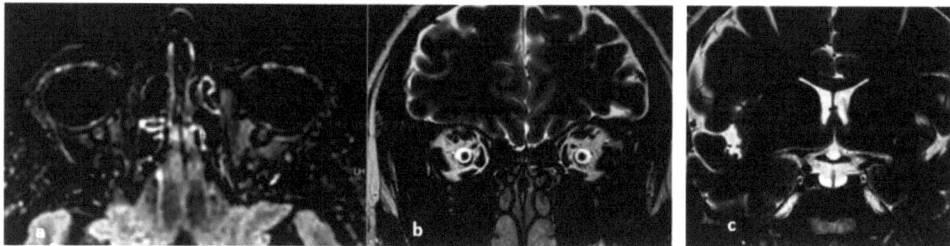

Figure 13. MRI signs of intracranial hypertension. They illustrate common findings in intracranial hypertension regardless of the presence of cerebral venous thrombosis. From left to right: (**a**) optic disc FLAIR hyperintensity, (**b**) dilation of the optic nerve sheaths, (**c**) empty sella turcica.

CE-MRV sequences should be differentiated from anatomical 3D T1 sequences such as SPGR, BRAVO, TFE, and FFE. These CE-MRV sequences are found in the manufacturers' catalogs of injected vascular sequences; they are optimized to visualize the enhanced circulating structures [Table 2]. Therefore, the parenchyma has a weak signal. Because of the short echo time (TE) and the possible use of masks, the fat is also erased. These CE-MRV sequences most often remain interpretable when using half doses of gadolinium. As with CT, with CE-MRV, the delay between injection and acquisition is from 35 to 45 s, and the injection flow rate 1 to 3 cc/s.

Table 2. Pitfalls of contrast-enhanced elliptical 3D sequences [8].

Risk	Solution
Acquisition too early: part of the venous system is not opacified	Immediately launch a new acquisition
	Using anatomical sequences: thrombus signal
	Complete with CT angiography
Missing a partial thrombosis on the MIP	Watch native images
Missing an old thrombosis (enhancement of the thrombus)	Do not use long and/or delayed injected sequences
Confusing Pacchionian granulation with thrombosis	Semiological knowledge

MR venography sequences allow for an initial positive diagnosis of cerebral venous thrombosis and also for monitoring the thrombus and visualizing its partial or complete recanalization. Complete recanalization is not necessary for symptom improvement.

MR venography sequences can be performed without contrast injection such as TOF or phase contrast or after the intravenous injection of gadolinium [19]. However, injected techniques are superior to TOF and phase contrast [Table 3].

Table 3. Advantages and disadvantages of techniques [8,20]. Gado: gadolinium, TOF: time of flight, PC: phase contrast. Elliptic 3D T1: CE-MRV.

Sequence	Gado	Duration	Advantages	Disadvantages
2D TOF	No	4 min	No contrast injection Arteries removed	Slow flow Cortical veins Spatial resolution
3D PC	No	6 min	No contrast injection Less sensitive to slow flows than 2DTOF	Slow flows Long Acquisition Spatial resolution
2D PC	No	2 min	No contrast injection Fast Acquisition No reconstructions	Slow flows Cortical vein Spatial resolution
Elliptic-centric 3D T1	Yes	1 min	Insensitive to slow flows (no false positives) Cortical veins	Not feasible if injection contraindicated Arteries not removed May contain fat interposition

Injected MR venography offers the same type of information as CT venography by showing the filling defect with similar sensitivities and specificities.

The vascular filling sequences with gadolinium are more reliable because of no risk of false positives on slow flows.

Additionally, 3D contrast-enhanced MR venography allows for better characterization of the intracranial venous anatomy [19]. If there is a contraindication to the injection, phase contrast is preferred to 2D TOF [9]. However, these CE-MRV sequences present some easily circumvented interpretation pitfalls.

What Is the Place of 3D Anatomical Sequences?

If we acquire 3D anatomical T1 sequences after the injection of gadolinium-based contrast agents [9], we must remember that in gradient echo, the venous sinuses are filled with gadolinium, whereas in spin echo, the sinus is naturally empty [Figure 14]. Therefore, the semiology of the poor filling of the vessel can only be retained on the T1 gradient-echo sequences after the injection of gadolinium.

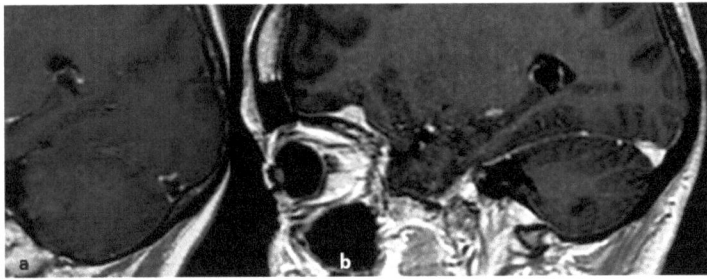

Figure 14. From left to right: (a) contrast-enhanced T1 spin echo, (b) contrast-enhanced T1 gradient echo.

Therefore, T1 spin echo is not a good technique for assessing the presence of a thrombus in a dural sinus.

Of note, old thrombi can be enhanced if the sequences are acquired too long after the injection. In chronic thrombosis, these sequences can be misinterpreted because of the possible enhancement of the clot, which can then mimic a permeable sinus.

The signal of the thrombus also evolves as a function of time, as shown in Table 4 [21].

Table 4. The evolution of the thrombus signal.

	Normal Sinus	Thrombus Less than 5 Days Old	Thrombus from D5 to D30	Thrombus Older than 1 Month
T1	Hyposignal	Isosignal	Hypersignal	Iso/Hypersignal
T2	Hyposignal	Hypo/Isosignal	Iso/Hypersignal	Iso/Hypersignal
Contrast-enhanced T1	Homogeneous because the fresh thrombus can be enhanced	Empty Delta sign	Empty Delta sign	Empty Delta

Along with vascular and parenchymal abnormalities, MRI signs of intracranial hypertension to look for include dilated optic nerve sheaths, papilledema, and empty sella turcica.

8. CT and Venous CT Scanning

Technique and Results

As well as MRI, CT can highlight parenchymal and vascular abnormalities. Because of its wide availability, CT is used in emergency departments as a triage examination for neurological symptoms not suggesting arterial ischemia. CT exposes the patient to significant ionizing radiation [19]. However, results remain normal in 30% of cases [13]. On nonenhanced CT [22], we can visualize direct and indirect signs of cerebral venous thrombosis.

Direct signs: a fresh thrombus spontaneously hyperdense in a dural sinus or a cortical vein usually called the "cord sign" [Figure 15] or dense clot sign [19,23–25]. The cord sign is best found in the first week of the disease, with estimated sensitivity of 64% and specificity of 97%. The spontaneous density of fresh blood gradually decreases after the first week. This sign is not very specific and can be falsely found in normal vessels with slow flow. Differential diagnoses are excessive visibility of circulating blood in venous structures in dehydrated patients, polycythemias, and increased hematocrit.

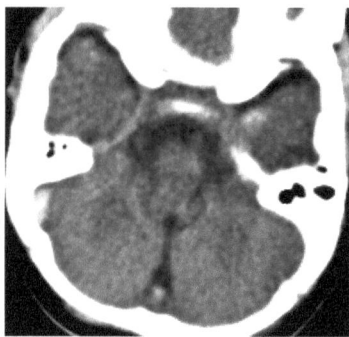

Figure 15. Nonenhanced CT. Spontaneous hyperdensity of the thrombus in the right lateral/sigmoid sinus junction.

Indirect signs: These occur in 60% to 80% of cases. The most common indirect signs evocative of cerebral venous thrombosis are multiple bilateral ischemic lesions or hematomas [Figure 16], bilateral thalamic edema, and temporo-occipital lesions [4,23]. Subarachnoid hemorrhage [10] or a herniation syndrome are also possibly seen.

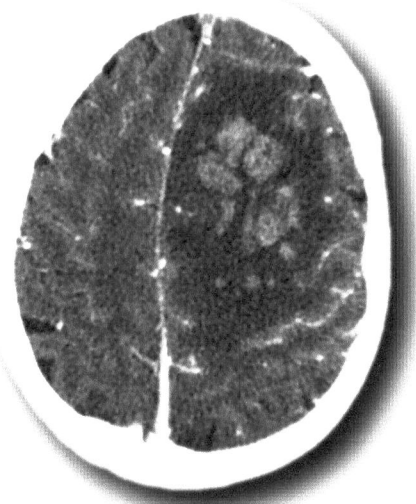

Figure 16. Left frontopolar venous hemorrhagic softening on CT.

The size of the ventricular cavities and good visibility of the sulci may be diminished in case of diffuse edema. Conversely, the volume of the ventricular cavities may sometimes be increased due to increased cerebrospinal fluid production and poor reabsorption. In these cases, the diagnosis of ventricular size change is greatly facilitated if the patient has previous neuroimaging findings.

The location of parenchymal abnormalities depends on the location of the thrombus and possible collateral supply routes. For example, deep abnormalities involving the internal capsule or thalami favor a deep venous thrombosis; temporo-occipital lesions suggest transverse sinus thrombosis and bilateral parasagittal hemispheric lesions of superior sagittal sinus thrombosis. The presence of a hemorrhagic focus or localized edema near a dural sinus favors a thrombosis of the sinus.

In case of suspected cerebral venous thrombosis on nonenhanced CT, the examination should be followed by CT venography or MR venography.

On iodinated contrast-enhanced CT, the injection is best performed with an automatic injector pushing 20 to 40 cc of iodinated contrast medium followed by physiological saline with an injection flow rate of 2 to 4 cc/sec. Volume acquisition starts from C1 to the vertex starting at 35 to 45 sec (or on the detection of arrival of the bolus in the right jugular vein) after the injection.

After intravenous injection [23], the most characteristic semiology is the empty delta sign [13], which results in a filling defect (corresponding to the thrombus) of contrast enhancement within a dural sinus enhanced in the periphery [6] [Figure 17]. To be positive, the sign of the empty delta must be visualized on several sections. The empty delta sign is most often visible between 5 days and 2 months after the event.

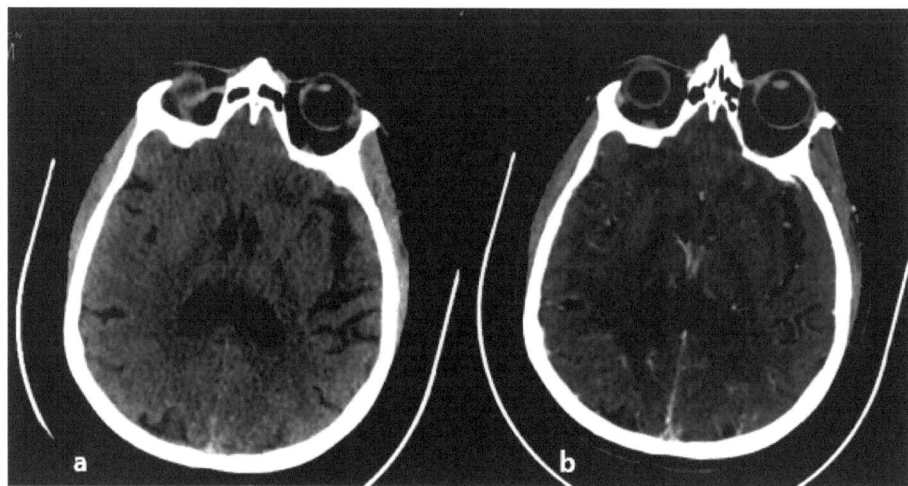

Figure 17. CT. From left to right: (**a**) nonenhanced CT: spontaneous hyperdensity of the superior sagittal sinus, (**b**) enhanced CT: empty delta sign testifying to the circulation of contrast around the thrombus, which appears as a defect of signal in the center of the superior sagittal sinus.

CT venography is less sensitive for the diagnosis of deep cortical venous thrombosis than for large dural sinus thrombosis; this can be improved by performing multiplanar reformations [Figure 18].

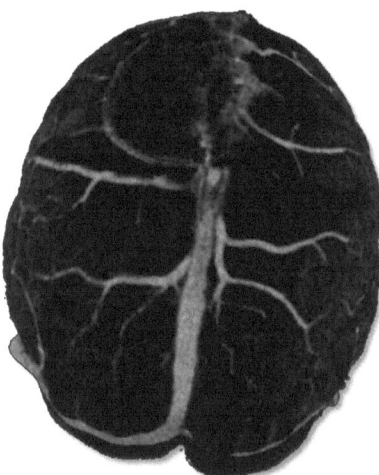

Figure 18. Volume rendering reconstructions of cerebral CT venography. Thrombosis of the anterior part of the superior sagittal sinus.

A false positive delta sign occurs when the superior sagittal sinus divides early. A split sinus or a septum within a sinus can also lead to a false positive diagnosis of cerebral venous thrombosis in an image with a pseudo empty delta sign. As in MRI, in CT, a chronic thrombus may enhance after iodinated contrast media injection and no longer give an empty delta sign.

The signs of intracranial hypertension, in particular the dilation of the optic nerve sheaths, are less well visualized than on MRI. The empty sella turcica remains clearly visible.

Again, normal CT results do not rule out cerebral venous thrombosis, and with any clinical doubt, complementary MRI should be performed.

9. Sensitivity and specificity

MRI: Several studies with evidence judged low compared MRI with MR venography with DSA acquisition. MR venography reliably demonstrated the large cerebral veins and sinus visualized on DSA. DSA was more sensitive than MR venography in evaluating the smaller cortical veins and the deep subcortical veins. In one study [26] of 20 patients with cerebral venous thrombosis, all documented by DSA, MRI with MR venography provided the diagnosis in all cases. When DSA was used as reference standard, CE-MRI had sensitivity and specificity 83% and 100%, respectively [27]. In another study of 92 patients [28], the sensitivity of MRI was 87%, specificity was 76.9%, positive predictive value was 94%, and negative predictive value was 58%.

The recommendation of the European Stroke Organization guidelines for the diagnosis of cerebral venous thrombosis is the use of MR venography as a reliable alternative to DSA for confirmation in patients with suspected cerebral venous thrombosis [5].

CT: Similarly, several studies with evidence judged low compared CT with CT venography with DSA. CT with CT venography was able to detect all cerebral venous thrombosis in patients with suspected cerebral venous thrombosis [29].

The recommendation of the European Stroke Organization guidelines for the diagnosis of cerebral venous thrombosis is the use of CT venography as a reliable alternative to DSA for the diagnosis of cerebral venous thrombosis [5].

In Xu's meta-analysis, published in 2018 [30], 24 eligible articles comprising 48 studies (4595 cases) were included. The pooled sensitivity of the CT-CVT (cerebral venous thrombosis)/CT-CVST (cerebral venous sinus thrombosis) groups was 0.79 and the specificity was 0.90, respectively. For the MRI-CVT/MRI-CVST groups, the pooled sensitivity was 0.82 and the pooled specificity was 0.92, respectively.

Digital Subtraction Angiography (DSA)

DSA for the positive diagnosis of cerebral venous thrombosis theoretically remains the most accurate method, but it has become exceptional because of noninvasive imaging. Cerebral angiography is performed only in cases of any doubt with CT venography or MR venography. The venous time must be visualized on at least two views. To improve diagnostic performance, the contralateral carotid artery is compressed. The diagnosis of cerebral venous thrombosis is easy with extensive thrombosis of the superior sagittal sinus, lateral sinus, or straight sinus [31]. The diagnosis is established on the typical presentation of a direct sign (absence of opacification of the thrombosed sinus) and indirect signs (presence of collateral circulation with venous dilatation and tortuous veins) but is more difficult when part of the sinus is not opacified or is irregular, in which case the indirect signs are more useful.

DSA is also used to guide exceptional therapeutic procedures such as endovascular mechanical thrombectomy used alone or combined with other techniques such as direct aspiration or pharmacological thrombolysis.

10. Summary of Imaging Support

If MRI is possible [13], 3D T1 turbo spin echo (TSE) without injection + 3D SWI + 3D FLAIR without injection + axial DWI, coronal T2 on the optical pathways; injection of gadolinium, then 3D CE-MR venography and 3D T1 gradient echo (for the veins) and spin echo if in doubt about an associated parenchymal or meningeal anomaly (e.g., meningioma), paying attention to the fact that the sinus is empty at the base in spin echo.

If MRI is impossible because not accessible or contraindicated, CT without injection can be followed by venous CT venography. However, CT exposes the patient to significant ionizing radiation [19].

11. Special Cases

11.1. Thrombosis of the Straight Sinus

Straight sinus thrombosis is a classical but rare type of cerebral venous thrombosis. It is difficult to diagnose. It appears as deep ischemic changes with or without hemorrhagic parenchymal changes that are often thalamic or even bi-thalamic [1] [Figures 19–21]. One of the differential diagnoses of straight sinus thrombosis is thrombosis of the artery of Percheron [31,32]. This artery is an anatomical variant. It is a single artery vascularizing the bi-thalamic territory. It usually arises from the first segment of one of the posterior cerebral arteries.

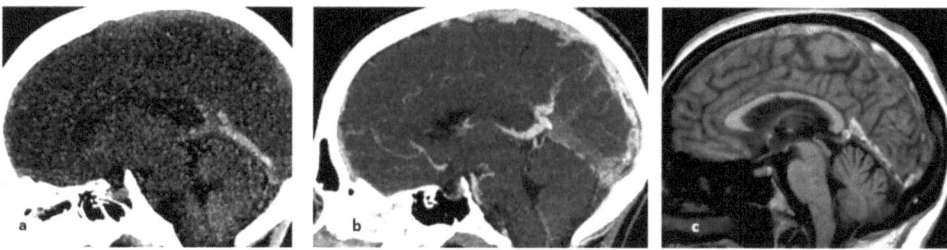

Figure 19. From left to right: (**a**) nonenhanced CT, sagittal plane; (spontaneous hyperdensity of the straight sinus); (**b**) after the injection of iodinated contrast media, absence of opacification of the straight sinus, thrombosis of the superior sagittal sinus above the torcular Herophili; (**c**) MRI, nonenhanced sagittal T1 sequence: spontaneous hypersignal of the thrombus.

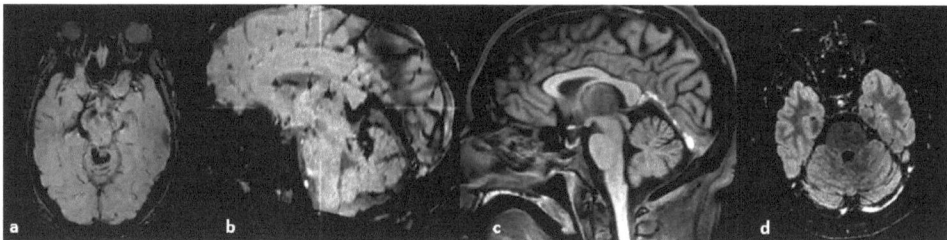

Figure 20. From left to right: (**a,b**) susceptibility-weighted imaging, axial (**a**) and sagittal (**b**) planes (thrombosis of the internal cerebral and basilar veins and straight sinus); (**c**) T1 sequence sagittal plane (spontaneous hypersignal of the thrombus in the straight sinus); (**d**) FLAIR image, axial plane (spontaneous hypersignal of the thrombus in the left lateral sinus).

Bi-thalamic disorders classically present a clinical triad associating paralysis of verticality, memory disorders, and confusion. This triad manifests the same in arterial (Percheron's artery) or venous (right sinus thrombosis) involvement.

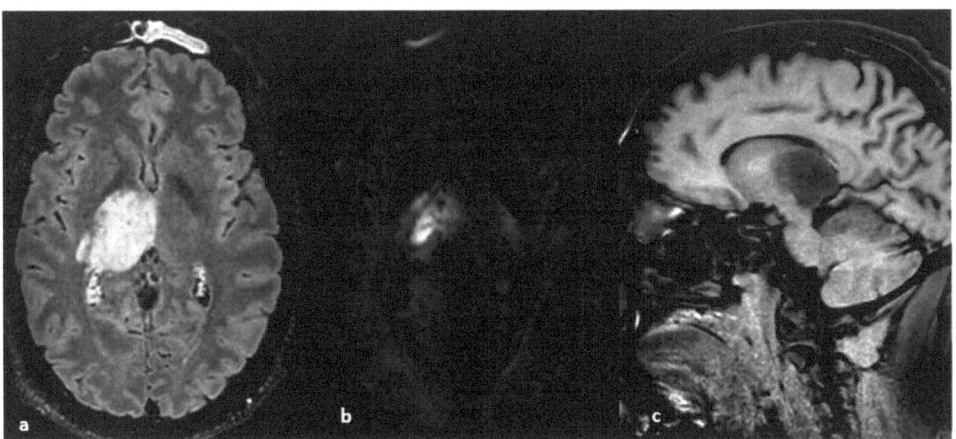

Figure 21. Ischemic lesion of the right thalamus. (**a**) FLAIR image, axial plane (spontaneous hypersignal of the right thalamus); (**b**) diffusion-weighted imaging; (hypersignal of the right thalamus); (**c**) nonenhanced T1 image, sagittal plane; (hyposignal of the right thalamus); (**d**) nonenhanced CT image (hypodensity of the right thalamus); (**e**) thrombosis of the right internal cerebral vein. Note the presence of left frontal sinusitis.

11.2. Thrombosis of Labbé's Vein

Labbé's vein, also known as the inferior anastomotic vein, is part of the superficial venous system of the brain. It connects the superficial middle cerebral to the lateral sinus. CT and MR reveal parenchymal temporal lesions ipsilateral to the thrombosis and a spontaneously hyperdense (CT) and hypersignal T1 (MRI) extra-axial band corresponding to the thrombosed vein of Labbé [33].

11.3. Differential Diagnoses

Hypoplasia of a lateral sinus: Attention must be paid to signal asymmetries linked to hypoplasia or aplasia of the lateral sinuses, particularly on the left side [Figure 22].

How to diagnose: With a hypoplastic lateral sinus, the groove of the lateral sinus, the jugular foramen, and the internal jugular vein are also hypoplastic on the same side, frequently with contralateral hypertrophy. In 3D FLAIR sequences, the asymmetry of the calibers of the two lateral sinuses can be visualized. The CE-MR venography sequences confirm the absence of a lacuna within the hypoplastic sinus. Finally, cases of frank hypoplasia frequently exhibit the presence of an occipital sinus, although it is not constant, especially with hypoplasia on the proximal third with a distal portion of the lateral sinus supplied by a large anastomotic vein.

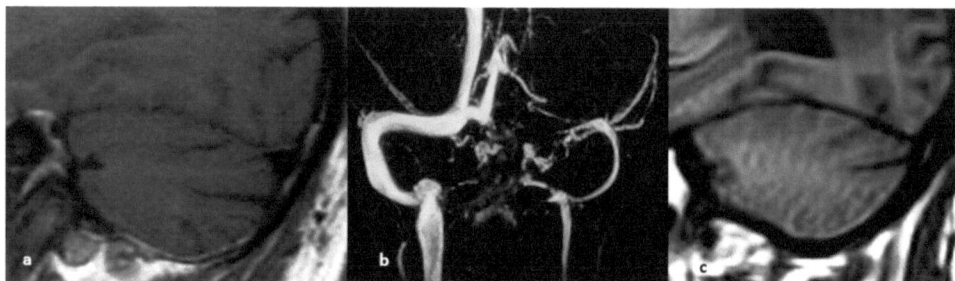

Figure 22. Left lateral sinus hypoplasia: (**a**) sagittal plane of the right lateral sinus; (**b**) phase contrast, lack of filling of the left lateral sinus; (**c**) sagittal plane of the right lateral sinus confirming its small caliber.

Pacchionian granulations [3,8]. Pacchionian arachnoid granulations are normal structures that protrude into the lumen of the dural sinus. When they are large, they can simulate a sinus thrombosis. They are most often seen in the transverse and superior sagittal sinuses. With the improvement in MRI spatial and contrast resolution, filling defects corresponding to arachnoid granulations are increasingly better visualized [Figure 23].

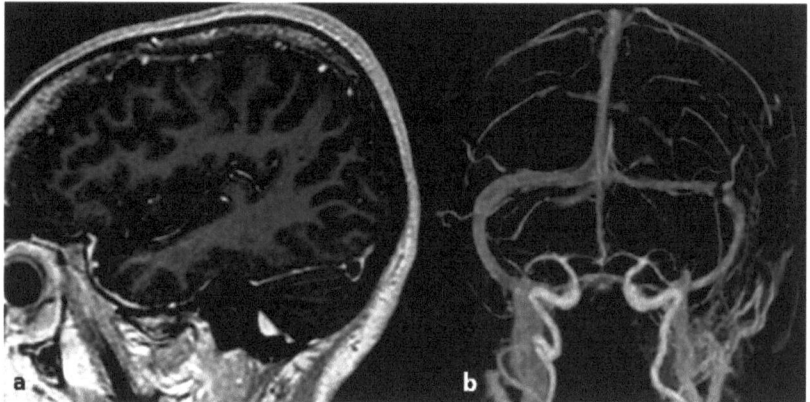

Figure 23. (**a**) Contrast-enhanced T1 image, sagittal plane (filling defect in the left lateral sinus); (**b**) CE-MRV confirms the typical round aspect of Pacchionian arachnoid granulations.

Arachnoid granulations must be differentiated from filling defects secondary to sinus thrombosis. Arachnoid granulations typically have a signal like that of cerebrospinal fluid and appear as focal filling defects with a characteristic anatomical distribution. They are often rounded and adherent to the wall of the dural sinus. After injection, they may present heterogeneous central enhancement.

Termination of the superior sagittal sinus above the torcular in the right lateral sinus. A high or asymmetric bifurcation may resemble an intra-sinus thrombus and induce a false empty delta sign [21]. The assessment of sequential images and the documentation of venous continuity are necessary to avoid this pitfall.

Conclusion: MRI and/or cerebral CT are reliable alternatives to DSA for imaging cerebral venous thrombosis. They are essential for the positive diagnosis of cerebral venous thrombosis. CT venography and MR venography are equally accurate for diagnosing cerebral venous thrombosis. The advantage of CT is the rapid acquisition, and the disadvantage is the significant exposure to ionizing radiation. MRI has the advantage of showing the thrombus itself and being more sensitive in detecting parenchymal lesions. Techniques may need to be combined to avoid pitfalls. The semiology of the nonenhanced CT should not be ignored because this examination remains widely practiced in cases of nonspecific neurological symptoms. Contrast-enhanced MRI is more accurate than non–contrast-enhanced MRI for diagnosing cerebral venous thrombosis and CT venography is more accurate than CT alone [23]. The radiologist must master the cerebral venous sinus anatomy and the different acquisitions to best orient the examination and avoid the pitfalls.

Funding: This research received no external funding.

Institutional Review Board Statement: The review did not require ethical approval.

Informed Consent Statement: Written informed consent has been obtained from the patient(s) to publish this paper.

Conflicts of Interest: Julien Savatovsky received honoraria for lectures and board participation from Bayer Healthcare. The other authors declare no conflict of interest.

References

1. Ulivi, L.; Squitieri, M.; Cohen, H.; Cowley, P.; Werring, D.J. Cerebral venous thrombosis: A practical guide. *Pract. Neurol.* **2020**, *20*, 356–367. [CrossRef] [PubMed]
2. Jianu, D.C.; Jianu, S.N.; Munteanu, G.; Flavius, T.D.; Brasan, C. *Ischemic Stroke of Brain*; IntechOpen: London, UK, 2018; Volume 1, pp. 45–76, ISBN 978-1-83881-709-1.
3. Stam, J. Thrombosis of the cerebral veins and sinuses. *N. Engl. J. Med.* **2005**, *352*, 1791–1798. [CrossRef]
4. Bousser, M.-G.; Ferro, J.M. Cerebral venous thrombosis: An update. *Lancet Neurol.* **2007**, *6*, 162–170. [CrossRef]
5. Ferro, J.M.; Bousser, M.; Canhão, P.; Coutinho, J.M.; Crassard, I.; Dentali, F.; di Minno, M.; Maino, A.; Martinelli, I.; Masuhr, F.; et al. European Stroke Organization guideline for the diagnosis and treatment of cerebral venous thrombosis—Endorsed by the European Academy of Neurology. *Eur. J. Neurol.* **2017**, *24*, 1203–1213. [CrossRef] [PubMed]
6. Li, A.Y.; Tong, E.; Yedavalli, V.S. A case-based review of cerebral venous infarcts with perfusion imaging and comparison to arterial ischemic stroke. *Front. Radiol.* **2021**, *1*, 687045. [CrossRef]
7. Arquizan, C. Thrombophlébites cérébrales: Aspects cliniques, diagnostic et traitement. *Réanimation* **2001**, *10*, 383–391. [CrossRef]
8. Canedo-Antelo, M.; Baleato-González, S.; Mosqueira, A.J.; Casas-Martínez, J.; Oleaga, L.; Vilanova, J.C.; Luna-Alcalá, A.; García-Figueiras, R. Radiologic clues to cerebral venous thrombosis. *RadioGraphics* **2019**, *39*, 1611–1628. [CrossRef]
9. Qu, H.; Yang, M. Early imaging characteristics of 62 cases of cerebral venous sinus thrombosis. *Exp. Ther. Med.* **2013**, *5*, 233–236. [CrossRef]
10. Gaikwad, A.B.; Mudalgi, B.A.; Patankar, K.B.; Patil, J.K.; Ghongade, D.V. Diagnostic role of 64-slice multidetector row CT scan and CT venogram in cases of cerebral venous thrombosis. *Emerg. Radiol.* **2008**, *15*, 325–333. [CrossRef]
11. Linn, J.; Ertl-Wagner, B.; Seelos, K.C.; Strupp, M.; Reiser, M.; Brückmann, H.; Brüning, R. Diagnostic value of multidetector-row CT angiography in the evaluation of thrombosis of the cerebral venous sinuses. *Am. J. Neuroradiol.* **2007**, *28*, 946–952.
12. Dmytriw, A.A.; Song, J.S.A.; Yu, E.; Poon, C.S. Cerebral venous thrombosis: State of the art diagnosis and management. *Neuroradiology* **2018**, *60*, 669–685. [CrossRef] [PubMed]
13. Saposnik, G.; Barinagarrementeria, F.; Brown, R.D.; Bushnell, C.D.; Cucchiara, B.; Cushman, M.; DeVeber, G.; Ferro, J.; Tsai, F.Y. Diagnosis and management of cerebral venous thrombosis: A statement for healthcare professionals from the American Heart Association/American Stroke Association. *Stroke* **2011**, *42*, 1158–1192. [CrossRef] [PubMed]
14. Hu, H.H.; Haider, C.R.; Campeau, N.G.; Huston, J., III; Riederer, S.J. Intracranial contrast-enhanced magnetic resonance venography with 6.4-fold sensitivity encoding at 1.5 and 3.0 Tesla. *J. Magn. Reson. Imaging* **2008**, *27*, 653–658. [CrossRef] [PubMed]
15. Bonneville, F. Imaging of cerebral venous thrombosis. *Diagn. Interv. Imaging* **2014**, *95*, 1145–1150. [CrossRef]
16. Lv, B.; Tian, C.-L.; Cao, X.-Y.; Liu, X.-F.; Wang, J.; Yu, S.-Y. Role of diffusion-weighted imaging in the diagnosis of cerebral venous thrombosis. *J. Int. Med. Res.* **2020**, *48*, 300060520933448. [CrossRef]
17. Lv, B.; Jing, F.; Tian, C.-L.; Liu, J.-C.; Wang, J.; Cao, X.-Y.; Liu, X.-F.; Yu, S.-Y. Diffusion-weighted magnetic resonance imaging in the diagnosis of cerebral venous thrombosis: A meta-analysis. *J. Korean Neurosurg. Soc.* **2021**, *64*, 418–426. [CrossRef]
18. Meckel, S.; Reisinger, C.; Bremerich, J.; Damm, D.; Wolbers, M.; Engelter, S.; Scheffler, K.; Wetzel, S. Cerebral venous thrombosis: Diagnostic accuracy of combined, dynamic and static, contrast-enhanced 4D MR venography. *Am. J. Neuroradiol.* **2010**, *31*, 527–535. [CrossRef] [PubMed]
19. Leach, J.L.; Fortuna, R.B.; Jones, B.V.; Gaskill-Shipley, M.F. Imaging of cerebral venous thrombosis: Current techniques, spectrum of findings, and diagnostic pitfalls. *RadioGraphics* **2006**, *26*, S19–S41. [CrossRef]
20. Oliveira, I.M.; Duarte, J.; Dalaqua, M.; Jarry, V.M.; Pereira, F.V.; Reis, F. Cerebral venous thrombosis: Imaging patterns. *Radiol. Bras.* **2022**, *55*, 54–61. [CrossRef]
21. Boukobza, M.; Crassard, I.; Bousser, M.; Chabriat, H. MR imaging features of isolated cortical vein thrombosis: Diagnosis and follow-up. *Am. J. Neuroradiol.* **2009**, *30*, 344–348. [CrossRef]

22. Linn, J.; Pfefferkorn, T.; Ivanicova, K.; Müller-Schunk, S.; Hartz, S.; Wiesmann, M.; Dichgans, M.; Brückmann, H. Noncontrast CT in deep cerebral venous thrombosis and sinus thrombosis: Comparison of its diagnostic value for both entities. *Am. J. Neuroradiol.* **2009**, *30*, 728–735. [CrossRef] [PubMed]
23. Van Dam, L.F.; van Walderveen, M.A.; Kroft, L.J.; Kruyt, N.D.; Wermer, M.J.; van Osch, M.J.; Huisman, M.V.; Klok, E. Current imaging modalities for diagnosing cerebral vein thrombosis—A critical review. *Thromb. Res.* **2020**, *189*, 132–139. [CrossRef] [PubMed]
24. Coutinho, J.M. Cerebral venous thrombosis. *J. Thromb. Haemost.* **2015**, *13*, S238–S244. [CrossRef] [PubMed]
25. Bousser, M.G.; Barnett, H.J.M. Chapter 12: Cerebral venous thrombosis. In *Stroke: Pathophysiology, Diagnosis, and Management*, 4th ed.; Mohr, J.P., Ed.; Churchill Livingstone: Philadelphia, PA, USA, 2004; pp. 301–325. ISBN 9780443066009.
26. Lafitte, F.; Boukobza, M.; Guichard, J.; Hoeffel, C.; Reizine, D.; Ille, O.; Woimant, F.; Merland, J. MRI and MRA for diagnosis and follow-up of cerebral venous thrombosis (CVT). *Clin. Radiol.* **1997**, *52*, 672–679. [CrossRef]
27. Liang, L.; Korogi, Y.; Sugahara, T.; Onomichi, M.; Shigematsu, Y.; Yang, D.; Kitajima, M.; Hiai, Y.; Takahashi, M. Evaluation of the intracranial dural sinuses with a 3D contrast-enhanced MP-RAGE sequence: Prospective comparison with 2D-TOF MR venography and digital subtraction angiography. *Am. J. Neuroradiol.* **2001**, *22*, 481–492.
28. Hatami, H.; Danesh, N.; Shojaei, M.; Hamedani, A.R. Evaluation of diagnostic values in NCCT and MRI of the patients with cerebral venous or sinus thrombosis in Loghman Hakim Hospital in Tehran 2014–2018. *Int. Clin. Neurosci. J.* **2019**, *6*, 17–21. [CrossRef]
29. Wong, G.K.C.; Siu, D.Y.W.; Abrigo, J.M.; Ahuja, A.T.; Poon, W.S. Computed tomographic angiography for patients with acute spontaneous intracerebral hemorrhage. *J. Clin. Neurosci.* **2012**, *19*, 498–500. [CrossRef]
30. Xu, W.; Gao, L.; Li, T.; Ramdoyal, N.D.; Zhang, J.; Shao, A. The performance of CT versus MRI in the differential diagnosis of cerebral venous thrombosis. *Thromb. Haemost.* **2018**, *118*, 1067–1077. [CrossRef]
31. Lazzaro, N.; Wright, B.; Castillo, M.; Fischbein, N.; Glastonbury, C.; Hildenbrand, P.; Wiggins, R.; Quigley, E.; Osborn, A. Artery of percheron infarction: Imaging patterns and clinical spectrum. *Am. J. Neuroradiol.* **2010**, *31*, 1283–1289. [CrossRef]
32. Kheiralla, O.; Alghamdi, S.; Aljondi, R.; Tajaldeen, A.; Bakheet, A. Artery of percheron infarction: A characteristic pattern of ischemia and variable clinical presentation: A literature review. *Curr. Med. Imaging* **2021**, *17*, 669–674. [CrossRef]
33. Shivaprasad, S.; Shroff, G.; Kumar, V. Vein of Labbe thrombosis by CT and MRI. *J. Neurol. Neurosurg. Psychiatry* **2012**, *83*, 1168–1169. [CrossRef] [PubMed]

Review

Epidemiology and Management of Cerebral Venous Thrombosis during the COVID-19 Pandemic

Natalia Novaes [1], Raphaël Sadik [2], Jean-Claude Sadik [3] and Michaël Obadia [1,*]

1 Hôpital Fondation Adolphe de Rothschild, Stroke Unit, 75019 Paris, France; natalianovaes.92@gmail.com
2 Hospital Riviera-Chablais, Unit of Geriatrics Rehabilitation, 1800 Vevey, Switzerland; raphael.sadik@hopitalrivierachablais.ch
3 Hôpital Fondation Adolphe de Rothschild, Radiology, 75019 Paris, France; jcsadik@for.paris
* Correspondence: mobadia@for.paris

Abstract: Cerebral venous thrombosis (CVT) is a rare type of stroke that may cause an intracranial hypertension syndrome as well as focal neurological deficits due to venous infarcts. MRI with venography is the method of choice for diagnosis, and treatment with anticoagulants should be promptly started. CVT incidence has increased in COVID-19-infected patients due to a hypercoagulability state and endothelial inflammation. CVT following COVID-19 vaccination could be related to vaccine-induced immune thrombotic thrombocytopenia (VITT), a rare but severe complication that should be promptly identified because of its high mortality rate. Platelet count, D-dimer and PF4 antibodies should be dosed. Treatment with non-heparin anticoagulants and immunoglobulin could improve recuperation. Development of headache associated with seizures, impaired consciousness or focal signs should raise immediate suspicion of CVT. In patients who received a COVID-19 adenovirus-vector vaccine presenting thromboembolic events, VITT should be suspected and rapidly treated. Nevertheless, vaccination benefits clearly outweigh risks and should be continued.

Keywords: cerebral venous thrombosis; COVID-19; adenovirus vaccine; vaccine-induced immune thrombotic thrombocytopenia (VITT)

1. Introduction

Cerebral venous thrombosis (CVT) is an uncommon type of stroke with an incidence around 3–4 cases per million adults, with a predominance in Caucasian females [1]. It may be associated with five major clinical syndromes:

- Increased intracranial pressure with newly onset headache in 70 to 90% of patients [2], and less frequently papilledema and palsy of the abducent nerve;
- Seizures, which may affect as much as 34% of patients [3];
- Focal neurological deficits [4];
- Encephalopathy or coma, usually in the context of multiple sinus or deep venous occlusions;
- Specific regional syndromes, including periorbital pain, ocular chemosis, palsies of oculomotor cranial nerves and the ophthalmic division of the fifth cranial nerve (in the case of cavernous sinus thrombosis).

The intracranial hypertension is due to increased venular and capillary pressure as well as decreased cerebrospinal fluid absorption.

There are several risk factors associated with CVT, such as pregnancy, postpartum and the use of oral contraceptives [5]. Other conditions such as hypercoagulability states in malignancy or genetic predisposition (mutation of Factor V Leiden, deficiency in proteins C or S, prothrombin mutation, hyperhomocysteinemia) may also be associated with this disease. Cancer treatment by tamoxifen, cisplatin or other chemotherapies is another rare cause of CVT. Specific neurological diseases such as cranial trauma, neurological intervention and bacterial meningitis are other possible causes of this disorder. In children particularly, acute head and neck infections (such as mastoiditis) are the primary causes of CVT. Finally, Behçet's disease and Systemic Lupus Erythematosus are the main systemic diseases associated with CVT [4].

By May 2022, COVID-19 had infected 513 million people worldwide and had caused over 6.2 million deaths [6]. Part of its morbidity and mortality has been related to the potential increase in thromboembolic events, such as CVT, described in several case reports [7]. A retrospective multicenter cohort study reported an incidence of 8.8 per 10,000 [8], versus 3–4 per million in previous publications before the pandemics [1,9–12]. Thus, its prevalence is higher in COVID-19-positive patients than in the general population, with a predominance of males (66%) and a mean age of 48 years. This was also suggested by other epidemiological studies that reported no predominance of young female patients, as is the case with classic CVT [13].

The aims of this study, therefore, are to report cases of patients with CVT related to COVID-19 who were hospitalized in the Neurovascular Unit of the Hôpital Fondation Adolphe de Rothschild in Paris and, afterwards, to review the literature concerning the management of CVT in the COVID-19 pandemic context.

2. Materials and Methods

A retrospective analysis of medical charts of the Neurovascular Unit of Hôpital Fondation Adolphe de Rothschild was performed. The number of hospitalizations due to cerebral venous thrombosis from 2018 to 2020 was compared with the period of 2020 to 2021. Cases in which COVID-19 infection was detected in relation to CVT were described.

Descriptive statistics were performed using JASP (JASP Team (2022), Version 0.16.3) (computer software), Eric-Jan Wagenmakers, University of Amsterdam. Amsterdam, The Netherlands.

A literature review was developed on the Pubmed database searching for the keywords "cerebral venous thrombosis", "COVID-19", "COVID vaccine", and "vaccine-induced thrombotic thrombocytopenia".

Patients and/or patients' families consented to the publication of images and data.

3. Results

During the period of 2018–2019, 39 individuals with CVT were hospitalized, while 47 patients were admitted during 2020–2021 (a 1.2-fold increase). However, COVID-19 PCR was positive in only 5 patients out of those 47 (10.6% of cases). Only one case of CVT was possibly related to a COVID-19 vaccine (Johnson & Johnson).

Table 1 shows the clinical and epidemiological data of patients presenting COVID-19 and CVT. All the patients were women, aged from 31 to 61 (mean 45.8, SD 13.9). Mean time from COVID-19 diagnosis to CVT was 18.6 days (SD 12.4), and the mean time from first CVT symptoms to diagnosis was 18.4 days (SD 11.8).

One patient had a history of breast cancer 5 years before evaluation. It was in remission, but still being treated by tamoxifen. Another individual was under oral contraception with an estrogen–progestogen combined pill for the treatment of menorrhagia and had an iron-deficiency anemia with a hemoglobin level of 7 g/dL. One patient was obese, with a Body Mass Index (BMI) of 34 kg/m^2 and had a previous history of five miscarriages, with anti-phospholipid syndrome ruled out.

Regarding neuroimaging features, three of our patients had transverse and sigmoid sinus thrombosis, one of which was also associated with a hemorrhagic venous infarct (Figure 1); one patient had superior sagittal and right transverse sinus thrombosis, and another had multiple sinuses, including the deep venous system. The latter also had venous infarct with hemorrhagic transformation (Figure 2) and underwent craniectomy and thrombectomy, but unfortunately died due to multiple neurological and respiratory complications.

Table 1. Clinical, radiological and epidemiological data of patients presenting CVT and COVID-19.

Gender	Age	Vaccination	Risk Factors	Time from COVID to CVT (Days)	Neuroimage	Treatment	Complications	Disclosure
F	61	No	No	15	Thrombosis in multiple sinuses (internal cerebral vein, Galen vein, right sinus, torcula, left lateral sinus)	LMWH, craniectomy, thrombectomy	Epilepsy	Death
F	54	No	Previous cancer, under Tamoxifen	0	Left transverse and sigmoid sinus thrombosis, with left temporal and parietal hemorrhagic infarct	LMWH	Neuropsychiatric alterations	Transferred to Psychiatry, not fully recovered. Persistence of cognitive disorders.
F	52	Yes (Astra Zeneca)	5 miscarriages, SAPL-negative	18	Right lateral and sigmoid sinus thrombosis	LMWH then apixaban	None	Discharged with no complications
F	31	No	No	30	Right lateral sinus and superior sagittal sinus thrombosis	LMWH	None	Discharged with no complications
F	31	No	Oral contraceptive, anemia Hb 7 g/dL	30	Right lateral and sigmoid sinus thrombosis	LMWH followed by Dabigatran	None	Discharged with no complications

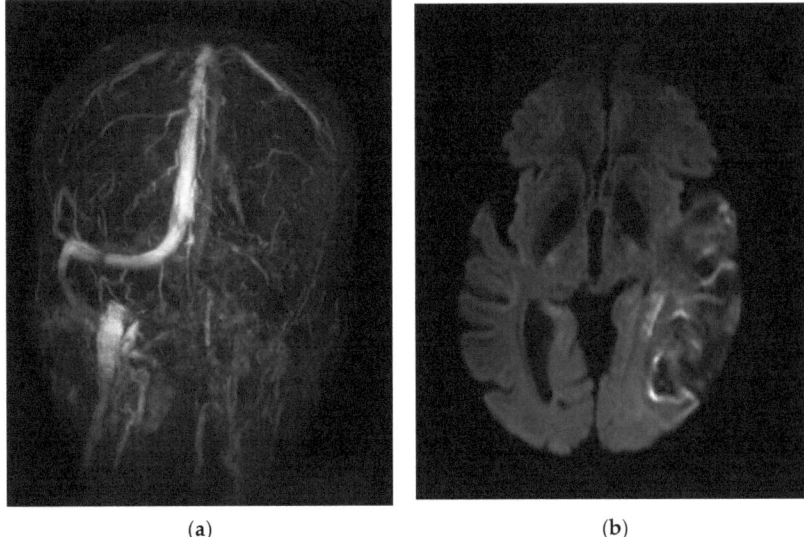

(a)   (b)

Figure 1. Cont.

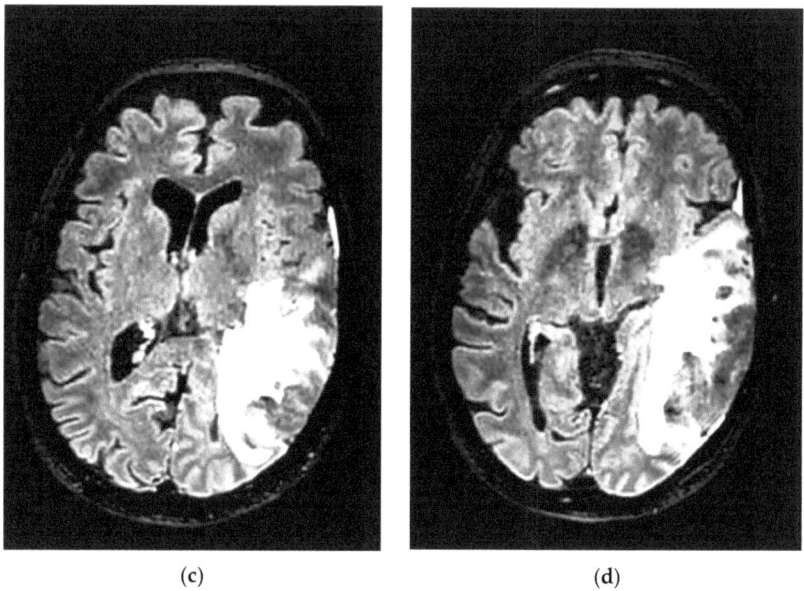

(c) (d)

Figure 1. (**a**) Venous MRI showing thrombosis of left transverse and sigmoid sinuses. (**b**) Diffusion-weighted image showing ischemia of left temporal region. (**c**,**d**) Fluid-attenuated inversion recovery (FLAIR) showing hypersignal in temporal and parietal regions.

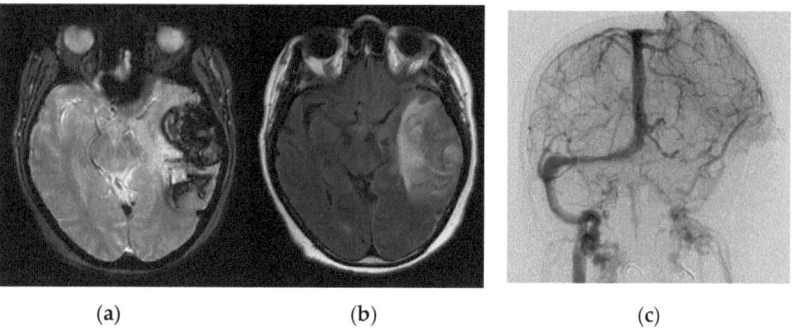

(**a**) (**b**) (**c**)

Figure 2. (**a**) Magnetic Resonance Imaging (T2* weighted image). (**b**) FLAIR, showing venous hemorrhagic infarct. (**c**) Venous angiogram showing extended thrombosis of the left transverse and sigmoid sinuses, after craniectomy.

A 70-year-old male patient was hospitalized for presenting CVT with involvement of the superior longitudinal sinus and the left transverse sinus (Figure 3). Such events took place three weeks after receiving a Johnson & Johnson vaccine. He had no other risk factors for thrombosis and presented a normal platelet count on diagnosis (246 G/L). He was treated with low-molecular-weight heparin (LMWH), later switched to Dabigatran, and had a favorable outcome.

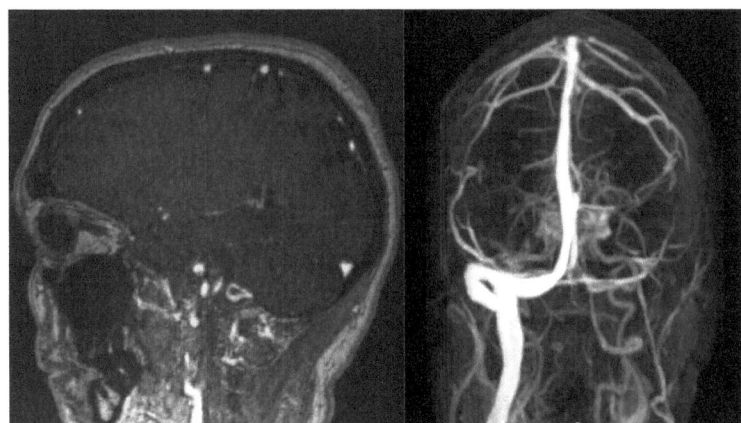

Figure 3. Venous MRI showing thrombosis of left transverse and sigmoid sinuses.

4. Discussion

CVT is a rare but potentially severe neurological disorder that may have a wide spectrum of clinical presentations.

The method of brain Magnetic Resonance Imaging (MRI) with contrast-enhanced venography is the one most commonly indicated to diagnose CVT. The diversity of radiological signs depends on the delay between symptom onset and MRI, but the typical finding consists of the visualization of the thrombus, a contrast-filling defect (empty delta sign), or the lack of flow signal. Venous strokes appear as an edematous region with mixed infarct, with possible hemorrhage in atypical locations, not compatible with arterial territories. If a venous MRI is not available, or for any reason contraindicated, a Computerized Tomography (CT) scan with venography is an alternative diagnostic modality.

Concerning treatment, it should consist of anticoagulation by low-molecular-weight heparin, warfarin or with Direct Oral Anticoagulants (DOACs). The RESPECT-CVT trial, which compared dabigatran versus warfarin in 120 randomized patients, reported no differences in the safety and efficacy between the groups [14]. Yaghi and colleagues [15] performed a retrospective multicentric international observational cohort including over 1000 patients. Real-world cases of CVT that were treated by either warfarin or DOACs were compared. Patients treated with DOACs presented similar rates of recanalization, death and recurrence, but with lower risk of major hemorrhage, than patients treated with warfarin [15]. Patients with a clear indication for warfarin (such as presence of anti-phospholipid antibody syndrome) were excluded.

A randomized trial compared Rivaroxaban versus warfarin or heparin in 114 children with CVT and found decreased bleeding risk with similar low recurrence rates and reduced thrombotic burden [16].

Endovascular treatment is mostly discussed in cases of thrombosis of multiple sinuses associated with severe intracranial hypertension and clinical deterioration. The American Heart Association guidelines recommend endovascular thrombolysis or thrombectomy in refractory patients who deteriorate despite anticoagulant treatment [17]. Systematic reviews published in 2015 and 2017 suggested that mechanical thrombectomy is safe [18] and effective in salvage therapy for refractory CVT [19]. A small case series of seven patients who presented clinical deterioration despite the best medical treatment reported good outcomes after such intervention [20]. A retrospective study including 30 patients with neurological deterioration or refractory seizures reported that combined endovascular mechanical thrombectomy and on-site chemical thrombolysis were reasonably safe and might be considered as an option for severe cases that are unresponsive to anticoagulation, especially for thrombosis of the superior sagittal sinus [21].

However, it is worth mentioning that a multicenter, randomized, open-label study (the TO-ACT study) that included 67 patients with CVT and at least one risk factor for poor outcome (coma, alteration in mental status, intracerebral hemorrhage or deep vein thrombosis) showed no difference in disability at 12 months between patients treated by a standard medical treatment versus those who underwent endovascular treatment [22]. The study was prematurely ended due to futility.

Decompressive craniectomy is a controversial procedure that can be performed in life-threatening situations. Two retrospective studies of medical records compared patients with malignant CVT treated by craniectomy versus medical treatment alone, and the results showed that craniectomy decreased mortality and improved functional outcomes [23,24]. A prospective small case series also suggested that this intervention can be lifesaving, with good clinical outcomes [25].

Antiepileptic drugs should not be used preventively, and corticoids have no benefit. Acetazolamide could eventually be useful in refractory intracranial hypertension [17].

Considering prognosis, it is largely variable depending on the site of thrombosis, the size of thrombus and also on the delay before clinical diagnosis and the start of treatment. The overall mortality is around 6% while circa 10% have permanent disability after one year of follow-up [26].

4.1. CVT Related to COVID-19 Infection: A Literature Review

The clinical presentation of CVT related to COVID-19 does not seem to be different from CVT which is not COVID-19-related: cephalalgia, seizures, encephalopathy, abducent palsies, papilledema and focal deficits such as hemiparesis or aphasia. In a multicenter study, headache was present in 50% of the cases, decreased level of consciousness in 12.5% and neurological focal deficits in 25% of patients. In another multicentric retrospective cohort, headache was present in 85% of cases. Focal symptoms such as hemiparesis or seizures were present in 42% of cases, and cortical signs such as aphasia or hemianopsia were present in 25% [8]. Possible complications, as in non-COVID-19-related CVT, were intracranial bleeding, seizures and decreased consciousness with intubation. A multicentric study reported intraparenchymal hemorrhage and subarachnoid hemorrhage in up to 25% of patients [27].

One study focused on neuro-ophthalmological complications of CVT related to COVID-19. The intracranial hypertension caused by CVT can lead to papilledema and direct ischemic injury of visual pathways and also to ocular motility impairment due to injury of oculomotor and abducent nerves with diplopia. For patients with papilledema and visual impairment, a lumbar puncture can be performed to rapidly lower intracranial pressure. Acetazolamide can also be used in this context. Severe cases should undergo cerebrospinal fluid shunt or optic nerve fenestration [28].

Thromboembolic events related to COVID-19 are frequent and can appear in later stages of infection and even after patients no longer have respiratory symptoms [7]. One study from Wuhan reported an incidence of deep venous thrombosis of 21% amongst COVID-19 patients [29]. Another paper reported that COVID-19 patients present higher levels of D-dimer and fibrinogen [30]. One review showed that 75% of patients had elevated D-dimers and 50% had increased CRP [13]. The presence of antiphospholipid antibodies was also described [31]. Also with regard to biological data, lumbar puncture was often performed, and was usually non-collaborative, showing mild protein elevation in cerebrospinal fluid [13].

It is worthy of mention that even "Long COVID-19 syndrome"—which refers to patients who present long-lasting inflammatory alterations and prolonged persistence of symptoms—can be associated with an increase in prothrombotic state. Some of the patients present persistent high levels of D-dimers with an increased risk of thromboembolic complications [32].

The literature reports 3 to 4 days as the mean time from neurological symptoms onset to CVT diagnosis and 7 to 11 days as the mean time from COVID-19 symptoms onset to

CVT diagnosis [8,13,27,33]. CVT also occurred in patients with mild respiratory symptoms, and no direct association between systemic severity and risk of CVT was found [27].

In a multicentric study, Abdalkader and colleagues [22] reported hypertension and diabetes as the most common comorbidities among patients. Risk factors such as obesity, intake of estrogen contraceptives and antiphospholipid syndrome were also present.

Regarding neuroimaging features, the transverse sinuses and the superior sagittal were most commonly affected; one patient also had deep venous thrombosis [27]. According to the International Study on Cerebral Vein and Dural Sinus Thrombosis, thrombosis of the deep venous system is an independent predictor of death [34].

Another case series showed that half of the patients presented multiple sinuses implicated [13]. One review suggested that there is a trend for COVID-19-related CVT patients to have hemorrhagic infarcts more often in the first admission neuroimage, although data were not statistically confirmed [35].

It has been well established in the literature that infections, in general, increase the risk of CVT, especially those related to the cranium, such as sinusitis, meningitis, mastoiditis, otitis and tonsillitis [28]. Viral infections were also associated with thromboembolic risk, such as Human Immunodeficiency Virus (HIV), Ebola, cytomegalovirus and varicella zoster [36]. These findings reinforce the link between infection and CVT.

The mechanisms which lead to the increase in thromboembolic events vary and include endothelial disfunction, cytokine storm, an increase in prothrombotic markers such as D-dimers and fibrinogen, as well as the rise of pro-inflammatory molecules such as interleukin-6 and C Reactive Protein (CRP), which would result in a hypercoagulability state [7]. The sepsis induced by the infection may also contribute to thromboembolic events [33].

COVID-19's interaction with angiotensin-converting enzyme (ACE) receptors may be the leading cause of endothelial damage, being associated with the coagulopathy caused by the increase in prothrombotic molecules such as D-dimers and fibrinogen, the dysregulation of inflammatory cascades as well as platelet dysfunction. The latter is characterized by increased platelet adherence and aggregation [37], which in turn would lead to an increase in thromboembolic events, which might be as severe as intravascular coagulation [35]. The increased viscosity can also potentialize endothelial damage, resulting in impaired microcirculation. The immune response to the virus can trigger complement activation, which culminates in prostaglandin and proinflammatory cytokines—the so-called cytokine storm—that also leads to altered coagulation. Antiphospholipid antibodies could also play a role in COVID-19-related CVT, as they were found in a few critical patients with COVID-19 and stroke [31].

Nevertheless, hypoxia, which is frequently present in COVID-19 patients, especially in the intensive care unit setting, is also associated with increased blood viscosity, the activation of genes related to hypoxia that interfere with coagulation and alterations in fibrinolysis [33].

Standard CVT treatment, with LMWH used in most cases, was associated with the treatment of complications, such as antiepileptic drugs when seizures were present or detected in the EEG of comatose patients. Very few patients were treated by endovascular thrombectomy or thrombolysis. A multicentric study already mentioned above recommends intravenous recombinant tissue plasminogen activator (rt-PA) and endovascular treatment as a last resort for refractory cases [27,38]. One multicentric retrospective cohort described two patients treated by endovascular thrombolysis, and craniectomy was also performed in two patients [8].

Concerning prognosis, one Asiatic review found a mortality rate in CVT related to COVID-19 as high as 45.5% [13]. CVT mortality in the non-COVID population is estimated to be below 10% [39]. In the same retrospective cohort mentioned above, mortality was 25%, 50% were transferred to a rehabilitation facility and 25% were discharged home [8].

4.2. CVT Associated with COVID-19 Vaccines

Not only COVID-19 infection but also COVID-19 vaccines were associated with thromboembolic episodes in many reports and reviews. To this date, 11.5 billion doses of COVID-19 vaccines have been administered worldwide [6], which has dramatically decreased morbidity and mortality related to the disease.

The rapid development of the vaccines was due, partially, to previous research on the technology of adenoviral vectors, which, along with m-RNA technology, accounts for the majority of vaccines that were administered during the pandemic period.

One of the most severe adverse effects attributed to the adenovirus-vector COVID-19 vaccine is immune thrombotic thrombocytopenia (VITT), which has already been associated with other adenoviral vector vaccines [26]. This condition can be similar to heparin-induced thrombocytopenia (HIT), as both are related to the presence of antibodies against platelet factor 4 (PF4), with thrombocytopenia and consequent thrombosis, although the antigenic target seems to be different in the two situations. In HIT, the heparin binds to PF4 and forms an antigen which triggers IgG autoantibodies, which, in their turn, will cause platelet activation and aggregation, leading to thrombosis. The antibody-covered platelets are then removed from circulation by the endothelial system and spleen, resulting in thrombocytopenia [40]. It has been speculated that in VITT, viral particles of the vaccine would bind to PF4 in a fashion similar to that in patients not previously exposed to heparin. This severe side effect was reported after vaccination with Astra Zeneca (ChAdOx1), Moderna (mRNA-1273) [41] and Johnson & Johnson (Ad26.COV2.S), occurring at a fourfold higher frequency with ChAdOx1 [26]. There have been three other reports of CVT after vaccination with the mRNA-type vaccine by Moderna [42], although patients presented normal platelet counts.

The fact that VITT occurs mainly after vaccination with ChAdOx1 suggests that VITT-induced antibodies against PF-4 do not react to the COVID-19 spike protein but probably react to the adenoviral vector [43].

One German multicentric vaccination study group found an incidence of CVT of 0.55/100,000 in patients after taking vaccines. They reported a total of 45 CVT cases within a month after vaccination, as well as nine ischemic strokes and four hemorrhagic strokes. There was a predominance of females (77.8%) and of patients younger than 60 years (80%); 85.5% of events occurred after ChAdOx1 vaccine, 14.5% after BNT162b2 vaccine; and none after mRNA-1273 vaccine. The adjusted incidence for the ChAdOx1 vaccine was 1.52 per 100,000, with an adjusted incidence of 3.14 for women [4,43,44]. This study pointed towards an increased risk of CVT after the ChAdOx1 vaccine, especially for young women.

One meta-analysis revealed that CVT represented 29% of total thromboembolic events following adenovirus-vector-based vaccination against COVID-19; 28% of patients who had CVT post vaccine died. The mean age of patients who presented CVT post vaccine was 45 years, with 75% of them being women; the mean time from vaccine to symptoms was 10 days, and 68% presented hemorrhagic infarcts [45].

The time of CVT symptoms onset after vaccine ranged from 6 to 15 days after the Ad26.COV2.S vaccine and 5 to 24 days after the ChAdOx1 vaccine [26,46]. The majority of patients did not have any history of thrombosis or coagulation disorders [47]. The outcomes of one case report of 12 patients who developed VITT after Ad26.COV2.S vaccine were 3 deaths, 3 continued ICU care, 2 continued non-ICU hospitalization, and 4 discharged home. Of the 12 patients, 7 developed intracranial hemorrhage (including the 3 individuals who died). The patients presented thrombocytopenia associated with increased D-dimers.

One large cohort study in the UK included 95 patients who presented CVT after COVID-19 vaccines, and it compared the group who fulfilled diagnostic criteria for VITT to the CVT without those criteria. It found that the mean age was lower in the VITT group (47 versus 57). The VITT group had more sinus thrombosed than the non-VITT group, more hemorrhagic infarcts and unfavorable outcomes. Outcomes were better amongst those who received non-heparin anticoagulants and immunoglobulin [48]. Another systematic review found that up to 49% of intracerebral hemorrhage or subarachnoid hemorrhage in CVT was associated with VITT [40]. One study also found VITT to be related to ischemic stroke [43].

There were also two cases of CVT reported after BNT162b2 vaccine, but with no evidence of VITT [49]. One of the patients had anemia and was under hormonal treatment.

A VITT risk score was developed, adapted from the HIT 4Ts scoring system which considers the number of thrombocytes, the timing post-vaccine, the presence of thrombosis or elevated D-dimers and the presence of other possible causes for thrombosis or thrombocytopenia. In the German study, CVTs with a score higher than two occurred after the ChAdOx1 vaccine, and 44% of these CVTs scored four points, meeting all criteria for likelihood of association with the vaccine [43]. The mortality of VITT is high, varying from 18.3% to 50% [26,43].

Clinicians should raise awareness of possible VITT, especially in young female patients presenting with CVT after exposure to COVID-19 vaccines, and they must dose PF4-antibodies if thrombocytopenia, preferentially by ELISA HIT assays (which were shown to have higher sensitivity for detection of these antibodies) [44]. Other techniques are platelet activation assays and serotonin release assays, but they are more influenced by technical aspects and the results are less uniform [26].

Treatment consists of anticoagulation by non-heparin anticoagulants (fondaparinux, argatroban, direct oral anticoagulants) and avoiding heparin and heparin products (including prothrombin complex concentrates) [26]. Warfarin should be avoided, especially in the beginning of treatment, due to its paradoxical induction to a hypercoagulability state. Anticoagulation should be continued for at least three months [26]. Fibrinolysis and mechanical thrombectomy should be restricted to cases with poor evolution despite anticoagulation [17]. Aspirin should also be avoided, due to an increased risk of bleeding, in addition to presenting no benefit.

Intravenous immunoglobulins, at a dose of 1 g/kg for at least 2 days, should be used in refractory cases [46,50]. For patients with a high antibody burden, plasma exchange can be performed in addition to immunoglobulins, for at least 5 days until platelet count improves. There is no consensus regarding the use of corticosteroids.

Platelet transfusions could be beneficial before invasive procedures or for patients with a high risk of bleeding [51]. In HIT, it was related to a fivefold increase in mortality, so it should be avoided [52]. The use of Eculizumab and rituximab are under investigation [26]. There is one case report of treatment of HIT by rituximab with favorable outcomes [53]. Eculizumab was given to two refractory patients who failed IVIG therapy, with improvement [54]. Nevertheless, the risk of CVT is much higher amongst patients infected by COVID-19 as opposed to patients who presented CVT secondary to the vaccine.

The main limitations of this study concern its small number of patients, as well as its retrospective nature. Although we have performed an extensive medical chart review to track patients who presented cerebral venous thrombosis in the context of a COVID-19 infection over the last two years, it is possible that some data are missing. One reason might be faulty medical chart completion. If the study had a prospective nature, medical staff could be made aware of more specific data that should be collected for all possible candidates. It is also possible that we have failed to diagnose COVID-19 in some patients with cerebral venous thrombosis due to fact that in the beginning of the pandemic not all individuals were screened for COVID-19.

5. Conclusions

CVT is a rare yet potentially severe complication of COVID-19 infection and also of COVID-19 vaccination. The development of headaches associated with seizures, impaired consciousness or focal signs should raise immediate suspicion of CVT, and neuroimaging should be obtained as soon as possible. In patients who received an adenovirus-vector vaccine and are presenting with thromboembolic events, platelet count, D-dimer and PF4 antibodies should be dosed, and if there is suspicion of VITT, non-heparin anticoagulation should be started in conjunction with immunoglobulins. Nevertheless, since COVID-19 infection itself is also related to thromboembolic events, the benefits of COVID-19 vaccination outweigh the risk of thrombosis and should not be interrupted [43,55]. A special consideration to bear in mind is that adenovirus-vector vaccines were mostly destined for low and middle income countries, since they are more easily stored and require only a single-dose regimen of immunization [8,47,55], so there might be a need to develop comparative ethnographic studies in the future in order to better understand such complex relations.

Author Contributions: Conceptualization, M.O. and J.-C.S.; writing—original draft preparation, N.N.; literature review N.N. and M.O.; writing—review and editing, R.S. and M.O. All authors have read and agreed to the published version of the manuscript.

Funding: This research received no external funding.

Institutional Review Board Statement: The study was conducted in accordance with the Declaration of Helsinki, and patients and/or their families consented to the publication of anonimized data. Ethical review and approval were waived due to its descriptive nature and the anonymization of data.

Informed Consent Statement: Informed consent was obtained from all subjects involved in the study.

Data Availability Statement: Data are available upon request.

Acknowledgments: We thank Rosana Novaes-Pinto for contributing to the English version of this manuscript.

Conflicts of Interest: The authors declare no conflict of interests.

References

1. Stam, J. Thrombosis of the cerebral veins and sinuses. *N. Engl. J. Med.* **2005**, *352*, 1791–1798. [CrossRef] [PubMed]
2. Wasay, M.; Kojan, S.; Dai, A.I.; Bobustuc, G.; Sheikh, Z. Headache in Cerebral Venous Thrombosis: Incidence, pattern and location in 200 consecutive patients. *J. Headache Pain.* **2010**, *11*, 137–139. [CrossRef] [PubMed]
3. Lindgren, E.; Silvis, S.M.; Hiltunen, S.; Heldner, M.R.; Serrano, F.; de Scisco, M.; Zelano, J.; Zuurbier, S.M.; van Kammen, M.S.; Mansour, M.; et al. Acute symptomatic seizures in cerebral venous thrombosis. *Neurology* **2020**, *95*, e1706–e1715. [CrossRef]
4. Ropper, A.H.; Klein, J.P. Cerebral Venous Thrombosis. *N. Engl. J. Med.* **2021**, *385*, 59–64. [CrossRef] [PubMed]
5. Coutinho, J.M.; Ferro, J.M.; Canhão, P.; Barinagarrementeria, F.; Cantú, C.; Bousser, M.G.; Stam, J. Cerebral venous and sinus thrombosis in women. *Stroke* **2009**, *40*, 2356–2361. [CrossRef]
6. WHO Coronavirus (COVID-19) Dashboard. 2022. Available online: https://covid19.who.int (accessed on 26 May 2022).
7. Dakay, K.; Cooper, J.; Bloomfield, J.; Overby, P.; Mayer, S.A.; Nuoman, R.; Sahni, R.; Gulko, E.; Kaur, G.; Santarelli, J.; et al. Cerebral Venous Sinus Thrombosis in COVID-19 Infection: A Case Series and Review of The Literature. *J. Stroke Cereb. Dis.* **2021**, *30*, 105434. [CrossRef] [PubMed]
8. Al-Mufti, F.; Amuluru, K.; Sahni, R.; Bekelis, K.; Karimi, R.; Ogulnick, J.; Cooper, J.; Overby, P.; Nuoman, R.; Tiwari, A.; et al. Cerebral Venous Thrombosis in COVID-19: A New York Metropolitan Cohort Study. *AJNR Am. J. Neuroradiol.* **2021**, *42*, 1196–1200. [CrossRef]
9. Devasagayam, S.; Wyatt, B.; Leyden, J.; Kleinig, T. Cerebral Venous Sinus Thrombosis Incidence Is Higher Than Previously Thought: A Retrospective Population-Based Study. *Stroke* **2016**, *47*, 2180–2182. [CrossRef]
10. Coutinho, J.M.; Zuurbier, S.M.; Aramideh, M.; Stam, J. The incidence of cerebral venous thrombosis: A cross-sectional study. *Stroke* **2012**, *43*, 3375–3377. [CrossRef]
11. Siegler, J.E.; Cardona, P.; Arenillas, J.F.; Talavera, B.; Guillen, A.N.; Chavarría-Miranda, A.; de Lera, M.; Khandelwal, P.; Bach, I.; Patel, P.; et al. Cerebrovascular events and outcomes in hospitalized patients with COVID-19: The SVIN COVID-19 Multinational Registry. *Int. J. Stroke* **2021**, *16*, 437–447. [CrossRef]
12. Taquet, M.; Husain, M.; Geddes, J.R.; Luciano, S.; Harrison, P.J. Cerebral venous thrombosis and portal vein thrombosis: A retrospective cohort study of 537,913 COVID-19 cases. *EClinicalMedicine* **2021**, *39*, 101061. [CrossRef] [PubMed]
13. Tu, T.M.; Goh, C.; Tan, Y.K.; Leow, A.S.; Pang, Y.Z.; Chien, J.; Shafi, H.; Pl Chan, B.; Hui, A.; Koh, J.; et al. Cerebral Venous Thrombosis in Patients with COVID-19 Infection: A Case Series and Systematic Review. *J. Stroke Cereb. Dis.* **2020**, *29*, 105379. [CrossRef] [PubMed]
14. Silvis, S.M.; Middeldorp, S.; Zuurbier, S.M.; Cannegieter, S.C.; Coutinho, J.M. Risk Factors for Cerebral Venous Thrombosis. *Semin. Thromb. Hemost.* **2016**, *42*, 622–631. [CrossRef] [PubMed]
15. Yaghi, S.; Shu, L.; Bakradze, E.; Salehi Omran, S.; Giles, J.A.; Amar, J.Y.; Henninger, N.; Elnazeir, M.; Liberman, A.; Moncrieffe, K.; et al. Direct Oral Anticoagulants Versus Warfarin in the Treatment of Cerebral Venous Thrombosis (ACTION-CVT): A Multicenter International Study. *Stroke* **2022**, *53*, 728–738. [CrossRef] [PubMed]

16. Male, C.; Lensing, A.W.A.; Palumbo, J.S.; Kumar, R.; Nurmeev, I.; Hege, K.; Bonnet, D.; Connor, P.; Hooimeijer, H.; Torres, M.; et al. Rivaroxaban compared with standard anticoagulants for the treatment of acute venous thromboembolism in children: A randomised, controlled, phase 3 trial. *Lancet Haematol.* **2020**, *7*, e18–e27. [CrossRef]
17. Saposnik, G.; Barinagarrementeria, F.; Brown, R.D.; Bushnell, C.D.; Cucchiara, B.; Cushman, M.; deVeber, G.; Ferro, J.M.; Tsai, F.Y. Diagnosis and management of cerebral venous thrombosis: A statement for healthcare professionals from the American Heart Association/American Stroke Association. *Stroke* **2011**, *42*, 1158–1192. [CrossRef]
18. Siddiqui, F.M.; Dandapat, S.; Banerjee, C.; Zuurbier, S.M.; Johnson, M.; Stam, J.; Coutinho, J. Mechanical thrombectomy in cerebral venous thrombosis: Systematic review of 185 cases. *Stroke* **2015**, *46*, 1263–1268. [CrossRef]
19. Ilyas, A.; Chen, C.J.; Raper, D.M.; Ding, D.; Buell, T.; Mastorakos, P.; Liu, K. Endovascular mechanical thrombectomy for cerebral venous sinus thrombosis: A systematic review. *J. Neurointerv. Surg.* **2017**, *9*, 1086–1092. [CrossRef]
20. Medhi, G.; Parida, S.; Nicholson, P.; Senapati, S.B.; Padhy, B.P.; Pereira, V.M. Mechanical Thrombectomy for Cerebral Venous Sinus Thrombosis: A Case Series and Technical Note. *World Neurosurg.* **2020**, *140*, 148–161. [CrossRef]
21. Liao, C.H.; Liao, N.C.; Chen, W.H.; Chen, H.C.; Shen, C.C.; Yang, S.F.; Tsuei, Y.S. Endovascular Mechanical Thrombectomy and On-Site Chemical Thrombolysis for Severe Cerebral Venous Sinus Thrombosis. *Sci. Rep.* **2020**, *10*, 4937. [CrossRef]
22. Coutinho, J.M.; Zuurbier, S.M.; Bousser, M.G.; Ji, X.; Canhão, P.; Roos, Y.B.; Crassard, I.; Paiva Nunes, A.; Uyttenboogaart, M.; Chen, J.; et al. Effect of Endovascular Treatment With Medical Management vs Standard Care on Severe Cerebral Venous Thrombosis: The TO-ACT Randomized Clinical Trial. *JAMA Neurol.* **2020**, *77*, 966–973. [CrossRef] [PubMed]
23. Baharvahdat, H.; Ahmadi, S.; Ganjeifar, B.; Etemadrezaie, H.; Zabyhian, S.; Sasannejad, P.; Bahadorkhan, G.; Mowla, A. Malignant Cerebral Venous Infarction: Decompressive Craniectomy versus Medical Treatment. *World Neurosurg.* **2019**, *128*, e918–e922. [CrossRef] [PubMed]
24. Ferro, J.M.; Crassard, I.; Coutinho, J.M.; Canhão, P.; Barinagarrementeria, F.; Cucchiara, B.; Derex, L.; Lichy, C.; Masjuan, J.; Massaro, A.; et al. Decompressive surgery in cerebrovenous thrombosis: A multicenter registry and a systematic review of individual patient data. *Stroke* **2011**, *42*, 2825–2831. [CrossRef] [PubMed]
25. Zuurbier, S.M.; Coutinho, J.M.; Majoie, C.B.; Coert, B.A.; van den Munckhof, P.; Stam, J. Decompressive hemicraniectomy in severe cerebral venous thrombosis: A prospective case series. *J. Neurol.* **2012**, *259*, 1099–1105. [CrossRef] [PubMed]
26. Rizk, J.G.; Gupta, A.; Sardar, P.; Henry, B.M.; Lewin, J.C.; Lippi, G.; Lavie, C. Clinical Characteristics and Pharmacological Management of COVID-19 Vaccine-Induced Immune Thrombotic Thrombocytopenia With Cerebral Venous Sinus Thrombosis: A Review. *JAMA Cardiol.* **2021**, *6*, 1451–1460. [CrossRef]
27. Abdalkader, M.; Shaikh, S.P.; Siegler, J.E.; Cervantes-Arslanian, A.M.; Tiu, C.; Radu, R.A.; Tiu, V.; Jillella, D.; Mansour, O.; Vera, V.; et al. Cerebral Venous Sinus Thrombosis in COVID-19 Patients: A Multicenter Study and Review of Literature. *J. Stroke Cereb. Dis.* **2021**, *30*, 105733. [CrossRef]
28. Medicherla, C.B.; Pauley, R.A.; de Havenon, A.; Yaghi, S.; Ishida, K.; Torres, J.L. Cerebral Venous Sinus Thrombosis in the COVID-19 Pandemic. *J. Neuroophthalmol.* **2020**, *40*, 457–462. [CrossRef]
29. Wang, W.; Sun, Q.; Bao, Y.; Liang, M.; Meng, Q.; Chen, H.; Li, J.; Wang, H.; Li, H.; Shi, Y.; et al. Analysis of Risk Factors for Thromboembolic Events in 88 Patients with COVID-19 Pneumonia in Wuhan, China: A Retrospective Descriptive Report. *Med. Sci. Monit.* **2021**, *27*, e929708. [CrossRef]
30. Han, H.; Yang, L.; Liu, R.; Liu, F.; Wu, K.L.; Li, J.; Liu, X.H.; Zhu, C.L. Prominent changes in blood coagulation of patients with SARS-CoV-2 infection. *Clin. Chem. Lab. Med.* **2020**, *58*, 1116–1120. [CrossRef]
31. Zhang, Y.; Xiao, M.; Zhang, S.; Xia, P.; Cao, W.; Jiang, W.; Chen, H.; Ding, X.; Zhao, H.; Zhang, H.; et al. Coagulopathy and Antiphospholipid Antibodies in Patients with Covid-19. *N. Engl. J. Med.* **2020**, *382*, e38. [CrossRef]
32. Acanfora, D.; Acanfora, C.; Ciccone, M.M.; Scicchitano, P.; Bortone, A.S.; Uguccioni, M.; Casucci, G. The Cross-Talk between Thrombosis and Inflammatory Storm in Acute and Long-COVID-19: Therapeutic Targets and Clinical Cases. *Viruses* **2021**, *13*, 1904. [CrossRef] [PubMed]
33. Cavalcanti, D.D.; Raz, E.; Shapiro, M.; Dehkharghani, S.; Yaghi, S.; Lillemoe, K.; Nossek, E.; Torres, J.; Jain, R.; Riin, H.A.; et al. Cerebral Venous Thrombosis Associated with COVID-19. *AJNR Am. J. Neuroradiol.* **2020**, *41*, 1370–1376. [CrossRef] [PubMed]
34. Girot, M.; Ferro, J.M.; Canhão, P.; Stam, J.; Bousser, M.G.; Barinagarrementeria, F.; Leys, D. Predictors of outcome in patients with cerebral venous thrombosis and intracerebral hemorrhage. *Stroke* **2007**, *38*, 337–342. [CrossRef] [PubMed]
35. Ghosh, R.; Roy, D.; Mandal, A.; Pal, S.K.; Chandra Swaika, B.; Naga, D.; Pandit, A.; Ray, B.K.; Benito-León, J. Cerebral venous thrombosis in COVID-19. *Diabetes. Metab. Syndr.* **2021**, *15*, 1039–1045. [CrossRef] [PubMed]
36. Goeijenbier, M.; van Wissen, M.; van de Weg, C.; Jong, E.; Gerdes, V.E.; Meijers, J.C.; Brandjes, D.P.M.; van Gorp, E.C.M. Review: Viral infections and mechanisms of thrombosis and bleeding. *J. Med. Virol.* **2012**, *84*, 1680–1696. [CrossRef]
37. Becker, R.C. COVID-19 update: Covid-19-associated coagulopathy. *J. Thromb. Thrombolysis* **2020**, *50*, 54–67. [CrossRef]
38. Eskey, C.J.; Meyers, P.M.; Nguyen, T.N.; Ansari, S.A.; Jayaraman, M.; McDougall, C.G.; DeMarco, J.K.; Gray, W.A.; Hess, D.C.; Higashida, R.T.; et al. Indications for the Performance of Intracranial Endovascular Neurointerventional Procedures: A Scientific Statement From the American Heart Association. *Circulation* **2018**, *137*, e661–e689. [CrossRef]
39. Bousser, M.G.; Ferro, J.M. Cerebral venous thrombosis: An update. *Lancet Neurol.* **2007**, *6*, 162–170. [CrossRef]
40. Sharifian-Dorche, M.; Bahmanyar, M.; Sharifian-Dorche, A.; Mohammadi, P.; Nomovi, M.; Mowla, A. Vaccine-induced immune thrombotic thrombocytopenia and cerebral venous sinus thrombosis post COVID-19 vaccination, a systematic review. *J. Neurol. Sci.* **2021**, *428*, 117607. [CrossRef]

41. Sangli, S.; Virani, A.; Cheronis, N.; Vannatter, B.; Minich, C.; Noronha, S.; Bhagavatula, R.; Speredelozzi, D.; Sareen, M.; Kaplan, R.B. Thrombosis With Thrombocytopenia After the Messenger RNA-1273 Vaccine. *Ann. Intern. Med.* **2021**, *174*, 1480–1482. [CrossRef]
42. Smadja, D.M.; Yue, Q.Y.; Chocron, R.; Sanchez, O.; Lillo-Le Louet, A. Vaccination against COVID-19: Insight from arterial and venous thrombosis occurrence using data from VigiBase. *Eur. Respir. J.* **2021**, *58*. [CrossRef] [PubMed]
43. Schulz, J.B.; Berlit, P.; Diener, H.C.; Gerloff, C.; Greinacher, A.; Klein, C.; Petzold, G.C.; Piccininni, M.; Poli, S.; Röhrig, R.; et al. COVID-19 Vaccine-Associated Cerebral Venous Thrombosis in Germany. *Ann. Neurol.* **2021**, *90*, 627–639. [CrossRef] [PubMed]
44. Franchini, M.; Liumbruno, G.M.; Pezzo, M. COVID-19 vaccine-associated immune thrombosis and thrombocytopenia (VITT): Diagnostic and therapeutic recommendations for a new syndrome. *Eur. J. Haematol.* **2021**, *107*, 173–180. [CrossRef] [PubMed]
45. Palaiodimou, L.; Stefanou, M.I.; Katsanos, A.H.; Aguiar de Sousa, D.; Coutinho, J.M.; Lagiou, P.; Michopoulos, I.; Naska, A.; Giannopoulos, S.; Vadikolias, K.; et al. Cerebral Venous Sinus Thrombosis and Thrombotic Events After Vector-Based COVID-19 Vaccines: A Systematic Review and Meta-analysis. *Neurology* **2021**, *97*, e2136–e2147. [CrossRef]
46. See, I.; Su, J.R.; Lale, A.; Woo, E.J.; Guh, A.Y.; Shimabukuro, T.T.; Streiff, M.B.; Rao, A.K.; Wheeler, A.P.; Beavers, S.F.; et al. US Case Reports of Cerebral Venous Sinus Thrombosis With Thrombocytopenia After Ad26.COV2.S Vaccination, March 2 to April 21, 2021. *JAMA* **2021**, *325*, 2448–2456. [CrossRef]
47. Gupta, A.; Sardar, P.; Cash, M.E.; Milani, R.V.; Lavie, C.J. Covid-19 vaccine- induced thrombosis and thrombocytopenia-a commentary on an important and practical clinical dilemma. *Prog. Cardiovasc. Dis.* **2021**, *67*, 105–107. [CrossRef]
48. Perry, R.J.; Tamborska, A.; Singh, B.; Craven, B.; Marigold, R.; Arthur-Farraj, P.; Yeo, J.M.; Zhang, L.; Hassan-Smith, G.; Jones, M.; et al. Cerebral venous thrombosis after vaccination against COVID-19 in the UK: A multicentre cohort study. *Lancet* **2021**, *398*, 1147–1156. [CrossRef]
49. Dias, L.; Soares-Dos-Reis, R.; Meira, J.; Ferrão, D.; Soares, P.R.; Pastor, A.; Gama, G.; Fonseca, L.; Fagundes, V.; Carvalho, M. Cerebral Venous Thrombosis after BNT162b2 mRNA SARS-CoV-2 vaccine. *J. Stroke Cerebrovasc. Dis.* **2021**, *30*, 105906. [CrossRef]
50. Warkentin, T.E. High-dose intravenous immunoglobulin for the treatment and prevention of heparin-induced thrombocytopenia: A review. *Expert Rev Hematol.* **2019**, *12*, 685–698. [CrossRef]
51. Scully, M.; Singh, D.; Lown, R.; Poles, A.; Solomon, T.; Levi, M.; Goldblatt, D.; Kotoucek, P.; Thomas, W.; Lester, W. Pathologic Antibodies to Platelet Factor 4 after ChAdOx1 nCoV-19 Vaccination. *N. Engl. J. Med.* **2021**, *384*, 2202–2211. [CrossRef]
52. Goel, R.; Ness, P.M.; Takemoto, C.M.; Krishnamurti, L.; King, K.E.; Tobian, A.A. Platelet transfusions in platelet consumptive disorders are associated with arterial thrombosis and in-hospital mortality. *Blood* **2015**, *125*, 1470–1476. [CrossRef] [PubMed]
53. Schell, A.M.; Petras, M.; Szczepiorkowski, Z.M.; Ornstein, D.L. Refractory heparin induced thrombocytopenia with thrombosis (HITT) treated with therapeutic plasma exchange and rituximab as adjuvant therapy. *Transfus. Apher. Sci.* **2013**, *49*, 185–188. [CrossRef] [PubMed]
54. Tiede, A.; Sachs, U.J.; Czwalinna, A.; Werwitzke, S.; Bikker, R.; Krauss, J.K.; Donnerstag, F.; WeiBenborn, K.; Hölinger, G.; Maasoumy, B.; et al. Prothrombotic immune thrombocytopenia after COVID-19 vaccination. *Blood* **2021**, *138*, 350–353. [CrossRef] [PubMed]
55. Thakur, K.T.; Tamborska, A.; Wood, G.K.; McNeill, E.; Roh, D.; Akpan, I.J.; Miller, E.; Bautista, A.; Classeen, J.; Kim, C.Y.; et al. Clinical review of cerebral venous thrombosis in the context of COVID-19 vaccinations: Evaluation, management, and scientific questions. *J. Neurol. Sci.* **2021**, *427*, 117532. [CrossRef] [PubMed]

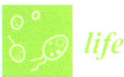

Case Report

Diagnosis and Management of Cerebral Venous Thrombosis Due to Polycythemia Vera and Genetic Thrombophilia: Case Report and Literature Review

Dragos Catalin Jianu [1,2,3,4], Silviana Nina Jianu [5], Nicoleta Iacob [6], Traian Flavius Dan [1,2,3,*], Georgiana Munteanu [1,2,3], Anca Elena Gogu [1,2,3], Raphael Sadik [7], Andrei Gheorghe Marius Motoc [2,8], Any Axelerad [2,9,*], Carmen Adella Sirbu [2,10], Ligia Petrica [2,4,11] and Ioana Ionita [12,13]

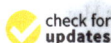

Citation: Jianu, D.C.; Jianu, S.N.; Iacob, N.; Dan, T.F.; Munteanu, G.; Gogu, A.E.; Sadik, R.; Motoc, A.G.M.; Axelerad, A.; Sirbu, C.A.; et al. Diagnosis and Management of Cerebral Venous Thrombosis Due to Polycythemia Vera and Genetic Thrombophilia: Case Report and Literature Review. *Life* 2023, *13*, 1074. https://doi.org/10.3390/life13051074

Academic Editor: Morayma Reyes Gil

Received: 24 February 2023
Revised: 15 April 2023
Accepted: 22 April 2023
Published: 24 April 2023

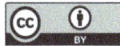

Copyright: © 2023 by the authors. Licensee MDPI, Basel, Switzerland. This article is an open access article distributed under the terms and conditions of the Creative Commons Attribution (CC BY) license (https://creativecommons.org/licenses/by/4.0/).

1. First Division of Neurology, Department of Neurosciences VIII, "Victor Babes" University of Medicine and Pharmacy, E. Murgu Sq., No. 2, 300041 Timisoara, Romania; jianu.dragos@umft.ro (D.C.J.); munteanu.georgiana@umft.ro (G.M.); anca.gogu@umft.ro (A.E.G.)
2. Centre for Cognitive Research in Neuropsychiatric Pathology (NeuroPsy-Cog), Department of Neurosciences VIII, "Victor Babes" University of Medicine and Pharmacy, 156 L. Rebreanu Ave., 300736 Timisoara, Romania; amotoc@umft.ro (A.G.M.M.); sircar13@yahoo.com (C.A.S.); petrica.ligia@umft.ro (L.P.)
3. First Department of Neurology, "Pius Brînzeu" Emergency County Hospital, 156 L. Rebreanu Ave., 300736 Timisoara, Romania
4. Centre for Molecular Research in Nephrology and Vascular Disease, Faculty of Medicine, "Victor Babes" University of Medicine and Pharmacy, 156 L. Rebreanu Ave., 300736 Timisoara, Romania
5. Department of Ophthalmology, "Dr. Victor Popescu" Military Emergency Hospital, 7 G. Lazar Ave., 300080 Timisoara, Romania; silvianajianu@yahoo.com
6. Department of Multidetector Computed Tomography and Magnetic Resonance Imaging, Neuromed Diagnostic Imaging Centre, 300218 Timisoara, Romania; nicoiacob@yahoo.co.uk
7. Department of Geriatrics-Rehabilitation, Riviera-Chablis Hospital, 3 Prairie Ave., 1800 Vevey, Switzerland; raphaelsadik@hopitalrivierachablais.ch
8. Department of Anatomy and Embryology, "Victor Babes" University of Medicine and Pharmacy, E. Murgu Sq., No. 2, 300041 Timisoara, Romania
9. Department of Neurology, General Medicine Faculty, Ovidius University, 900470 Constanta, Romania
10. Department of Neurology, Central Military Emergency University Hospital, Clinical Neuroscience Department, "Carol Davila" University of Medicine and Pharmacy, 020021 Bucharest, Romania
11. Division of Nephrology, Department of Internal Medicine II, "Victor Babes" University of Medicine and Pharmacy, E. Murgu Sq., No. 2, 300041 Timisoara, Romania
12. Division of Hematology, Department V, "Victor Babes" University of Medicine and Pharmacy, E. Murgu Sq., No. 2, 300041 Timisoara, Romania; ionita.ioana@umft.ro
13. Multidisciplinary Research Center for Malignant Hemopathies (CMCHM), "Victor Babes" University of Medicine and Pharmacy, E. Murgu Sq., No. 2, 300041 Timisoara, Romania
* Correspondence: traian.dan@umft.ro (T.F.D.); axelerad.docu@365.univ-ovidius.ro (A.A.)

Abstract: (1) Background: Cerebral venous and dural sinus thrombosis (CVT) rarely appears in the adult population. It is difficult to diagnosis because of its variable clinical presentation and the overlapping signal intensities of thrombosis and venous flow on conventional MR images and MR venograms. (2) Case presentation: A 41-year-old male patient presented with an acute isolated intracranial hypertension syndrome. The diagnosis of acute thrombosis of the left lateral sinus (both transverse and sigmoid portions), the torcular Herophili, and the bulb of the left internal jugular vein was established by neuroimaging data from head-computed tomography, magnetic resonance imaging (including Contrast-enhanced 3D T1-MPRAGE sequence), and magnetic resonance venography (2D-TOF MR venography). We detected different risk factors (polycythemia vera-PV with *JAK2 V617F* mutation and inherited low-risk thrombophilia). He was successfully treated with low-molecular-weight heparin, followed by oral anticoagulation. (3) Conclusions: In the case of our patient, polycythemia vera represented a predisposing risk factor for CVT, and the identification of *JAK2 V617F* mutation was mandatory for the etiology of the disease. Contrast-enhanced 3D T1-MPRAGE sequence proved superior to 2D-TOF MR venography and to conventional SE MR imaging in the diagnosis of acute intracranial dural sinus thrombosis.

Keywords: cerebral venous thrombosis (CVT); polycythemia vera (PV); inherited (genetic) thrombophilia; intracranial hypertension syndrome; lateral sinus thrombosis; contrast enhanced three-dimensional T1 magnetization-prepared rapid acquisition gradient-echo (3D T1-MPRAGE) imaging

1. Introduction

Cerebral venous thrombosis (CVT), including thrombosis of cerebral veins and intracranial dural sinuses, represents an underdiagnosed and less common cause of stroke (0.5–1% of all strokes in adults), but it is much more frequent than previously assumed [1–5].

In adults, CVT has a higher frequency among cases with inherited thrombophilia, mostly women (due to oral contraceptives, pregnancy, postpartum, or post-abortion) and patients with malignancy or infections [6–12].

Different Philadelphia-negative myeloproliferative neoplasms (MPNs) (including Polycythemia Vera–PV, essential thrombocythemia, and primary myelofibrosis) have an increased risk of venous thrombosis. However, previous studies indicate that CVT is rarely associated with MPNs (especially PV) [6,13].

Polycythemia vera (PV) is a *BCR::ABL1* negative, chronic MPN characterized by the proliferation and accumulation primarily of erythroid mass due to an abnormal clone of hematopoietic stem cells. This uncontrolled proliferation leads to an increase in hemoglobin (Hb) and hematocrit (HCT) levels and can be associated with an augmentation in the production of myeloid leukocyte cells and megakaryocytes [14].

The Janus kinase 2 V617F *(JAK2V617F)* mutation led to the diagnosis of PV, which rarely determines CVT [15].

This report describes an extremely rare case of thrombosis of multiple intracranial dural sinuses due to PV and genetic thrombophilia in an adult. The thrombosis affected the left lateral sinus (LS) (both transverse and sigmoid portions), the torcular Herophili, and the bulb of the left internal jugular vein (IJV). The patient clinically developed an isolated intracranial hypertension syndrome. He presented a history of PV with *JAK2V617F* mutation and a genetic low-risk thrombophilia (MTHFR A1298C heterozygote, Factor XIII homozygote, PAI 1 4G/5G heterozygote mutation). The clinical, neuroimaging, laboratory features, treatment, and the short outcome of our patient with CVT were presented and compared with those described in the literature.

2. Case Presentation

A 41-year-old male patient initially came to our Hematology Department in 2018, reporting mild asthenia and fatigue. He presented a history of grade II essential hypertension, right sub-segmental pulmonary thromboembolism (2017), venous thrombosis of the left lower limb (affecting popliteal and posterior tibial vein), and inherited low-risk thrombophilia (MTHFR A1298C heterozygote, Factor XIII homozygote, PAI 1 4G/5G heterozygote mutation).

During the clinical examination, plethoric facies, aquagenic pruritus, and erythromelalgia were noted. Physical examination revealed splenomegaly: spleen was palpable 1 cm below the rib cage. The neurological exam was also normal.

2.1. Laboratory Results

A complete blood count (CBC) noted leucocytosis: high white blood cell count (15.62×10^9/L (normal range, 3.5–9.5×10^9/L)), neutrophilia, thrombocytosis (362×10^9/L (normal range, 135–350×10^9/L)), increased red cell count (7.31×10^{12}/L (normal range 4.35–5.65×10^{12}/L)), a raised haemoglobin (Hb 185 g/L (normal range 132–166 g/L, grams per liter)), and increased hematocrit level (HCT 55.5% (normal range, 38.3–48.6%)).

Abdominal ultrasonography noted splenomegaly (with a maximum spleen length of 14.7 cm; normal values between 8.9 to 11.3 cm).

Bone marrow biopsy revealed age-adjusted hyper-cellularity with trilineage growth, including prominent erythroid, granulocytic, and megakaryocytic proliferation with pleomorphic, mature megakaryocytes, which suggested a histological aspect compatible with PV. The bone marrow biopsies performed in November 2017 and January 2022 (histopathological and immunohistochemistry exam) showed results of histopathological aspect compatible with PV. Additionally, the molecular biology from peripheral blood (genomic DNA isolation, ARMS-PCR amplification) revealed the presence of *JAK2 V617F* mutation homozygote (50% mutant clone); he also presented a subnormal serum erythropoietin level of 2.5 mU/mL (normal range, 3.1–16.5 milliunits per milliliter (mU/mL)).

Electrocardiography and cardiac ultrasonography showed the presence of sinus tachycardia, mitral valve prolapse, and low-grade mitral insufficiency.

Correlating the anamnestic, clinical, and laboratory data, the diagnosis of MPN PV with positive *JAK2V617F* mutation was established. In addition, based on personal thrombotic antecedents, the patient was included in the high-risk class. Risk-adapted therapy was considered. The treatment followed consisted of Alpha interferon (Intron A) (3×3 million UI/week), associated with periodic venesections, antiplatelet medication (Aspirin 75 mg/day, continuous), anticoagulant medication (Dabigatran etexilate 150×2/day, continuous), and specific cardiovascular treatment (Ramipril 5 mg/day, continuous).

In January 2022, the patient was readmitted to the Hematology department for reevaluation. Laboratory data revealed leukocytosis with neutrophilia, increased Hb and HCT levels, and thrombocytosis. The coagulation parameter measures noted an activated partial prothrombin time (APTT) of 73.6 s; thrombin officially standardized ratio (INR) of 1.07; prothrombin time (PT) of 13.5 s; fibrinogen content of 291 mg/dL; and quantitative D-dimer level of 138 ng/mL. No other relevant abnormalities were found.

Abdominal ultrasonography was performed in which splenomegaly (spleen = 14/5.5 cm) was detected. Bone marrow biopsy was reassessed and described a histopathological appearance compatible with PV. Based on the inadequate disease response described through splenomegaly presence, bone marrow alteration, progressive erythrocytosis, thrombocytosis, and leukocytosis, FDA-approved Ropeginterferon alfa-2b (100 µg) treatment was initiated in March 2022. We raised the dose every two weeks. The hematological parameters stabilized at 250 µg. We maintained this dose. Treatment was well tolerated without any presence of significant adverse effects.

In September 2022, the patient came to the emergency department (ED) of our hospital with acute onset (12 h) of severe (8/10) headache, initially associated with vomiting. The headache was generalized, augmenting gradually, and becoming permanent.

Upon physical examination, the patient presented redness of the skin, tachycardia, and moderate hypertension (HR = 92 bpm, BP = 155/100 mmHg), without fever.

Neurological examination was unremarkable.

Direct ophthalmoscopy and color fundus photography revealed bilateral papilledema but without visual complaints.

The ear-nose-throat (ENT) examination findings were normal.

His clinical diagnosis was established as isolated intracranial hypertension syndrome.

2.2. Neuroimaging Data

Unenhanced head CT realized in the ED of our hospital revealed hyperdensities along the left tentorium. We did not observe any parenchymal lesions or any air sinus abnormalities. He was admitted to our Department of Neurology with a probable diagnosis of CVT with a modified Rankin Scale (mRS) score of 1.

The patient underwent magnetic resonance imaging (MRI) combined with MR venography (MRV) with a 1.5-T MR unit in the first 12 h of admission in our Department of Neurology. The brain protocol included Sagittal T1W-weighted sequences; Axial diffusion-DWI sequences; Axial T2W; Axial fluid-attenuated inversion recovery-FLAIR; Axial T1W; post-contrast Axial T1W; and post-contrast 3DT1W.

We also used fast spoiled gradient-echo (FSPGR) and magnetization-prepared rapid acquisition gradient-echo (MPRAGE), both pulse sequence types belonging to the GRE family. We also used T2 star-weighted angiography (SWAN) sequence and advanced sequences, such as PROPELLER (Periodically Rotated Overlapping ParallEL Lines with Enhanced Reconstruction).

For post-contrast 3D T1W imaging, we used a 3D T1-weighted (3D-T1W) FSPGR sequence and a 3D T1-MPRAGE sequence.

The absence of parenchymal lesions was noted on the non-enhanced CT scan and the MRI (T1, T2, FLAIR, DWI, 3DT1-MPRAGE, 3DT1 FSPGR, and SWAN sequences). The diagnosis of acute thrombosis of the left LS (both transverse and sigmoid portions), the torcular Herophili, and the bulb of the left IJV was obtained based on the association of positive signs (definite spontaneous left LS hyperdensity on nonenhanced CT and hypointense signal of left LS, the torcular Herophili, and the bulb of left IJV on MRI sequences), and negative signs (filling defects with no visualization/absence of flow-related signal within the entire left LS, the torcular Herophili, and the bulb of the left IJV at MR venography (2D-TOF), denoting their occlusion) (Figures 1–4).

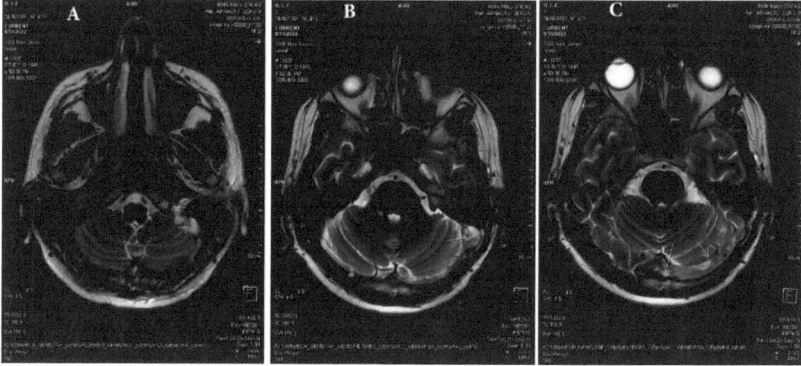

Figure 1. (A–C) Axial T2 PROPELLER: reduced flow in the left jugular bulb, left sigmoid sinus, left transverse sinus, and torcular Herophili (white arrows).

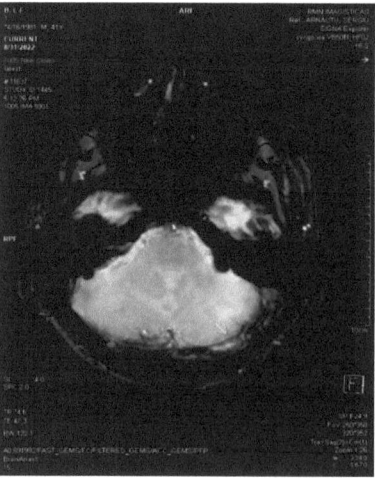

Figure 2. 3D Axial SWAN shows acute thrombosis in the left transverse sinus (white arrow).

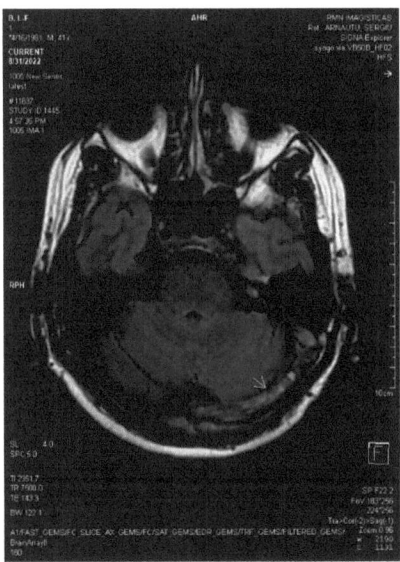

Figure 3. 2D axial FLAIR shows reduced flow in the left transverse sinus (white arrow).

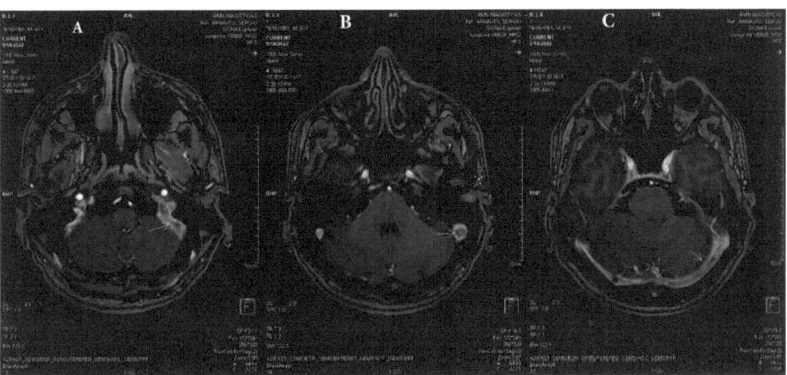

Figure 4. (**A–C**) Axial 3DT1 fast spoiled gradient-echo (FSPGR) post-contrast magnetic resonance demonstrates extensive filling defects throughout the dural sinuses (white arrows: left transverse sinus, left sigmoid sinus, left jugular bulb, and torcular Herophili).

2.3. Laboratory Tests

Laboratory tests revealed increased Hb and HCT levels, increased red cell count, leukocytosis with neutrophilia, and thrombocytosis. The coagulation parameter measures noted an activated partial prothrombin time (APTT) of 72 s, thrombin officially standardized ratio (INR) of 1.03, prothrombin time (PT) of 13.8 s, fibrinogen content of 284 mg/dL and quantitative D-dimer level of 142 ng/mL. No other relevant laboratory abnormalities were observed.

2.4. Treatment in the Acute Phase

Considering the CVT diagnosis, he immediately received low-molecular-weight heparin (LMWH) (Enoxaparin sodium-6000 IU twice a day).

Meanwhile, after three days of treatment with LMWH, the symptoms of headache and vomiting were gradually relieved, and he was discharged having recovered completely (MRS = 0).

2.5. Treatment after the Acute Phase

At discharge, due to his prothrombotic condition of PV with *JAK2V617F* mutation, and a genetic low-risk thrombophilia, we recommended oral anticoagulation (with dabigatran etexilate-150 mg twice daily) for an indefinite duration.

Neurological and imaging follow-ups were done at 30 days and three months after discharge, respectively.

We did not observe any recurrence (he did not present any other neurological symptoms/signs), deep vein thrombosis, or pulmonary embolism during this period of time.

The follow-up MRI/MRV demonstrated unchanged filling defects through the dural sinuses (Figures 5–7).

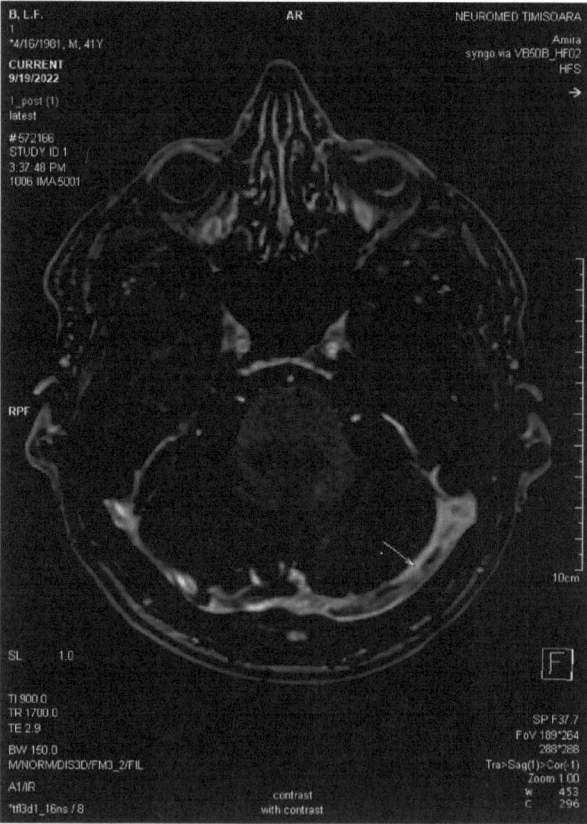

Figure 5. Axial 3DT1 MPRAGE post-contrast magnetic resonance after three weeks demonstrates unchanged filling defects throughout the dural sinuses (white arrows: left transverse sinus and torcular Herophili).

Further testing was undertaken, so contrast-enhanced 3D T1-MPRAGE imaging was done on the patient. The images obtained more clearly revealed a hypointense signal of the left LS, the torcular Herophili, and the bulb of the left IJV (Figure 5).

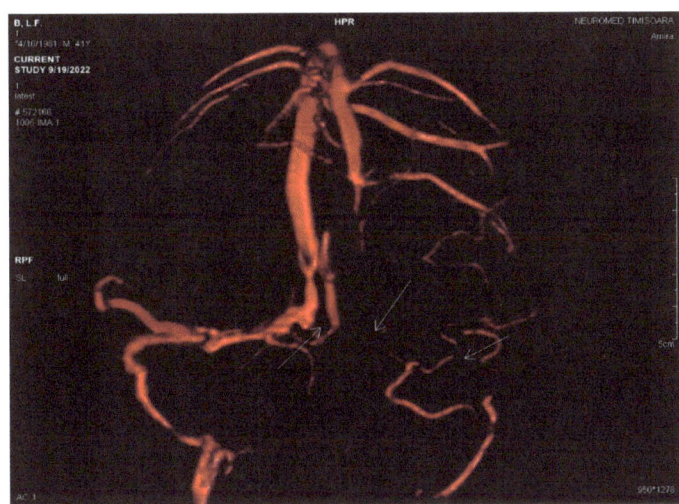

Figure 6. VRT reconstruction by PC 3DVENO sequence after three weeks: absent flow in the left jugular bulb, left sigmoid sinus, left transverse sinus, and torcular Herophili (white arrows).

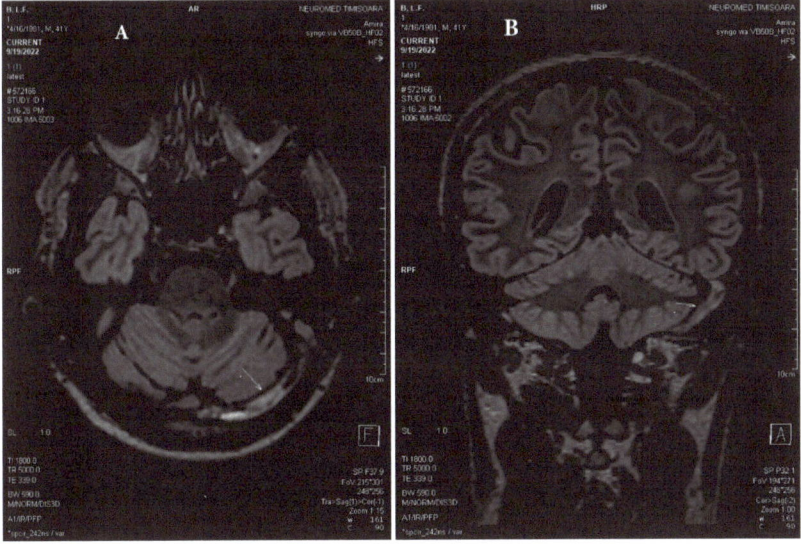

Figure 7. (**A**) Axial and (**B**) coronal MPR T2 spc_ir_dark_fl performed after three weeks shows unchanged reduced flow in the left jugular bulb, left sigmoid sinus, left transverse sinus, and torcular Herophili (white arrows).

3. Discussion

Clinical and imaging diagnosis of CVT is frequently difficult because of its nonspecific and variable clinical presentation and the overlapping signal intensities of thrombosis and venous flow on conventional MR images and MR venograms [10,11].

The clinical aspects of CVT are influenced by the following factors: site and number of occluded venous vessels, the functionality of collateral pathways, associated parenchymal lesions (vasogenic or cytotoxic edema, hemorrhage), age, gender, etiology, and interval from clinical onset to the beginning of the treatment [7,10,11]. A wide range of clinical presentations appears in patients with CVT. In adults, the most common clinical syndromes observed in combination or as isolated syndromes are intracranial hypertension, focal neurological deficits, seizures, and encephalopathy [1–3,16–19].

Isolated intracranial hypertension represents the most common clinical syndrome noted in CVT (nearly 40% of patients in the International Study on Cerebral Vein and Dural Sinus Thrombosis (ISCVT) cohort)) [6,7]. It is represented by headaches associated with vomiting, papilledema, visual symptoms, and sixth nerve palsy [20]. Headache is an extremely frequent neurological symptom of CVT (nearly 90% of patients in the -ISCVT cohort). It may be localized or diffused [20]. Papilledema is noted on funduscopy in 25–40% of CVT patients [6–8].

The patient in the current report presented with isolated intracranial hypertension with severe diffuse headache associated with vomiting and bilateral papilledema.

Two main pathophysiological mechanisms are implied in the genesis of CVT clinical spectrum: the first is represented by the diminution of cerebrospinal fluid (CSF) absorption, and the second by the progressive increase of venular and capillary pressure [12,21–23].

In our case, the isolated intracranial hypertension was produced by the complete thrombosis of different intracranial dural sinuses (left transverse sinus, left sigmoid sinus, left jugular bulb, and torcular Herophili), due to PV with *JAK2V617F* mutation, and to a genetic low-risk thrombophilia (MTHFR A1298C heterozygote, Factor XIII homozygote, PAI 1 4G/5G heterozygote mutation), with the consecutive diminution of CSF absorption [12,24,25].

According to the 2016 WHO classification, diagnostic criteria for PV are divided into two groups: major and minor [26]. On the one hand, the major criteria are defined by elevated Hb (>16.5 g/dL for men/>16.0 g/dL in women), HCT (>49% in men/>48% in women), or red cell mass level (>25% above mean normal predicted value); bone marrow pleomorphic changes such as panmyelosis and hypercellularity; and presence of *JAK2V617F* mutation, as in our case. On the other hand, the minor criterion for PV comprises a subnormal erythropoietin level. At least two major criteria plus the minor criterion are required for PV diagnosis [26].

PV is characterized by the clonal proliferation of hematopoietic stem cells, which determines the abnormal rise and accumulation of different circulating blood cells [27].

Consequently, PV produces hyperviscosity with stasis of blood (decreasing blood flow velocities) and eventually the appearance of thrombosis in different arterial and venous vessels.

The link between leukocytosis and thrombosis has been analyzed in different experimental studies based on the fact that in MPNs chronic and subclinical systemic inflammation presents an essential role in the pathogenesis of vascular events [28–31].

However, strong arguments supporting leukocytosis as an inflammatory biomarker potentially helping to differentiate prognostic categories in PV were still missing until recent studies noted that the neutrophil-to-lymphocyte ratio (NLR) represents an inexpensive and convenient predictor of venous thrombosis in PV [28–31].

Several groups of authors observed that arterial (AT) and venous (VT) thrombotic events are the most common complications in cases with PV and are the most important causes of morbidity and mortality [32–34].

In this context, these authors established that JAK2V617F VAF (variant allele frequency) >50% represented an independent strong predictor of VT (identifying patients with PV at high risk for VT), proving that AT and VT are different aspects which might require distinct management [32–34].

Thrombosis of intracranial dural sinuses affects CSF absorption, thus augmenting the intracranial pressure and producing the clinical syndrome of intracranial hypertension [5,35,36].

In addition, our patient had a *JAK2V617F* mutation, which represents an independent risk factor for thrombosis [15,37].

Inherited thrombophilias are the most important risk factors linked to CVT. Three mutations have been highly associated with CVT: factor V, Leiden; factor II, the prothrombin variant (PT 20210A); and the homozygosity for MTHFR C677T (severe genetic risk thrombophilia). These mutations were not relevant to our case because our patient presented only a low genetic risk of thrombophilia (MTHFR A1298C heterozygote, Factor XIII homozygote, PAI 1 4G/5G heterozygote mutation) [6,38,39].

Comprehensive knowledge of different anatomical variants of intracranial dural sinuses and cerebral veins is mandatory to identify CVT.

Each lateral sinus (LS) is located between the torcular Herophili and the IJV and contains two parts: the transverse segment (which lies on the attached border of the tentorium) and the sigmoid segment (which runs on the internal side of the mastoid process). The LSs collect venous blood from the posterior portions of the cerebral hemispheres, brainstem, and cerebellum. LSs also receive some of the diploic veins and some small veins from the middle ear, thus explaining their thrombosis in patients with mastoiditis or otitis media [1–6,12]. Frequently (in 50–80% of the cases), the two transverse sinuses are asymmetric, hypoplastic, or aplastic, transverse sinuses (usually the left one) being a relatively common variation (between 15% to 30% of all the patients) [1–6,12]. Therefore, the absence of a signal within a sinus, most commonly the left transverse sinus, may not always indicate thrombosis. It is usually suggestive of hypoplasia or aplasia, which was not present in our case [1,2,40–42].

Due to the great anatomic variability (in location, number, and anastomoses) of cortical veins and the posterior fossa veins, it is very difficult to identify their isolated occlusion [1–6]. In contrast to these two groups of veins, the deep cerebral veins are constant, and, in consequence, they are always identified at venography, thus any occlusion at their level being accurately detected, which was not our case [1,2,12,42].

Conventional MRI sequences, two-dimensional time-of-flight (2D-TOF) MR Venography, contrast-enhanced CT projection venography, and digital subtraction angiography (DSA) are common techniques in the diagnosis of dural sinus thrombosis [42].

On conventional MRI sequences, the dilated collaterals of the cerebral veins and dural sinuses and cerebral venous thrombosis are easily diagnosed in the subacute stage, but usually, they are not detected at the acute stage of CVT because the venous clot and the venous flow can produce overlapping signal intensities, as in our case [43].

With 2D-TOF MR Venography alone, it is very difficult to differentiate a hypoplastic or atretic dural sinus from its thrombosis. However, dural sinus thrombosis was presumed indirectly in our case by the absence of normal flow in the left lateral sinus since the thrombosis was usually isointense with the brain parenchyma [44]. A second pitfall of 2D-TOF MR Venography is represented by the signal loss of intracranial vessels, in which the direction of intracranial blood flow is within the imaging plane. This so-called saturation may resemble thrombotic occlusion [44–46].

According to different authors, high-resolution CT Venography has been considered superior to MR Venography (2DTOF or phase-contrast); however, we did not use this technique in our case because it presents a few disadvantages, including exposure to X-rays, the use of iodinated contrast material, poor delineation of skull base structures, and complex post-processing work [46,47].

Therefore, a noninvasive and more accurate diagnostic imagistic technique, the 3D contrast-enhanced T1 MPRAGE sequence, was used in our case for the acute diagnosis of intracranial dural sinus thrombosis [46,47].

According to different studies, this sequence is better than 2D-TOF MR Venography and conventional spin-echo (SE) imaging in the detection of both normal dural sinuses and cerebral venous anatomy and cerebral venous thrombosis, respectively, because it is not influenced by the angle between the cerebral vessel and the scan slab plane or flow velocities. For this reason, the MPRAGE sequence can excellently delineate cerebral veins and dural sinuses with good contrast and resolution between dural sinuses and neighboring cerebral lesions. The hypo-intense to intermediately-intense thrombosis was identified in our case because of excellent contrast of the thrombosis, the intensely enhanced sinus, and the adjacent brain parenchyma [48,49].

On the one hand, MPRAGE sequence makes possible the accurate diagnosis of an acute stage of CVT. Supplementary, the concomitant identification of dilated collateral veins and cerebral venous infarcts it is mandatory to predict prognosis with great confidence. Because of its superior ability to detect DSA, 3D contrast-enhanced MPRAGE represents an alternative as an efficient, noninvasive technique for the diagnosis and short-term follow-up of cases with acute CVT, as in our case [48,49].

On the other hand, this sequence may not be suitable in cases with chronic CVT due to organized and subsequently vascularized chronic venous clots because the enhanced thrombosis decreases the contrast with the normal intracranial dural sinus. Consequently, DSA and 2D-TOF MR Venography may be superior to 3D contrast-enhanced T1 MPRAGE in such cases [48].

The T2 star-weighted angiography (SWAN), or susceptibility-weighted angiography, is a high-resolution 3D multi-echo gradient echo (GRE) sequence that is more sensitive than GRE in the detection of cerebral hemorrhage and calcifications, which were not detected in our case. The SWAN sequence clearly identifies small blood vessels, microbleeds, and large vascular structures in the brain. SWAN also achieves larger images than GRE with a significantly higher contrast difference between the lesion and the healthy parenchyma, as in our case [50].

Head motion represents the main problem in magnetic resonance imaging (MRI). According to different authors, PROPELLER (Periodically Rotated Overlapping ParallEL Lines with Enhanced Reconstruction) MRI determines a sure means of quantifying and compensating for head motion, reducing motion artifact, and improving image quality compared with standard TSE sequences; thus intracranial pathology, including CVT, is better demonstrated with this technique, as in our case [51].

Therapeutic approaches for PV are predominantly targeting the clinical manifestation control increasing the quality of life by preventing the associated complications such as thrombotic events, secondary myelofibrosis, or acute leukemia transformation. Current treatment recommendations are adapted according to patient risk-adapted classification, so patients 60 years old or younger without prior history of thrombotic events are included as low-risk, while patients over 60 years old or with a history of thrombosis are considered high-risk, as the patient in our case was [52]. Cytoreductive therapy such as Hydroxyurea (HU), along with aspirin or phlebotomies, are generally accepted as first-line therapies in PV patients, but because of the frequency of HU intolerance, adverse effects, and disease progression, there was an increased need for modifying-disease agents. Interferons (INFs) and recombinant pegylated interferons have been studied as alternative therapeutic agents to HU. Recently, the usage of recombinant pegylated interferon alfa 2b in PV has been approved by the FDA with promising results, as in our case [53–55].

Given the confirmed CVT, anticoagulation was conducted in our case as the first-line therapy using initially body-weight-adjusted subcutaneous low-molecular-weight heparin, followed by oral anticoagulation (with dabigatran etexilate) [8,10].

Consistently, the clinical course of CVT was very good at three months. Several authors have suggested that recanalization of the occluded intracranial dural sinuses appears in 40–90% of CVT cases, the majority within the first four months of evolution, being reduced thereafter [6–8]. On the one hand, the cavernous sinus and the deep cerebral veins present a higher rate of recanalization; instead, the lowest rates were noted in LS occlusion, as in our case. On the other hand, recanalization of the thrombosed intracranial dural sinus is not related to the outcome after CVT, as in our case [6–8].

4. Conclusions

In our case, PV represented a predisposing factor for CVT, and the *JAK2V617F* mutation was helpful for diagnosis. Contrast-enhanced 3D T1-MPRAGE was superior to 2D-TOF

MR venography and conventional SE MR imaging in the diagnosis of acute intracranial dural sinus thrombosis.

Author Contributions: Conceptualization, D.C.J. and I.I.; methodology, D.C.J., I.I., T.F.D., A.A. and N.I.; software, G.M. and R.S.; validation, D.C.J., S.N.J., N.I., T.F.D., G.M., A.E.G., R.S., A.G.M.M., A.A., C.A.S., L.P. and I.I.; formal analysis, D.C.J., N.I. and I.I.; investigation, D.C.J., S.N.J., N.I. and I.I.; resources, D.C.J.; data curation, T.F.D.; writing—original draft preparation, D.C.J. and I.I.; writing-review and editing, D.C.J. and T.F.D.; visualization, D.C.J., S.N.J., N.I., T.F.D., G.M., A.E.G., R.S., A.G.M.M., A.A., C.A.S., L.P. and I.I.; supervision, D.C.J.; project administration, D.C.J. All authors have read and agreed to the published version of the manuscript.

Funding: This research received no external funding.

Institutional Review Board Statement: The study was conducted according to the guidelines of the Declaration of Helsinki and approved by the Institutional Review Board (or Ethics Committee) of "Pius Brinzeu" Emergency County Hospital, Timisoara, Romania (protocol code 382/21.02.2023).

Informed Consent Statement: Informed consent was obtained from the patient included in the study.

Data Availability Statement: First Department of Neurology, "Pius Brinzeu" Emergency County Hospital, Timisoara, Romania; Department of Multidetector Computed Tomography and Magnetic Resonance Imaging, Neuromed Diagnostic Imaging Centre, Timisoara, Romania.

Conflicts of Interest: The authors declare no competing interest.

References

1. Bousser, M.G.; Barnett, H.J.M. Chapter Twelve: Cerebral Venous Thrombosis. In *Stroke (Pathophysiology, Diagnosis, and Management)*, 4th ed.; Mohr, J.P., Choi, D.W., Grotta, J.C., Weir, B., Wolf, P.A., Eds.; Churchill Livingstone: London, UK, 2004; pp. 301–325.
2. Ferro, J.M.; Canhão, P. Chapter 45: Cerebral Venous Thrombosis. In *Stroke (Pathophysiology, Diagnosis, and Management)*, 6th ed.; Grotta, J.C., Albers, G.W., Broderick, J.P., Kasner, S.E., Lo, E.H., Mendelow, A.D., Sacco, R.L., Wong, L.K.S., Eds.; Elsevier: Amsterdam, The Netherlands, 2016; pp. 716–730.
3. Stam, J. Thrombosis of the cerebral veins and sinuses. *N. Engl. J. Med.* **2005**, *352*, 1791–1798. [CrossRef] [PubMed]
4. Coutinho, J.M.; Zurbier, S.M.; Aramideh, M.; Stam, J. The Incidence of Cerebral Venous Thrombosis A Cross-Sectional Study. *Stroke* **2012**, *43*, 3375–3377. [CrossRef] [PubMed]
5. Devasagayam, S.; Wyatt, B.; Leyden, J.; Kleinig, T. Cerebral Venous Sinus Thrombosis Incidence Is Higher Than Previously Thought: A Retrospective Population-Based Study. *Stroke* **2016**, *47*, 2180. [CrossRef]
6. Ferro, J.M.; Canhao, P.; Stam, J.; Bousser, M.G.; Barinagarrementeria, F. Prognosis of cerebral vein and dural sinus thrombosis: Results of the International Study on Cerebral Vein and Dural Sinus Thrombosis (ISCVT). *Stroke* **2004**, *35*, 664–670. [CrossRef]
7. Ferro, J.M.; Canhão, P. Cerebral Venous Thrombosis: Etiology, Clinical Features, and Diagnosis. Available online: https://www.uptodate.com/contents/cerebral-venous-thrombosis-etiology-clinical-features-and-diagnosis (accessed on 15 October 2021).
8. Saposnik, G.; Barinagarrementeria, F.; Brown, R.D.; Bushnell, C.D.; Cucchiara, B.; Cushman, M.; de Veber, G.; Ferro, J.M.; Tsai, F.Y.; on behalf of the American Heart Association Stroke Council and the Council on Epidemiology and Prevention. Diagnosis and management of cerebral venous thrombosis: A statement for healthcare professionals from the American Heart Association/American Stroke Association. *Stroke* **2011**, *42*, 1158–1192. [CrossRef]
9. Coutinho, J.M.; Ferro, J.M.; Canhão, P.; Barinagarrementeria, F.; Bousser, M.G.; Stam, J. Cerebral Venous and Sinus Thrombosis in Women. *Stroke* **2009**, *40*, 2356–2361. [CrossRef]
10. Dmytriw, A.A.; Song, J.S.A.; Yu, E.; Poon, C.S. Cerebral venous thrombosis: State of the art diagnosis and management. *Neuroradiology* **2018**, *60*, 669–685. [CrossRef] [PubMed]
11. Jianu, D.C.; Jianu, S.N.; Dan, T.F.; Munteanu, G.; Copil, A.; Birdac, C.D.; Motoc, A.G.M.; Docu Axelerad, A.; Petrica, L.; Arnautu, S.F.; et al. An Integrated Approach on the Diagnosis of Cerebral Veins and Dural Sinuses Thrombosis (a Narrative Review). *Life* **2022**, *12*, 717. [CrossRef]
12. Piazza, G. Cerebral Venous Thrombosis. *Circulation* **2012**, *125*, 1704–1709. [CrossRef]
13. Dentali, F.; Ageno, W.; Rumi, E.; Casetti, I.; Poli, D.; Scoditti, U.; Maffioli, M.; di Minno, M.N.D.; Caramazza, D.; Pietra, D.; et al. Cerebral venous thrombosis and myeloproliferative neoplasms: Results from two large databases. *Thromb. Res.* **2014**, *134*, 41–43. [CrossRef] [PubMed]
14. Iurlo, A.; Cattaneo, D.; Bucelli, C.; Baldini, L. New Perspectives on Polycythemia Vera: From Diagnosis to Therapy. *Int. J. Mol. Sci.* **2020**, *21*, 5805. [CrossRef]
15. Godeneche, G.; Gaillard, N.; Roy, L.; Mania, A.; Tondeur, S.; Chomel, J.; Lavabre, T.; Arquizan, C.; Neau, J. JAK2 V617F Mutation Associated with Cerebral Venous Thrombosis: A Report of Five Cases. *Cerebrovasc. Dis.* **2010**, *29*, 206–209. [CrossRef] [PubMed]

16. Jianu, D.C.; Jianu, S.N.; Munteanu, G.; Dan, F.T.; Barsan, C. Chapter 3—Cerebral Vein and Dural Sinus Thrombosis. In *Ischemic Stroke of Brain*; Sanchetee., P., Ed.; Intech Open: London, UK, 2018; pp. 45–76. Available online: https://www.intechopen.com/chapters/61125 (accessed on 15 November 2021).
17. Munteanu, G.; Motoc, A.G.M.; Dan, T.F.; Gogu, A.E.; Jianu, D.C. Aphasic Syndromes in Cerebral Venous and Dural Sinuses Thrombosis-A Review of the Literature. *Life* **2022**, *12*, 1684. [CrossRef]
18. Jianu, D.C.; Jianu, S.N.; Dan, T.F.; Iacob, N.; Munteanu, G.; Motoc, A.G.M.; Baloi, A.; Hodorogea, D.; Axelerad, A.D.; Ples, H.; et al. Diagnosis and Management of Mixed Transcortical Aphasia Due to Multiple Predisposing Factors, including Postpartum and Severe Inherited Thrombophilia, Affecting Multiple Cerebral Venous and Dural Sinus Thrombosis: Case Report and Literature Review. *Diagnostics* **2021**, *11*, 1425. [CrossRef] [PubMed]
19. Dan, T.F.; Jianu, S.N.; Iacob, N.; Motoc, A.G.M.; Munteanu, G.; Baloi, A.; Albulescu, N.; Jianu, D.C. Management of an old woman with cavernous sinus thrombosis with two different mechanisms: Case report and review of the literature. *Rom. J. Morphol. Embryol.* **2020**, *61*, 1329–1334. [CrossRef] [PubMed]
20. Biousse, V.; Ameri, A.; Bousser, M.G. Isolated intracranial hypertension as the only sign of cerebral venous thrombosis. *Neurology* **1999**, *53*, 1537. [CrossRef] [PubMed]
21. Schaller, B.; Graf, R. Cerebral Venous Infarction-The Pathophysiological Concept. *Cerebrovasc. Dis.* **2004**, *18*, 179–188. [CrossRef] [PubMed]
22. Gotoh, M.; Ohmoto, T.; Kuyama, H. Experimental study of venous circulatory disturbance by dural sinus occlusion. *Acta Neurochir.* **1993**, *124*, 120. [CrossRef]
23. Lövblad, K.O.; Bassetti, C.; Schneider, J.; Guzman, R.; El-Koussy, M.; Remonda, L.; Schroth, G.S.O. Diffusion-weighted mr in cerebral venous thrombosis. *Cereb. Dis.* **2001**, *11*, 169. [CrossRef]
24. Tefferi, A.; Vannucchi, A.M.; Barbui, T. Polycythemia vera: Historical oversights, diagnostic details, and therapeutic views. *Leukemia* **2021**, *35*, 3339–3351. [CrossRef]
25. Wen, H.; Jin, D.; Chen, Y.; Cui, B.; Xiao, T. Cerebellar venous thrombosis mimicking a cerebellar tumor due to polycythemia vera: A case report. *BMC Neurol.* **2021**, *21*, 225. [CrossRef]
26. Barbui, T.; Thiele, J.; Gisslinger, H.; Kvasnicka, H.M.; Vannucchi, A.M.; Guglielmelli, P.; Orazi, A.; Tefferi, A. The 2016 WHO classification and diagnostic criteria for myeloproliferative neoplasms: Document summary and in-depth discussion. *Blood Cancer J.* **2018**, *8*, 15. [CrossRef] [PubMed]
27. Spivak, J.L. Polycythemia vera. *Curr. Treat. Option Oncol.* **2018**, *19*, 12. [CrossRef] [PubMed]
28. Carobbio, A.; Vannucchi, A.M.; De Stefano, V.; Masciulli, A.; Guglielmelli, P.; Loscocco, G.G.; Ramundo, F.; Rossi, E.; Kanthi, Y.; Tefferi, A.; et al. Neutrophil-to-lymphocyte ratio is a novel predictor of venous thrombosis in polycythemia vera. *Blood Cancer J.* **2022**, *12*, 28. [CrossRef]
29. Farrukh, F.; Guglielmelli, P.; Loscocco, G.G.; Pardanani, A.; Hanson, C.A.; De Stefano, V.; Barbui, T.; Gangat, N.; Vannucchi, A.M.; Tefferi, A. Deciphering the individual contribution of absolute neutrophil and monocyte counts to thrombosis risk in polycythemia vera and essential thrombocythemia. *Am. J. Hematol.* **2022**, *97*, E35–E37. [CrossRef] [PubMed]
30. Wang, X.; Tu, Y.; Cao, M.; Jiang, X.; Yang, Y.; Zhang, X.; Lai, H.; Tu, H.; Li, J. The Predictive Value of Neutrophil-Lymphocyte Ratio in Patients with Polycythemia Vera at the Time of Initial Diagnosis for Thrombotic Events. *BioMed Res. Int.* **2022**, *2022*, 9343951. [CrossRef]
31. Carobbio, A.; Ferrari, A.; Masciulli, A.; Ghirardi, A.; Barosi, G.; Barbui, T. Leukocytosis and thrombosis in essential thrombocythemia and polycythemia vera: A systematic review and meta-analysis. *Blood Adv.* **2019**, *3*, 1729–1737. [CrossRef]
32. Guglielmelli, P.; Loscocco, G.G.; Mannarelli, C.; Rossi, E.; Mannelli, F.; Ramundo, F.; Coltro, G.; Betti, S.; Maccari, C.; Ceglie, S.; et al. JAK2V617F variant allele frequency >50% identifies patients with polycythemia vera at high risk for venous thrombosis. *Blood Cancer J.* **2021**, *11*, 199. [CrossRef]
33. Soudet, S.; Le Roy, G.; Cadet, E.; Michaud, A.; Morel, P.; Marolleau, J.P.; Sevestre, M.A. JAK2 allele burden is correlated with a risk of venous but not arterial thrombosis. *Thromb. Res.* **2022**, *211*, 1–5. [CrossRef]
34. Moliterno, A.R.; Kaizer, H.; Reeves, B.N. $JAK2^{V617F}$ Allele Burden in Polycythemia Vera: Burden of Proof. *Blood* **2023**, *141*, 1934–1942. [CrossRef]
35. Sirin, N.G.; Yesilot, N.; Ekizoğlu, E.; Keles, N.; Tuncay, R.; Coban, O.; Bahar, S.Z. A case report of cerebral venous thrombosis in polycythemia vera presenting with intracranial and spinal subdural hematoma. *Case Rep. Neurol.* **2010**, *2*, 37–45. [CrossRef] [PubMed]
36. Eliaçik, S.; Savas, Ö.Ö.; Komut, E.; Tan, F.U. Partial status epilepticus in cerebral venous sinus thrombosis, initial manifestation of polycythemia vera. *Ann. Indian Acad Neurol.* **2019**, *22*, 536–537. [PubMed]
37. Radia, D.; Geyer, H.L. Management of symptoms in polycythemia vera and essential thrombocythemia patients. *Hematology* **2015**, *2015*, 340–348. [CrossRef] [PubMed]
38. Gogu, A.E.; Motoc, A.G.; Stroe, A.Z.; Docu Axelerad, A.; Docu Axelerad, D.; Petrica, L.; Jianu, D.C. Plasminogen Activator Inhibitor-1 (PAI-1) Gene Polymorphisms Associated with Cardiovascular Risk Factors Involved in Cerebral Venous Sinus Thrombosis. *Metabolites* **2021**, *11*, 266. [CrossRef] [PubMed]
39. Gogu, A.E.; Jianu, D.C.; Dumitrascu, V.; Ples, H.; Stroe, A.Z.; Docu Axelerad, D.; Docu Axelerad, A. MTHFR Gene Polymorphisms and Cardiovascular Risk Factors, Clinical-Imagistic Features and Outcome in Cerebral Venous Sinus Thrombosis. *Brain Sci.* **2021**, *11*, 23. [CrossRef]

40. Jianu, D.C.; Jianu, S.N.; Motoc, A.G.M.; Poenaru, M.; Petrica, L.; Vlad, A.; Ursoniu, S.; Gogu, A.E.; Dan, T.F. Diagnosis and management of a young woman with acute isolated lateral sinus thrombosis. *Rom. J. Morphol. Embryol.* **2017**, *58*, 1515–1518.
41. Jianu, D.C.; Jianu, S.N.; Dan, T.F.; Motoc, A.G.M.; Poenaru, M. Pulsatile tinnitus caused by a dilated left petrosquamosal sinus. *Rom. J. Morphol. Embryol.* **2016**, *57*, 319–322.
42. Sadik, J.-C.; Jianu, D.C.; Sadik, R.; Purcell, Y.; Novaes, N.; Saragoussi, E.; Obadia, M.; Lecler, A.; Savatovsky, J. Imaging of Cerebral Venous Thrombosis. *Life* **2022**, *12*, 1215. [CrossRef]
43. Zimmerman, R.D.; Ernst, R.J. Neuroimaging of cerebral venous thrombosis. *Neuroimaging Clin. N. Am.* **1992**, *2*, 463–485.
44. Ayanzen, R.H.; Bird, C.R.; Keller, P.J.; McCully, F.J.; Theobald, M.R.; Heiserman, J.E. Cerebral MR venography: Normal anatomy and potential diagnostic pitfalls. *AJNR Am. J. Neuroradiol.* **2000**, *21*, 74–78.
45. Vogl, T.J.; Bergman, C.; Villringer, A.; Einhäupl, K.; Lissner, J.; Felix, R. Dural sinus thrombosis: Value of venous MR angiography for diagnosis and follow-up. *AJR Am. J. Roentgenol.* **1994**, *162*, 1191–1198. [CrossRef]
46. Ozsvath, R.R.; Casey, S.O.; Lustrin, E.S.; Alberico, R.A.; Hassankhani, A.; Patel, M. Cerebral venography: Comparison of CT and MR projection venography. *AJR Am. J. Roentgenol.* **1997**, *169*, 1699–1707. [CrossRef] [PubMed]
47. Casey, S.O.; Alberico, R.A.; Patel, M.; Jimenez, J.M.; Ozsvath, R.R.; Maguire, W.M.; Taylor, M.L. Cerebral CT venography. *Radiology* **1996**, *198*, 163–170. [CrossRef] [PubMed]
48. Liang, L.; Korogi, Y.; Sugahara, T.; Onomichi, M.; Shigematsu, Y.; Yang, D.; Kitajima, M.; Hiai, Y.; Takahashi, M. Evaluation of the intracranial dural sinuses with a 3D contrast enhanced MP-RAGE sequence: Prospective comparison with 2D-TOF MR venography and digital subtraction angiography. *Am. J. Neuro-Radiol.* **2001**, *22*, 481–492.
49. Stevenson, J.; Knopp, E.A.; Litt, A.W. MP-RAGE subtraction venography: A new technique. *J. Magn. Reson. Imaging* **1995**, *5*, 239–241. [CrossRef]
50. Docampo, J.; Gonzalez, N.; Bravo, F.; Sarroca, D.; Morales, C.; Bruno, C. Susceptibility-Weighted Angiography of Intracranial Blood Products and Calcifications Compared to Gradient Echo Sequence. *Neuroradiol. J.* **2013**, *26*, 493–500. [CrossRef]
51. Forbes, K.P.; Pipe, J.G.; Bird, C.R.; Heiserman, J.E. PROPELLER MRI: Clinical testing of a novel technique for quantification and compensation of head motion. *J. Magn. Reson. Imaging* **2001**, *14*, 215–222. [CrossRef]
52. Tefferi, A.; Barbui, T. Polycythemia vera and essential thrombocythemia: 2021 update on diagnosis, risk-stratification and management. *Am. J. Hematol.* **2020**, *95*, 1599–1613. [CrossRef]
53. Yacoub, A.; Mascarenhas, J.; Kosiorek, H.; Prchal, J.T.; Berenzon, D.; Baer, M.R.; Ritchie, E.; Silver, R.T.; Kessler, C.; Winton, E.; et al. Pegylated interferon alfa-2a for polycythemia vera or essential thrombocythemia resistant or intolerant to hydroxyurea. *Blood* **2019**, *134*, 1498–1509. [CrossRef]
54. Kiladjian, J.-J.; Klade, C.; Georgiev, P.; Krochmalczyk, D.; Gercheva-Kyuchukova, L.; Egyed, M.; Dulicek, P.; Illes, A.; Pylypenko, H.; Sivcheva, L.; et al. Long-term outcomes of polycythemia vera patients treated with ropeginterferon Alfa-2b. *Leukemia* **2022**, *36*, 1408–1411. [CrossRef]
55. Petrica, L.; Vlad, A.; Gluhovschi, G.; Gadalean, F.; Dumitrascu, V.; Vlad, D.; Popescu, R.; Velciov, S.; Gluhovschi, C.; Bob, F.; et al. Glycated peptides are associated with the variability of endothelial dysfunction in the cerebral vessels and the kidney in type 2 diabetes mellitus patients: A cross-sectional study. *J. Diabetes Complicat.* **2015**, *29*, 230–237. [CrossRef] [PubMed]

Disclaimer/Publisher's Note: The statements, opinions and data contained in all publications are solely those of the individual author(s) and contributor(s) and not of MDPI and/or the editor(s). MDPI and/or the editor(s) disclaim responsibility for any injury to people or property resulting from any ideas, methods, instructions or products referred to in the content.

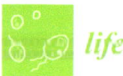 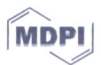

Article

The Burden of Cerebral Venous Thrombosis in a Romanian Population across a 5-Year Period

Adina Stan [1,2,3,†], Silvina Ilut [1,2,3,†], Hanna Maria Dragos [1,2,3,*], Claudia Bota [2,3], Patricia Nicoleta Hanghicel [2,3], Alexander Cristian [2,3], Irina Vlad [1,2], Diana Mocanu [3], Stefan Strilciuc [1,2,†], Paul Stefan Panaitescu [4], Horatiu Stan [1] and Dafin F. Muresanu [1,2,3]

1. Department of Neurosciences, Iuliu Hatieganu University of Medicine and Pharmacy, No. 8 Victor Babes Street, 400012 Cluj-Napoca, Romania
2. RoNeuro Institute for Neurological Research and Diagnostic, No. 37 Mircea Eliade Street, 400364 Cluj-Napoca, Romania
3. Neurology Department, Emergency County Hospital Cluj-Napoca, 400347 Cluj-Napoca, Romania
4. Department of Microbiology, Iuliu Hatieganu University of Medicine and Pharmacy, No. 8 Victor Babes Street, 400012 Cluj-Napoca, Romania
* Correspondence: dragos.hanna.maria@elearn.umfcluj.ro; Tel.: +40-773991273
† These authors contributed equally to this work.

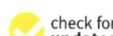

Citation: Stan, A.; Ilut, S.; Dragos, H.M.; Bota, C.; Hanghicel, P.N.; Cristian, A.; Vlad, I.; Mocanu, D.; Strilciuc, S.; Panaitescu, P.S.; et al. The Burden of Cerebral Venous Thrombosis in a Romanian Population across a 5-Year Period. *Life* **2022**, *12*, 1825. https://doi.org/10.3390/life12111825

Academic Editor: Hieronim Jakubowski

Received: 12 October 2022
Accepted: 7 November 2022
Published: 9 November 2022

Publisher's Note: MDPI stays neutral with regard to jurisdictional claims in published maps and institutional affiliations.

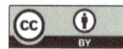

Copyright: © 2022 by the authors. Licensee MDPI, Basel, Switzerland. This article is an open access article distributed under the terms and conditions of the Creative Commons Attribution (CC BY) license (https:// creativecommons.org/licenses/by/ 4.0/).

Abstract: Health policies in transitioning health systems are rarely informed by the social burden and the incidence shifts in disease epidemiology. Cerebral venous thrombosis (CVT) is a type of stroke more often affecting younger adults and women, with higher incidences being reported in recent studies. A retrospective, hospital-based population study was conducted at Cluj-Napoca Emergency County Hospital across a 5-year period between 2017 and 2021. The overall incidence and the rates in distinctive gender and age groups were assessed. Length of hospital stay (LHS), modified Rankin score (mRS) and mortality at discharge and at 3 months were calculated. Fifty-three patients were included. The median age was 45 years, and 64.2% were women. In our population of 3,043,998 person-years, 53 CVT cases resulted in an incidence of 1.74 per 100,000 (95% CI 1.30–2.27). CVT incidence was higher in women (2.13 per 100,000, 95% CI 1.47–2.07). There was a statistically significant difference in LHS between patients with different intracranial complications (Kruskal–Wallis, $p = 0.008$). The discharge mRS correlated with increasing age ($r_s = 0.334$, $p = 0.015$), transient risk factors (Fisher's exact test, $p = 0.023$) and intracranial complications (Fisher's exact test, $p = 0.022$). In addition, the mRS at 3 months was statistically associated with increasing age ($r_s = 0.372$, $p = 0.006$) and transient risk factors (Fisher's exact test, $p = 0.012$). In-hospital mortality was 5.7%, and mortality at follow up was 7.5%, with higher rates in women (5.9% and 8.8%, respectively). Our findings may provide insight regarding the epidemiological features of certain patient groups more prone to developing CVT and its complications, informing local and central stakeholders' efforts to improve standards of care.

Keywords: cerebral venous thrombosis; incidence; mortality; length of stay

1. Introduction

Cerebral venous thrombosis (CVT) is an uncommon type of stroke that affects younger adults and women more often than ischemic and hemorrhagic stroke [1–3]. CVT incidence was previously estimated at around 0.2 to 0.5 per 100,000 per year [4,5], but higher incidences of 1.57 or 1.32 per 100,000 have been reported in recent studies [3,6,7]. Whether the accessibility to neuroimaging diagnosis and methodological differences between studies may explain these findings or a true increase in incidence was identified in the last decade is not clear. No studies on CVT incidence in Romanian populations were found.

First estimates of mortality in CVT patients are derived from autopsy studies performed several decades ago [8]. In the past, CVT was associated with poor prognosis and high mortality rate [8]. In recent studies [6,7,9–12], the prognosis became more favorable; a mortality of 4% to 5% in the acute phase and a declining trend in overall mortality among patients with CVT have been described [3,13]. The majority of data on CVT patients was derived from reference cohorts such as the multicenter prospective and retrospective VENOST study [14] and the International Study on Cerebral Vein and Dural Sinus Thrombosis (ISCVT) [1], where a discharge mortality of 4.3% and a mortality of 8.3% at follow up were reported [1]. Inconsistent with previous studies [6,7,9,10,15,16], no fatal events were reported among a Romanian cohort of 43 patients in 2014 [11].

Our study was designed to address these inconsistencies as well as the lack of local epidemiological data. The primary aim was to investigate the incidence and the social burden of CVT on a Romanian-hospital-based population, by assessing the length of hospital stay (LHS), modified Rankin scale (mRS) and mortality at discharge and at three months. The secondary aim was to perform a literature review, comparing our findings with those reported by other hospital-based population studies on incidence and mortality in CVT patients.

2. Materials and Methods

A retrospective hospital-population-based study was conducted at Cluj-Napoca Emergency County Hospital (CNECH), the second largest tertiary stroke center in Romania. Patients were identified through electronic charts based on the relevant International Classification of Diseases, Tenth Revision (ICD-10) codes for CVT cases during a 5-year period between 2017 and 2021. Only inhabitants living in the hospital's catchment area (Cluj County) were included. The hospital had a catchment area of around 608,800 habitants/year between 2017 and 2021. All CVT cases in this area are in contact with our hospital at the initial admission as part of acute management and follow up. Thus, it is possible to estimate population-based rates for CVT. Population figures for the incidence rates were obtained from the Romanian National Institute of Statistics [17].

The hospital's electronic database was searched to identify patients over 18 years old with a new CVT diagnosis between 1 January 2017 and 31 December 2021. The following ICD-10 codes were searched for: I63.6, I67.6, O22.5 and O87.3. All clinical and neuroradiological assessments for the identified CVT cases were reassessed and confirmed by a senior neurologist. Patients with repeated presentations due to chronic CVT during the study period were counted as one case in the analysis. Demographic, clinical, radiological and potential risk factors were investigated for all patients.

To calculate the overall incidence, the observed CVT cases admitted to CNECH were used as the numerator and the population of Cluj County aged ≥ 18 years as the denominator. The adult population of Cluj County was 604,635 in 2017, 606,485 in 2018, 608,739 in 2019, 611,508 in 2020 and 612,631 in 2021 [17], resulting in 3,043,998 person-years across the 5-year period. In addition, the CVT incidences depending on gender and different age groups were also assessed. Incidence rates were expressed per 100,000 person-years, and 95% confidence intervals (95% CI) were displayed.

To assess the burden of CVT at the regional level, LHS, mRS and mortality at discharge and at three months were calculated. The influence of the main predictive factors for outcome in CVT [1] was also investigated.

Since the sample size was narrow, determining the distribution of continuous variables was important for choosing an appropriate statistical method. As the LHS variable showed a positively skewed distribution (Shapiro–Wilk test, $p = 0.001$), the median and the interquartile range were used to describe these data. Logarithmic transformations [18] for LHS were performed, but the data became more skewed, departing from normal distribution (Shapiro–Wilk test, $p < 0.001$); therefore, non-parametric tests were selected. Spearman correlation was used to investigate the association between age and LHS, mRS at discharge or mRS at three months. Categorical data were presented as counts and percentages. The differences between groups of categorical data were assessed using chi-square or Fisher's exact test, and the effect size was described using Crammer's V values. The significance level alpha was 0.05. Statistical analyses were performed using IBM SPSS Statistics, version 26.0. The study protocol was approved by the Independent Ethics Committee of CNECH.

3. Results

3.1. Study Population

Among the 53 patients included, the median age was 45 years (range: 18–89), and 64.2% were women. Table 1 shows the demographics, risk factors and clinical and radiological findings among all included patients. In all, 60.4% of patients presented with acute onset. The most prevalent symptom was headache, followed by motor weakness, seizures and nausea/vomiting. Most patients developed CVT involving two or more sinuses/veins. Among those with only one sinus involved, the most frequent sites were the transverse sinus and the superior sagittal sinus. CVT risk factors were found in 75.47% of the patients, and most patients had at least one identified risk factor. The most frequent transient risk factors in women were pregnancy or puerperium and oral contraceptive use, whereas head trauma and local infections were the only transient risk factors encountered in men. Thrombophilia was by far the most common persistent risk factor in all patients. No transient or persistent risk factors were found in thirteen patients. Furthermore, 18.8% of patients presented at least two intracranial lesions on CT or MRI. Venous infarction was the most common radiological finding among all patients. Parenchymal hemorrhage was more frequent in men and subarachnoid hemorrhage in women.

Table 1. Demographic, clinical, radiological and risk factor data presented as total and percentage.

Patient Characteristics	Total, N = 53	Female, N = 34, 64.2%	Male, N = 19, 35.8%
Median age (interquartile range), years	45 (29)	45 (22)	44 (40)
Type of onset, N (%)			
Acute	32 (60.4%)	20 (58.8%)	12 (63.2%)
Subacute	16 (30.2%)	10 (29.4%)	6 (31.6%)
Chronic	5 (9.4%)	4 (11.8%)	1 (5.2%)
Clinical presentation, N (%)			
Headache	31 (58.5%)	22 (64.7%)	9 (47.4%)
Nausea/vomiting	10 (18.9%)	6 (17.6%)	4 (21.1%)
Motor weakness	19 (35.8%)	14 (41.2%)	5 (26.3%)
Seizures	14 (26.4%)	6 (17.6%)	8 (42.1%)
Coma	9 (17%)	6 (17.6%)	3 (15.8%)
Speech disturbances	6 (11.3%)	6 (17.6%)	0
Cranial nerve palsies	5 (9.43%)	2 (5.8%)	3 (15.8%)
Cerebellar signs	4 (7.5%)	4 (11.8%)	0
Sinus/vein involved, N (%)			
Transverse sinus	8 (15.1%)	6 (17.6%)	2 (10.5%)
Superior sagittal sinus	5 (9.4%)	2 (5.9%)	3 (15.8%)
Cavernous sinus	3 (5.7%)	0	3 (15.8%)
Cortical veins	3 (5.7%)	3 (8.8%)	0
Two or more sinuses/veins involved	34 (64.1%)	23 (67.7%)	11 (57.9%)

Table 1. Cont.

Patient Characteristics	Total, N = 53	Female, N = 34, 64.2%	Male, N = 19, 35.8%
Transient risk factors, N (%)			
Pregnancy and puerperium	4 (7.5%)	4 (11.8%)	0
Oral contraceptives	4 (7.5%)	4 (11.8%)	0
Head trauma	6 (11.3%)	3 (8.8%)	3 (15.8%)
Local infections	4 (7.5%)	2 (5.9%)	2 (10.5%)
SARS-CoV-2 infection	1 (1.88%)	1 (2.94%)	0
Adenoviral-vector-based SARS-CoV-2 vaccination	1 (1.88%)	0	1 (5.2%)
Two or more transient risk factors	2 (3.8%)	2 (5.9%)	0
Persistent risk factors, N (%)			
Prior thromboembolism	3 (5.7%)	2 (5.9%)	1 (5.3%)
Thrombophilia	13 (24.5%)	7 (20.6%)	6 (31.6%)
Neoplasia	4 (7.5%)	4 (11.7%)	0
Two or more persistent risk factors	7 (13.2%)	5 (14.7%)	2 (10.5%)
Without transient or persistent risk factors, N (%)	13 (24.52%)	7 (20.56%)	6 (31.6%)
Complications, N (%)			
Venous infarct	9 (17%)	7 (20.6%)	2 (10.5%)
Subarachnoid hemorrhage	3 (5.7%)	2 (5.9%)	1 (5.3%)
Parenchymal hemorrhage	3 (5.7%)	0	3 (15.7%)
Two or more complications	10 (18.8%)	9 (26.4%)	1 (5.3%)
Without complications	28 (52.8%)	16 (47.1%)	12 (63.2%)

3.2. The Incidence of CVT

In our population of 3,043,998 person-years, 53 identified cases resulted in an incidence of 1.74 per 100,000 (95% CI 1.30–2.27). The incidence of CVT across a 5-year period and incidence figures for different gender and age groups are depicted in Figure 1 and in Table 2, respectively. CVT incidence was higher in women compared to men. The highest incidence of CVT was found in 2021 (3.59 per 100,000, 95% CI 2.25–5.43). Across the 5-year period, CVT incidence seems to follow a general ascending trend; although, in 2020, a decline in incidence was registered. The CVT incidence in patients between 18 and 49 years old increased 4.5-fold in 2021 compared to 2017. The highest overall incidence among all gender and age groups was found for women in the 18–49 age group (2.43 per 100,000, 95% CI 1.43–3.62). Only in the 50–69 age group, the incidence rates for men and women were similar.

3.3. The Burden of CVT

The median LHS was 10 days (interquartile range 7). There was a statistically significant difference in LHS between patients with different intracranial lesions (Kruskal–Wallis, $\chi^2(4) = 13.906$, $p = 0.008$), with a mean rank of LHS of 17.44 for venous infarct patients, 24 for subarachnoid hemorrhage patients, 41.83 for intracranial hemorrhage patients and 39.6 in patients who had developed multiple complications. No associations between LHS and age ($r_s = 0.077$, $p > 0.05$), gender (Mann–Whitney, $p > 0.05$), CVT location, risk factors or mRS were found (Kruskal–Wallis, $p > 0.05$).

The median of mRS at discharge was 2 (interquartile range 2). A positive moderate relationship between discharge mRS and age was seen ($r_s = 0.334$, $p = 0.015$), indicating that 11.15% of the variation of discharge mRS was explained by age ($r_s^2 = 0.1115$). Moreover, there was a significant difference in discharge mRS between patients with different transient risk factors (Fisher's exact test, $p = 0.023$, Cramer's V of 0.473, medium effect size). Women in pregnancy/puerperium or using oral contraceptive had an mRS between 0 and 3. Patients with traumatic brain injury presented a higher mRS of 2–4, and 50% of patients with infections died during hospitalization. A significant association was found between discharge mRS and intracranial lesions (Fisher's exact test, $p = 0.022$, Cramer's V of 0.434, medium effect size). Most patients with venous infarction had an mRS of 0–2, while those who developed multiple lesions had an mRS > 2 at discharge. Meanwhile, 66.7% of patients with intraparenchymal hemorrhage had a discharge mRS of 4. No statistical associations between mRS and gender, CVT location or persistent risk factors were found (chi-square, $p > 0.05$).

The median of mRS at follow up was 1 (interquartile range 2). A positive moderate relationship between 3-month mRS and age was seen ($r_s = 0.372$, $p = 0.006$), indicating that 13.83% of the variation of 3-month mRS was explained by age ($r_s^2 = 0.1383$). A significant association between mRS and transient risk factors was found (Fisher's exact test, $p = 0.012$, Cramer's V of 0.461, medium effect size). Most patients without transient risk factors had a 3-month mRS between 0 and 2. No statistical associations between 3-month mRS and gender, CVT location, intracranial lesions or persistent risk factors were found (chi-square, $p > 0.05$). Figure 2 depicts the distribution of mRS at discharge and at three months among different age groups.

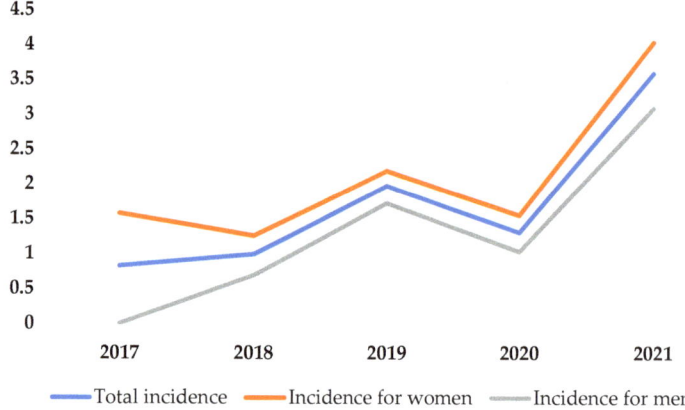

Figure 1. Incidence of CVT across 5-year period.

In-hospital mortality was 5.7% for the total sample, with higher rates in women compared to males. The >70 age group showed the highest discharge mortality (16.7%). Mortality at follow up was 7.5%. Three-month mortality was higher for women. A significant association between mortality at follow up and age groups was found (Fisher's exact test, $p = 0.003$, Cramer's V of 0.577, strong effect size). Overall, 50% of patients over 70 years old died at 3 months after CVT compared to 3.3% of patients between 18 and 49 years old. No patients from the 50–69 years age group died in the first three months.

Table 3 displays our results regarding the incidence and mortality of CVT in relation to previous hospital-based population studies in different countries. Based on the country of origin, studies were classified as coming from high-, upper- or lower-middle-income countries using the definition of the World Bank [19]. Among high-income countries, an increasing trend in incidence and a decline in mortality at discharge and follow up were identified across the last 40 years. A tendency for increased age at CVT diagnosis could be observed. Fewer and heterogenous data from upper- and lower-middle-income countries were found. The median age and proportion of women from our study were similar to those reported by the VENOST study [14], but the overall incidence found in our cohort was comparable to recent incidences observed in studies in high-income countries.

Table 2. Incidence of CVT across the 5-year period regarding gender and age groups (95% CI).

	2017	2018	2019	2020	2021	Overall Incidence
Incidence/year	0.82 (0.26–1.92)	0.98 (0.36–2.15)	1.97 (1.09–3.44)	1.30 (0.56–2.57)	3.59 (2.25–5.43)	1.74 (1.30–2.27)
Women	1.57 (0.51–3.68)	1.25 (0.34–3.22)	2.19 (0.88–4.51)	1.55 (0.50–3.63)	4.04 (2.12–6.91)	2.13 (1.47–2.97)
Men	0	0.69 (0.08–2.50)	1.72 (0.56–4.03)	1.03 (0.21–3.01)	3.09 (1.41–5.87)	1.31 (0.79–2.04)
Incidence/18–49 y	0.86 (0.17–2.52)	1.75 (0.64–3.81)	1.77 (0.65–3.85)	0.59 (0.07–2.15)	3.89 (2.07–6.66)	1.76 (1.19–2.53)
Women	1.72 (0.35–5.04)	2.32 (0.63–5.95)	1.76 (0.36–5.15)	0.59 (0.01–3.29)	5.36 (2.45–10.1)	2.43 (1.43–3.62)
Men	0	1.17 (0.01–4.23)	1.77 (0.03–5.19)	0.59 (0.01–3.33)	2.41 (0.06–6.17)	1.18 (0.05–2.17)
Incidence/50–69 y	0.57 (0.01–3.20)	0	2.18 (0.05–5.58)	2.67 (0.08–6.25)	3.71 (1.49–7.64)	1.86 (1.08–2.08)
Women	1.09 (0.02–6.07)	0	2.07 (0.02–7.47)	4.07 (1.11–10.4)	2.01 (0.02–7.29)	1.87 (0.08–3.56)
Men	0	0	2.30 (0.02–8.32)	1.13 (0.02–6.29)	5.58 (1.82–13.0)	1.85 (0.80–3.65)
Incidence/>70 y	1.18 (0.03–6.61)	0	2.31 (0.28–8.34)	1.12 (0.28–6.26)	2.20 (0.26–7.98)	1.37 (0.50–2.99)
Women	1.95 (0.49–10.8)	0	3.80 (0.46–13.7)	0	3.64 (0.44–13.1)	1.89 (0.61–4.44)
Men	0	0	0	2.85 (0.72–15.8)	0	0.58 (0.14–3.25)

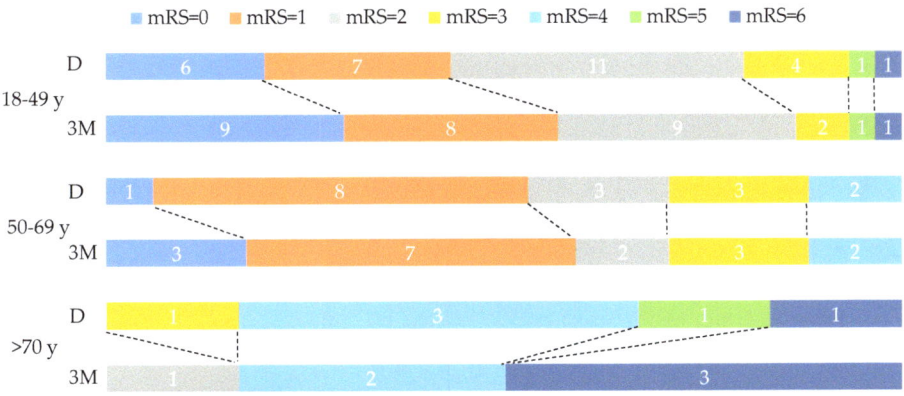

Figure 2. Discharge (D) and three-month (3M) mRS distribution on age groups. Data labels represent number of patients per mRS group.

Table 3. Different studies reporting the incidence and the mortality of CVT on local populations compared to ISCVT.

	ISCVT [1]	High-Income Countries							Upper-Middle-Income Countries			Lower-Middle-Income Countries
Country	21 Countries	Portugal [15]	Hong Kong [16]	Australia [6]	Netherlands [7]	France [10]	Norway [9]	Italy [12]	Mexico [20]	VENOST [14], Turkey	Romania (Our Study)	Iran [21]
Time interval	1998–2002	1980–1998	1995–1998	2005–2011	2008–2010	2011–2016	2011–2017	2012–2019	1999–2008	2000–2015	2017–2021	2001–2004
Sample size	624	142	13	105	94	194	62	32	24	1144	53	122
Incidence per 100,000	NR	0.22	0.34	1.57	1.32	NR	1.75	1.6	NR	NR	1.74	1.23
Median age	37 (16–86)	35	30	49	41	40	46	41	30	40	45	26
Women, %	74.5%	72%	77%	52%	72%	68.4%	53%	75%	83%	67.9%	64.2%	75%
LHS, median	17	NR	NR	NR	NR	10	NR	20	22	NR	10	NR
Discharge mortality	4.3%	6%	8%	9%	1%	2.9%	3%	0%	8%	NR	5.7%	NR
Mortality at follow up	8.3%	NR	NR	12%	3%	3.4%	3%	0%	NR	NR	7.5%	NR

ISCVT = International Study on Cerebral Vein and Dural Sinus Thrombosis, NR = not reported.

4. Discussion

4.1. The Incidence of CVT

The overall incidence of CVT found in this study corroborates those of other recent studies from Norway [9], Italy [12], Australia [6] and two Dutch [7] provinces, reporting higher annual CVT incidence than previous studies [15,16,21].

CVT incidence varies in distinct parts of the world due to distinctive socioeconomic and demographic features or risk factors [9]. A cohort derived from four prospective international studies [22] showed that the incidence of venous thromboembolism was higher in high-income countries compared to upper-middle-income countries and lower-middle-/low-income countries. The diagnosis of thrombosis events seems to be affected by reduced access to hospital and diagnostic facilities in low-income countries [22]. Regarding Romania, the increasing accessibility to CT and MRI venography may explain the higher incidence comparable to that reported by high-income countries.

In our study, the incidence for women was higher compared with other studies (2.13 per 100,000 person-years, 95% CI 1.47–2.97) [6,9,10,12,21]. It was shown that the CVT risk in women using oral contraceptives is 7.59 times higher compared to that in women not taking oral contraception [23]. Combined oral contraceptives (COCs) represented 8.8% of contraceptive use prevalence, reaching 15.4% or more in high-income countries [24]. A cross-sectional survey [25] on COC use conducted in 2014 on women in community pharmacies in Cluj-Napoca revealed that 38.9% of women had used COCs for more than two years, out of which more than half bought the pills without prescription from a pharmacy at least once [25], raising concerns about harmful use.

A recent meta-analysis [23] on pregnancy-related strokes reported an incidence of 9.1 cases of CVT per 100,000 pregnancies, with CVT accounting for from 9% up to 48% of total pregnancy-related strokes. In our study, 11.8% of patients presented pregnancy-related CVT, half of them occurring in the first two postpartum weeks. Interestingly, the other half of patients developed CVT in the first trimester, which is exceedingly rare. Incongruent with other studies [23,26], the patients had associated complications such as bilateral thalamic infarction and parenchymal hemorrhages.

In the 50–69 age group, the incidence rates for men and women were equal, similar to other studies reporting no predilection toward women in elderly CVT patients [2,27–29]. This finding could be explained by a decreasing trend in CVT incidence in women aged 50–69, attributed to the absence of gender-specific risk factors, especially COCs and pregnancy/puerperium state.

The lowest incidence of CVT was found in men over 70 years old probably due to a poor life expectancy in men compared to women (70 years old versus 79 years old) and an overrepresentation of women among all age groups (171,104 men compared to 264,374 women reported across the 5-year analyzed period) [17]. An important clinical finding in multiple studies [27,29] on CVT in older patients is the absence of headache in patients over 55 years old, but in our study, no significant difference between different age groups and the presence of headache or other CVT symptoms was found (chi-square, $p > 0.05$).

4.2. The Burden of CVT

In our study, the median LHS was 10 days, which was similar to the median LHS found in a French study [10], but much lower compared to that in the ISCVT [1] study probably due to different study periods (1998–2002 in ISCVT versus 2017–2021 in our study). A decreased LHS was reported by recent American studies (median LHS = 4) [30,31], with longer LHS being associated with age and male gender. In our study, no association between LHS and age, gender, CVT location, risk factors or outcome was found.

Discharge mRS increased with age, which is similar to the case in previous studies [1,14]. Half of the patients who had any infections (nose, throat, ear or extracranial) as the cause of their CVT died, and patients who developed CVT after previous cranial trauma had an mRS of 2 to 4 at discharge (Fisher's exact test, $p = 0.023$). These findings are similar to those of the ISCVT cohort [1] that reported a 3.34-fold increased risk of death or dependency in patients with infections and CVT. Patients with two or more intracranial complications had an mRS > 2 at discharge. Furthermore, 66.7% of patients with parenchymal hemorrhage presented an mRS of 4; these results are also similar to those reported by ISCVT investigators [1].

Risk factors associated with poor prognosis at 3 months were similar to those found in acute phase: age, infections and cranial trauma. Neither parenchymal hemorrhage nor persistent risk factors such as cancer influenced the outcome at 3 months (chi-square, $p > 0.05$), which is different from ISCVT [1] and VENOST [14] studies, which found that any malignancy is associated with a 2.9 increased risk of death or dependency [1].

The in-hospital mortality rate was 5.7%, similar to that in previous hospital-based studies [6,7,9,10,15,16,20,21]. In the ISCVT [1], a discharge mortality rate of 4.3% and mortality of 8% at follow up were reported. Among high-income countries [6,7,9,10,15,16] (Table 3), a trend in declining mortality in adult patients diagnosed with CVT was observed at least in the last decade. A significant inverse correlation between mortality and year of patient recruitment ($r = -0.72$, $p < 0.001$) was reported [13]. The sensitivity analysis of the studies from high-income countries reported a similar inverse correlation ($r = -0.70$, $p < 0.001$) [13]. Interestingly, after the exclusion of studies published before 1990, the inverse correlation persisted ($r = -0.51$, $p < 0.001$), but when all studies published before 2000 were excluded, the correlation disappeared ($r = -0.06$, $p = 0.67$) [13].

Part of the decline in mortality is due to the general improvement of hospital care and increasing availability of neuroimaging techniques and recent therapeutic strategies. Before the implementation of cerebral angiography, CVT was diagnosed with certainty only at surgery or autopsy, with the selection bias of patients in severe clinical condition [13,32] being common in the first mortality studies. The severity of CVT cases has also decreased over time, with fewer cases of coma or severe neurological deficits being identified [7,13,21]. Moreover, the introduction of anticoagulation [33] and decompressive hemicraniectomy [34] improved the survival of patients. A shift in risk factors associated with CVT may also explain the decline in mortality and increase in incidence. Across the years, traumatic and septic CVT have decreased, while the number of women using oral contraceptives increased [13]. It is known that trauma- or sepsis-related CVT has a worse prognosis [35] compared to a favorable outcome in patients using oral contraceptives [2] as was found in our cohort.

It is important to observe shifts in the pattern of incidence and mortality in patients with CVT, also considering the pre-pandemic and pandemic periods. CVT is a rare but severe complication after SARS-CoV-2 infection [36–38], and CVT has been reported following immunization [39], especially with adenovirus-vector-based [40] and ChAdOx1-S vaccines [41]. Our sample included a patient with a moderate form of COVID-19 infection–associated CVT and a patient who developed CVT after 10 days from adenovirus-vector-based SARS-CoV-2 vaccination. CVT occurring after adenoviral-vector-based COVID-19 vaccination is usually associated with vaccine-induced immune thrombotic thrombocytopenia and the presence of antibodies against platelet factor 4 (PF4) [42,43], but the platelet counts of our patient were normal across multiple blood tests, and PF4 antibodies were not evaluated.

4.3. Limitations

The demographics, clinical features and associated risk factors suggest that our study included a sample of patients that is representative for CVT [1]. The sample size may be regarded as narrow with 53 cases, but the study extended across five years and screened all acute cerebrovascular presentations at the second-largest stroke center in Romania. Another limitation is the retrospective design of the study, but because an extensive assessment of the anonymized electronic medical records was performed, it is unlikely that this design might have introduced bias.

5. Conclusions

This study investigated the burden of CVT in a Romanian-hospital-based population and compared regional findings with cross-sectional studies from different countries. These results have clinical practice implications concerning additional investigations and the management and prognosis of CVT. The diagnosis of one subsequent disease or risk factor in CVT patients should not limit the search for additional comorbidities or risk factors. Furthermore, as infections, cranial trauma and intracranial hemorrhage are potential predictors of poor outcome, patients showing these features should be thoroughly investigated and monitored. CVT shows an increasing incidence particularly in the 18–49 age group in the Romanian population across the last five years. In the presence of suggestive CVT symptoms in this age group, a CT angiography at the emergency department should be considered to exclude CVT. Further multicenter prospective studies on Romanian populations should be conducted to assess the incidence and the burden of CVT.

Author Contributions: Conceptualization, A.S., S.I., S.S. and D.F.M.; methodology, A.S., S.I., S.S., H.S., H.M.D. and D.F.M.; software, S.S., H.M.D. and P.S.P.; validation, A.S., S.I., S.S., H.S. and D.F.M.; formal analysis, A.S., S.S., H.M.D. and P.S.P.; investigation, A.S., S.I., S.S., H.S. and D.F.M.; data curation, C.B., P.N.H., A.C., I.V. and D.M.; writing—original draft preparation, H.M.D., C.B., P.N.H., A.C., I.V. and D.M.; writing—review and editing, A.S., S.I., S.S., H.S. and D.F.M.; visualization, A.S., H.M.D. and P.S.P.; supervision, A.S., S.I., S.S. and D.F.M. All authors have read and agreed to the published version of the manuscript.

Funding: This research received no external funding.

Institutional Review Board Statement: The study was conducted in accordance with the Declaration of Helsinki and approved by the Independent Ethics Committee of CNECH (No. 51214, 6 December 2021).

Informed Consent Statement: Not applicable.

Data Availability Statement: Data available on request due to privacy or ethical issues. The data presented in this study are available on request from the corresponding author.

Conflicts of Interest: The authors declare no conflict of interest.

References

1. Ferro, J.M.; Canhão, P.; Stam, J.; Bousser, M.-G.; Barinagarrementeria, F.; ISCVT Investigators. Prognosis of Cerebral Vein and Dural Sinus Thrombosis: Results of the International Study on Cerebral Vein and Dural Sinus Thrombosis (ISCVT). *Stroke* **2004**, *35*, 664–670. [CrossRef] [PubMed]
2. Coutinho, J.M.; Ferro, J.M.; Canhão, P.; Barinagarrementeria, F.; Cantú, C.; Bousser, M.-G.; Stam, J. Cerebral Venous and Sinus Thrombosis in Women. *Stroke* **2009**, *40*, 2356–2361. [CrossRef] [PubMed]
3. Silvis, S.M.; de Sousa, D.A.; Ferro, J.M.; Coutinho, J.M. Cerebral Venous Thrombosis. *Nat. Rev. Neurol.* **2017**, *13*, 555–565. [CrossRef] [PubMed]
4. Stam, J. Thrombosis of the Cerebral Veins and Sinuses. *N. Engl. J. Med.* **2005**, *352*, 1791–1798. [CrossRef]
5. Bousser, M.-G.; Ferro, J.M. Cerebral Venous Thrombosis: An Update. *Lancet Neurol.* **2007**, *6*, 162–170. [CrossRef]
6. Devasagayam, S.; Wyatt, B.; Leyden, J.; Kleinig, T. Cerebral Venous Sinus Thrombosis Incidence Is Higher Than Previously Thought. *Stroke* **2016**, *47*, 2180–2182. [CrossRef]
7. Coutinho, J.M.; Zuurbier, S.M.; Aramideh, M.; Stam, J. The Incidence of Cerebral Venous Thrombosis: A Cross-Sectional Study. *Stroke* **2012**, *43*, 3375–3377. [CrossRef]
8. Kalbag, R.; Woolf, A. *Cerebral Venous Thrombosis*; Oxford University Press: London, UK, 1967.
9. Kristoffersen, E.S.; Harper, C.E.; Vetvik, K.G.; Zarnovicky, S.; Hansen, J.M.; Faiz, K.W. Incidence and Mortality of Cerebral Venous Thrombosis in a Norwegian Population. *Stroke* **2020**, *51*, 3023–3029. [CrossRef]
10. Triquenot Bagan, A.; Crassard, I.; Drouet, L.; Barbieux-Guillot, M.; Marlu, R.; Robinet-Borgomino, E.; Morange, P.-E.; Wolff, V.; Grunebaum, L.; Klapczynski, F.; et al. Cerebral Venous Thrombosis: Clinical, Radiological, Biological, and Etiological Characteristics of a French Prospective Cohort (FPCCVT)—Comparison with ISCVT Cohort. *Front. Neurol.* **2021**, *12*, 753110. [CrossRef]
11. Bălașa, R.; Daboczi, M.; Costache, O.; Maier, S.; Bajko, Z.; Moțățaianu, A.; Bălașa, A. Risk factors and diagnosis of cerebral venous thrombosis: Data from a cohort of 45 Romanian patients. *Acta Marisiensis-Ser. Med.* **2014**, *60*, 207–214. [CrossRef]

12. Foschi, M.; Pavolucci, L.; Rondelli, F.; Amore, G.; Spinardi, L.; Rinaldi, R.; Favaretto, E.; Favero, L.; Russo, M.; Pensato, U.; et al. Clinicoradiological Profile and Functional Outcome of Acute Cerebral Venous Thrombosis: A Hospital-Based Cohort Study. *Cureus* **2021**, *13*, e17898. [CrossRef] [PubMed]
13. Coutinho, J.M.; Zuurbier, S.M.; Stam, J. Declining Mortality in Cerebral Venous Thrombosis: A Systematic Review. *Stroke* **2014**, *45*, 1338–1341. [CrossRef] [PubMed]
14. Duman, T.; Uluduz, D.; Midi, I.; Bektas, H.; Kablan, Y.; Goksel, B.K.; Milanlioglu, A.; Necioglu Orken, D.; Aluclu, U.; VENOST Study Group. A Multicenter Study of 1144 Patients with Cerebral Venous Thrombosis: The VENOST Study. *J. Stroke Cerebrovasc. Dis.* **2017**, *26*, 1848–1857. [CrossRef] [PubMed]
15. Ferro, J.M.; Correia, M.; Pontes, C.; Baptista, M.V.; Pita, F.; Cerebral Venous Thrombosis Portuguese Collaborative Study Group (Venoport). Cerebral Vein and Dural Sinus Thrombosis in Portugal: 1980–1998. *Cerebrovasc. Dis.* **2001**, *11*, 177–182. [CrossRef] [PubMed]
16. Mak, W.; Mok, K.Y.; Tsoi, T.H.; Cheung, R.T.; Ho, S.L.; Chang, C.M. Cerebral Venous Thrombosis in Hong Kong. *Cerebrovasc. Dis.* **2001**, *11*, 282–283. [CrossRef] [PubMed]
17. TEMPO Online. Available online: http://statistici.insse.ro:8077/tempo-online/#/pages/tables/insse-table (accessed on 30 September 2022).
18. Feng, C.; Wang, H.; Lu, N.; Chen, T.; He, H.; Lu, Y.; Tu, X.M. Log-Transformation and Its Implications for Data Analysis. *Shanghai Arch. Psychiatry* **2014**, *26*, 105–109. [CrossRef] [PubMed]
19. World Bank Open Data | Data. Available online: https://data.worldbank.org/ (accessed on 1 October 2022).
20. Rodríguez-Rubio, L.R.; Medina-Córdova, L.L.; Andrade-Ramos, M.A.; González-Padilla, C.; Bañuelos-Becerra, L.J.; Chiquete, E.; Coronado-Magaña, H.; Pérez-Flores, G.; Rojas-Andrews, A.; González-Cornejo, S.; et al. Cerebral venous thrombosis at the Hospital Civil de Guadalajara "Fray Antonio Alcalde". *Rev. Mex. Neurocienc.* **2009**, *10*, 177–183.
21. Janghorbani, M.; Zare, M.; Saadatnia, M.; Mousavi, S.A.; Mojarrad, M.; Asgari, E. Cerebral Vein and Dural Sinus Thrombosis in Adults in Isfahan, Iran: Frequency and Seasonal Variation. *Acta Neurol. Scand.* **2008**, *117*, 117–121. [CrossRef]
22. Siegal, D.M.; Eikelboom, J.W.; Lee, S.F.; Rangarajan, S.; Bosch, J.; Zhu, J.; Yusuf, S.; the Venous Thromboembolism Collaboration. Variations in Incidence of Venous Thromboembolism in Low-, Middle-, and High-Income Countries. *Cardiovasc. Res.* **2021**, *117*, 576–584. [CrossRef]
23. Swartz, R.H.; Cayley, M.L.; Foley, N.; Ladhani, N.N.N.; Leffert, L.; Bushnell, C.; McClure, J.A.; Lindsay, M.P. The Incidence of Pregnancy-Related Stroke: A Systematic Review and Meta-Analysis. *Int. J. Stroke* **2017**, *12*, 687–697. [CrossRef]
24. Christin-Maitre, S. History of Oral Contraceptive Drugs and Their Use Worldwide. *Best Pract. Res. Clin. Endocrinol. Metab.* **2013**, *27*, 3–12. [CrossRef] [PubMed]
25. Farca, A.; Popa, A.D.; Mardale, S.; Leucu, D.-C.; Mogo, C. Counselling, Knowledge and Attitudes towards Combined Oral Contraceptives: A Cross-sectional Survey among Romanian Women. *Farmacia* **2017**, *65*, 954–961.
26. Axelerad, A.D.; Zlotea, L.A.; Sirbu, C.A.; Stroe, A.Z.; Axelerad, S.D.; Cambrea, S.C.; Muja, L.F. Case Reports of Pregnancy-Related Cerebral Venous Thrombosis in the Neurology Department of the Emergency Clinical Hospital in Constanta. *Life* **2022**, *12*, 90. [CrossRef] [PubMed]
27. Zuurbier, S.M.; Hiltunen, S.; Lindgren, E.; Silvis, S.M.; Jood, K.; Devasagayam, S.; Kleinig, T.J.; Silver, F.L.; Mandell, D.M.; Putaala, J.; et al. Cerebral Venous Thrombosis in Older Patients. *Stroke* **2018**, *49*, 197–200. [CrossRef]
28. Dentali, F.; Poli, D.; Scoditti, U.; Di Minno, M.N.D.; De Stefano, V.; Stefano, V.D.; Siragusa, S.; Kostal, M.; Palareti, G.; Sartori, M.T.; et al. Long-Term Outcomes of Patients with Cerebral Vein Thrombosis: A Multicenter Study. *J. Thromb. Haemost.* **2012**, *10*, 1297–1302. [CrossRef] [PubMed]
29. Ferro, J.M.; Canhão, P.; Bousser, M.-G.; Stam, J.; Barinagarrementeria, F.; ISCVT Investigators. Cerebral Vein and Dural Sinus Thrombosis in Elderly Patients. *Stroke* **2005**, *36*, 1927–1932. [CrossRef]
30. Holcombe, A.; Mohr, N.; Farooqui, M.; Dandapat, S.; Dai, B.; Zevallos, C.B.; Quispe-Orozco, D.; Siddiqui, F.; Ortega-Gutierrez, S. Patterns of Care and Clinical Outcomes in Patients with Cerebral Sinus Venous Thrombosis. *J. Stroke Cerebrovasc. Dis.* **2020**, *29*, 105313. [CrossRef]
31. Birnbaum, J.A.; Labagnara, K.F.; Unda, S.R.; Altschul, D.J. Analyzing the Effect of Weekend and July Admission on Patient Outcomes Following Non-Pyogenic Intracranial Venous Thrombosis. *Interdiscip. Neurosurg.* **2020**, *22*, 100797. [CrossRef]
32. Bousser, M.-G. Cerebral Venous Thrombosis. *Stroke* **1999**, *30*, 481–483. [CrossRef]
33. Coutinho, J.; de Bruijn, S.F.; Deveber, G.; Stam, J. Anticoagulation for Cerebral Venous Sinus Thrombosis. *Cochrane Database Syst. Rev.* **2011**, CD002005. [CrossRef]
34. Ferro, J.M.; Crassard, I.; Coutinho, J.M.; Canhão, P.; Barinagarrementeria, F.; Cucchiara, B.; Derex, L.; Lichy, C.; Masjuan, J.; Massaro, A.; et al. Decompressive Surgery in Cerebrovenous Thrombosis: A Multicenter Registry and a Systematic Review of Individual Patient Data. *Stroke* **2011**, *42*, 2825–2831. [CrossRef] [PubMed]
35. Nasr, D.M.; Brinjikji, W.; Cloft, H.J.; Saposnik, G.; Rabinstein, A.A. Mortality in Cerebral Venous Thrombosis: Results from the National Inpatient Sample Database. *Cerebrovasc. Dis.* **2013**, *35*, 40–44. [CrossRef] [PubMed]
36. Tu, T.M.; Goh, C.; Tan, Y.K.; Leow, A.S.; Pang, Y.Z.; Chien, J.; Shafi, H.; Chan, B.P.; Hui, A.; Koh, J.; et al. Cerebral Venous Thrombosis in Patients with COVID-19 Infection: A Case Series and Systematic Review. *J. Stroke Cerebrovasc. Dis.* **2020**, *29*, 105379. [CrossRef]

37. Hameed, S.; Wasay, M.; Soomro, B.A.; Mansour, O.; Abd-Allah, F.; Tu, T.; Farhat, R.; Shahbaz, N.; Hashim, H.; Alamgir, W.; et al. Cerebral Venous Thrombosis Associated with COVID-19 Infection: An Observational, Multicenter Study. *Cerebrovasc. Dis. Extra* **2021**, *11*, 55–60. [CrossRef] [PubMed]
38. Al-Mufti, F.; Amuluru, K.; Sahni, R.; Bekelis, K.; Karimi, R.; Ogulnick, J.; Cooper, J.; Overby, P.; Nuoman, R.; Tiwari, A.; et al. Cerebral Venous Thrombosis in COVID-19: A New York Metropolitan Cohort Study. *AJNR Am. J. Neuroradiol.* **2021**, *42*, 1196–1200. [CrossRef]
39. Tu, T.M.; Yi, S.J.; Koh, J.S.; Saffari, S.E.; Hoe, R.H.M.; Chen, G.J.; Chiew, H.J.; Tham, C.H.; Seet, C.Y.H.; Yong, M.H.; et al. Incidence of Cerebral Venous Thrombosis Following SARS-CoV-2 Infection vs MRNA SARS-CoV-2 Vaccination in Singapore. *JAMA Netw. Open* **2022**, *5*, e222940. [CrossRef] [PubMed]
40. See, I.; Su, J.R.; Lale, A.; Woo, E.J.; Guh, A.Y.; Shimabukuro, T.T.; Streiff, M.B.; Rao, A.K.; Wheeler, A.P.; Beavers, S.F.; et al. US Case Reports of Cerebral Venous Sinus Thrombosis with Thrombocytopenia After Ad26.COV2.S Vaccination, 2 March to 21 April 2021. *JAMA* **2021**, *325*, 2448–2456. [CrossRef]
41. Pottegård, A.; Lund, L.C.; Karlstad, Ø.; Dahl, J.; Andersen, M.; Hallas, J.; Lidegaard, Ø.; Tapia, G.; Gulseth, H.L.; Ruiz, P.L.-D.; et al. Arterial Events, Venous Thromboembolism, Thrombocytopenia, and Bleeding after Vaccination with Oxford-AstraZeneca ChAdOx1-S in Denmark and Norway: Population Based Cohort Study. *BMJ* **2021**, *373*, n1114. [CrossRef]
42. Muir, K.-L.; Kallam, A.; Koepsell, S.A.; Gundabolu, K. Thrombotic Thrombocytopenia after Ad26.COV2.S Vaccination. *N. Engl. J. Med.* **2021**, *384*, 1964–1965. [CrossRef]
43. Greinacher, A.; Thiele, T.; Warkentin, T.E.; Weisser, K.; Kyrle, P.A.; Eichinger, S. Thrombotic Thrombocytopenia after ChAdOx1 NCov-19 Vaccination. *N. Engl. J. Med.* **2021**, *384*, 2092–2101. [CrossRef]

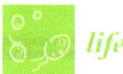

Review

Aphasic Syndromes in Cerebral Venous and Dural Sinuses Thrombosis—A Review of the Literature

Georgiana Munteanu [1,2,3], Andrei Gheorghe Marius Motoc [2,4], Traian Flavius Dan [1,2,3,*], Anca Elena Gogu [1,2,3] and Dragos Catalin Jianu [1,2,3]

1. First Division of Neurology, Department of Neurosciences, "Victor Babeș" University of Medicine and Pharmacy, 300041 Timișoara, Romania
2. Centre for Cognitive Research in Neuropsychiatric Pathology (NeuroPsy-Cog), "Victor Babeș" University of Medicine and Pharmacy, 300736 Timișoara, Romania
3. First Department of Neurology, "Pius Brînzeu" Emergency County Hospital, 300736 Timișoara, Romania
4. Department of Anatomy and Embryology, "Victor Babeș" University of Medicine and Pharmacy, 300041 Timișoara, Romania
* Correspondence: traian.dan@umft.ro; Tel.: +40-745035178

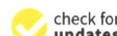

Citation: Munteanu, G.; Motoc, A.G.M.; Dan, T.F.; Gogu, A.E.; Jianu, D.C. Aphasic Syndromes in Cerebral Venous and Dural Sinuses Thrombosis—A Review of the Literature. *Life* 2022, *12*, 1684. https://doi.org/10.3390/life12111684

Academic Editor: Alexey V. Polonikov

Received: 2 October 2022
Accepted: 20 October 2022
Published: 24 October 2022

Publisher's Note: MDPI stays neutral with regard to jurisdictional claims in published maps and institutional affiliations.

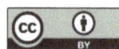

Copyright: © 2022 by the authors. Licensee MDPI, Basel, Switzerland. This article is an open access article distributed under the terms and conditions of the Creative Commons Attribution (CC BY) license (https://creativecommons.org/licenses/by/4.0/).

Abstract: Aphasia is an acquired central disorder of language that affects a person's ability to understand and/or produce spoken and written language, caused by lesions situated usually in the dominant (left) cerebral hemisphere. On one hand aphasia has a prevalence of 25–30% in acute ischemic stroke, especially in arterial infarcts. On the other hand, cerebral venous and dural sinuses thrombosis (CVT) remains a less common and underdiagnosed cause of ischemic stroke (0.5–1% of all strokes). Aphasia has been observed in almost 20% of patients who suffered CVT. The presence of aphasia is considered a negative predictive factor in patients with stroke, severe language disorders corresponding to arduous recovery. Taking into consideration data from the literature, aphasia is also considered a predictive factor for patients with CVT; its absences, together with the absence of worsening after admission, are determinants of complete recovery after CVT. This review has as the principal role of gathering current information from the literature (PubMed database 2012–2022) regarding the clinical features of aphasic syndromes and its incidence in patients with CVT. The main conclusion of this review was that aphasic syndromes are not usually the consequence of isolated thrombosis of dural sinuses or cerebral veins thrombosis. The most frequent form of CVT that determines aphasia is represented by the left transverse sinus thrombosis associated with a posterior left temporal lesion (due to left temporal cortical veins thrombosis), followed by the superior sagittal sinus thrombosis associated with a left frontal lesion (due to left frontal cortical veins thrombosis). Only a few cases are presenting isolated cortical veins thrombosis and left thalamus lesions due to deep cerebral vein thrombosis. We also concluded that the most important demographic factor was the gender of the patients, women being more affected than men, due to their postpartum condition.

Keywords: aphasia; cerebral venous thrombosis; intracranial dural sinus thrombosis; CVT

1. Introduction

On one hand, aphasia, which is an acquired central disorder of language, is one of the most common focal neurologic deficits observed in CVT, being noticed in 19–24% of cases [1,2]. On the other hand—CVT represents a less common and underdiagnosed cause of stroke (0.5–1% of all strokes) [3]. Unlike older studies that showed an incidence of 0.2–0.5/100,000 person/year [4], recent studies show a higher incidence (1.32–1.57/100,000 person/year) [5]. This might be the consequence of greater accessibility to imaging technologies as well as an increased interest and awareness in diagnosing CVT. Aphasia is usually the consequence of left lateral sinus (LS) and tributaries cortical veins thrombosis from the dominant hemisphere. In 2009, Damak et al. conducted a study with 195 patients with CVT. Among those patients, 157 (80.51%) suffered from lateral sinus thrombosis. The researchers evaluated the percentage of patients with lateral sinus thrombosis who had suffered aphasia and concluded that ~13% were presenting language disturbances, being the most common focal sign [6]. The presence of aphasia in stroke is well known as being a negative predictive factor in the evolution of patients: the more severe the language disorder, the more difficult the recovery of these patients. Furthermore, Ferro et al. concluded in one of theirs studies in 2002 that the determinants of complete recovery after CVT were: the absence of aphasia and the absence of worsening after admission [7].

CVT is a special category of cerebrovascular disease, encountered especially in children and younger adults rather than in arterial ischemic strokes (frequently in those with pro-thrombotic conditions, such as inherited thrombophilia), mostly women (oral contraceptives, pregnancy, postpartum or post-abortion). Early acquaintance of CVT's clinical features (including language disturbances) may improve the prognosis of this potentially fatal pathology.

1.1. Definition of Aphasia

The term of aphasia includes the inability of a person to understand and/or produce spoken language, sometimes also accompanied by the incapacity of reading (alexia) and writing (agraphia). It is always the consequence of an acquired central disorder, meaning that it occurs after the language has already been developed. Aphasia should be differentiated from a peripheral disorder of language (such as weakness or discoordination of phonatory musculature) that may easily simulate aphasia [8].

1.2. Language Localization

The organization of language networks has not been yet fully elucidated, despite the technological advances made in past years. Using complex techniques, especially functional neuroimaging, scientists have proven that language production is the result of neural activation from a vast network scattered in different structures of the brain: the cortex, the basal ganglia, the cerebellum and even the brainstem. This is the reason a disruption of this network determines spectrum of clinical signs. Functional neuroimaging studies suggested that the core of language operates in the left perisylvian regions in most individuals (95% right-handed and 75% left-handed), and there are two principal pathways in the language network: the dorsal fronto-parietal pathway (which is responsible for articulatory and syntactic tasks) and the ventral temporal pathway (which is responsible for decoding sounds to lexical representations and a word's significance) [8,9]:

Anterior areas (so called expressive/motor areas) are represented by:

a. Broca's area—the posterior part of the left third frontal gyrus (F3)—Brodmann areas 44 and 45;
b. Left insula's cortex and the underlying white matter;
c. Left Rolandic operculum—the lower part of the motor area (Fa);
d. Left premotor and prefrontal areas (forward and superior of Broca's area);
e. The supplementary motor area;

Posterior areas (so called comprehensive/sensorial areas) are represented by:

a. Wernicke's area: the posterior part of the first two temporal gyri-T1/T2 (Brodmann area 22);
b. The inferior parietal lobes: the angular gyrus (Brodmann area 39), and the supramarginal gyrus (Brodmann area 40);
c. The anterior part of the temporal lobe.

1.3. Types of Aphasic Syndromes

The most important determining factors of aphasias are the etiology, the site, and the magnitude of the causative lesion/lesions [10]. Age and sex of the patient are also determinant factors for the aphasia secondary to ischemic stroke: younger male patients are more predisposed to develop non-fluent aphasias rather than older patients and female patients.

Taking into consideration the clinical features of aphasia, there are seven types of aphasic syndromes [9–12]:

i. Broca's aphasia (10–15%);
ii. Wernicke's aphasia (15%);
iii. Conduction aphasia (15%);
iv. Transcortical aphasias:
  a. Transcortical motor aphasia (15–20%);
  b. Transcortical sensory aphasia;
  c. Mixed transcortical aphasia.
v. Global aphasias (24–38%);
vi. Anomic plus aphasias (20%);
vii. Atypical aphasias: mixed aphasias, thalamic aphasias, and capsulo-striatal aphasias (10%).

More than 10% of aphasic syndromes remain unclassifiable, particularly in patients with ischemic stroke history.

1.4. Etiology of Aphasia

Regarding the etiology of aphasic syndromes, there are various cerebral lesions (acute/chronic, progressive/intermittent/long-lasting, localized/diffuse) that can disturb language networks usually situated in right-handed individuals in the dominant hemisphere (rarely, in the non-dominant hemisphere in right-handed subjects—the so called "crossed aphasia") [8]. The most commonly involved pathologies that are producing aphasic syndromes are: the cerebro-vascular pathology—"vascular aphasias" (ischemic stroke, hemorrhagic stroke, cerebral veins and dural sinuses thrombosis), post-traumatic brain injuries, brain tumors (left frontal and temporal lobes), cerebral infections (especially viral encephalitis secondary to Herpes simplex virus), neurodegenerative diseases (Alzheimer disease, primary progressive aphasia), multiple sclerosis (rarely). There are also situations when different pathologies reproduce an acute stroke— "stroke mimics": migraine with aura, focal epilepsy, hypoglycemic coma, encephalopathies (hepatic, uremic, hypoxic, hyponatremic).

2. Materials and Methods

We achieved a literature search in the PubMed database [cerebral phlebothrombosis aphasia-Search Results-PubMed (nih.gov)], from 2012 to 2022 (in the present), using the following search terms: "aphasia" and "cerebral phlebothrombosis". Our main objective was to identify the incidence of aphasic syndrome, the main characteristics of those syndromes and correlation between clinical picture and localization of cerebral veins or dural sinuses thrombosis. After identifying the articles, we reviewed the abstracts of the papers and made a preliminary evaluation of their eligibility. After this stage, all potentially eligible papers were accessed and read. We included only those papers which met the eligibility criteria and were relevant to our review (Figure 1).

We applied the following eligibility/including criteria:

(1) Presence of language disturbances (aphasia, dysphasia) and description of aphasia 's type or characteristics;
(2) Case-report studies published between 2012–2022;
(3) Adult human studies;
(4) Articles written in English;
(5) The patients included in the study were diagnosed based on an imaging examination: computed tomography (CT), computed tomography venography (CTV), magnetic resonance imaging (MRI), magnetic resonance venography (MRV), intra-arterial angiography (Digital Substraction Angiography—DSA);
(6) Detailed, reliable medical history, physical examination, results of laboratory and imaging examinations were required.

The principal exclusion criteria were the absence of aphasia or lack of information regarding aphasia (N = 21), not being a case-report study (N = 15), absence of CVT and presence of other causes of stroke (N = 5).

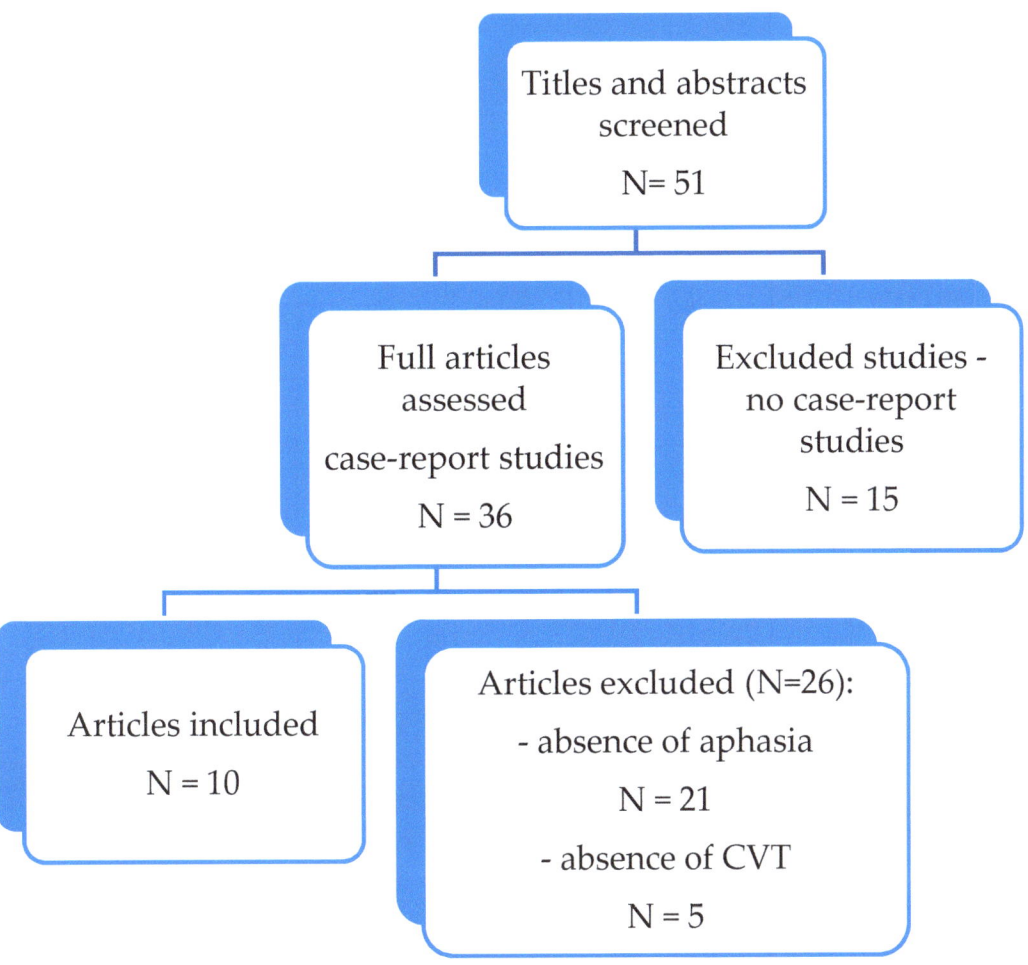

Figure 1. Flowchart of the articles search, N-number of studies.

3. Results

After carefully analyzing all these studies (Table 1), we noted these results.

The first is that the interest for characterizing the distinctive features of aphasic syndromes is extremely poor. The authors usually specify only the term of "dysphasia", "aphasia" or "language disturbances", without fitting into a certain aphasia type. This fact explains the difficult identification of eligible articles for our study and consecutively their small number.

The second result is that the most frequent site of CVT that determines aphasia is represented by the left transverse sinus thrombosis associated with a posterior left temporal lesion (due to left temporal cortical veins thrombosis), with a percentage of 90% ($n = 9/10$), followed by the superior sagittal sinus thrombosis associated with a left frontal lesion (due to left frontal cortical veins thrombosis), with a percentage of 40% ($n = 4/10$). Only 20% of cases were presenting isolated cortical veins thrombosis ($n = 2/10$) and 10% ($n = 1/10$)

left thalamus lesions due to deep cerebral vein thrombosis. Our results are comparable to recent data from the literature. According to International Study on Cerebral Vein and Dural Sinus Thrombosis, aphasia is commonly the consequence of left transverse sinus thrombosis, followed by the superior sagittal sinus thrombosis [3,13,14].

Table 1. Distribution on age, gender, associated pathologies, site of thrombosis and types of aphasia in CVT patients-case-report studies 2012–2022 Pub-Med data [15–24].

Study	First Author and Year of Publication	Age	Gender	Associated Pathologies	Site of CVT	Type of Aphasia
Reversible anomia and cerebral venous thrombosis: A case report and review of the literature	Biniyam A. Ayele et al. (2022) [15]	30	F	two months after dead fetus birth	left transverse, sigmoid sinus (lateral sinus), corresponding cortical veins.	non-fluent aphasia, anomic aphasia
Diagnosis and Management of Mixed Transcortical Aphasia Due to Multiple Predisposing Factors, including Postpartum and Severe Inherited Thrombophilia, Affecting Multiple Cerebral Venous and Dural Sinus Thrombosis: Case Report and Literature Review	Dragos, Catalin Jianu et al. (2021) [16]	38	F	inherited thrombophilia 18 days postpartum	superior sagittal sinus, the straight sinus, the vein of Galen, the deep venous system on the left, the lateral sinus left internal jugular vein	mixed transcortical aphasia (isolation aphasia)
Bilateral thalamic lesion presenting as Broca's type subcortical aphasia in cerebral venous thrombosis: Index case report	Shambaditya Das et al. (2021) [17]	35	M	multiple substances abuse (alcohol, tobacco, and cannabis), thrombophilia—decreased levels of protein C, protein S and antithrombin III	superior sagittal sinus bilateral transverse sinus (lateral sinus)	non-fluent aphasia–Broca's aphasia
Cerebral Venous Thrombosis and Its Clinical Diversity	Giovana Ennis et al. (2021) [18]	75	F	immune thrombocytopenic purpura, arterial hypertension, and pulmonary embolism	superior sagittal sinus the left lateral sinus	global aphasia
Cerebral venous sinus thrombosis associated with spontaneous heparin-induced thrombocytopenia syndrome after total knee arthroplasty	Steven R Hwang et al. (2020) [19]	56	F	hypertension degenerative osteoarthritis	left transverse and sigmoid sinuses (lateral sinus) left internal jugular vein	unspecified type
The ugly duckling of aphasia: cerebral venous sinus thrombosis as a mimic of TIA and stroke	Alexander Engelmann et al. (2020) [20]	86	M	colon adenocarcinoma (status post resection); recent surgery for right sphenoid wing meningioma	left transverse (lateral) sinus	fluent aphasia
Bilateral corpus callosum and corona radiata infarction due to cerebral venous sinus thrombosis presenting as headache and acute reversible aphasia: A rare case report	Rui Lan et al. (2020) [21]	30	F	20 days post-partum	superior sagittal sinus the left transverse (lateral) sinus	non-fluent aphasia–Broca's aphasia
Ipsilateral Dural Thickening and Enhancement: A Sign of Isolated Cortical Vein Thrombosis? A Case Report and Review of the Literature	Davide Marco Croci et al. (2016) [22]	30	F	14 days postpartum	left cortical veins thrombosis	global aphasia
Anomia and mild headache: A subtle presentation of cerebral venous thrombosis	WS Kuan (2014) [23]	52	F	thrombophilia: low levels of protein C activity of 64% expected range 70–130%), protein S activity of 50% (expected range 55–140%) and anti-thrombin III level of 62% (expected range 80–120)	left transverse and sigmoid (lateral) sinuses, the left internal jugular vein	non-fluent aphasia, anomic aphasia
Broca's aphasia due to cerebral venous sinus thrombosis following chemotherapy for small cell lung cancer: A case report and review of literature	Tolga Tuncel et al. (2014) [24]	27	M	advanced-stage small cell lung cancer cisplatin-based chemotherapy	left transverse (lateral) sinus thrombosis	non-fluent aphasia, anomic aphasia

The third result is that the most frequent type of aphasias found in patients with CVT are: the non-fluent type (Broca's aphasia and anomic aphasia) with a percentage of 50% ($n = 5/10$) and the global/mixed aphasia (percentage of 30%). Only one case of fluent aphasia (10%, $n = 1/10$) was described in the case-report studies included in our research.

The fourth result is that young female patients (especially in the first 8 weeks postpartum, with/without thrombophilia), oncological cases and severe medical conditions (immune pathologies, toxic substances abuse) are having a higher risk in developing CVT. From our statistical data, the mean age of female patients was 44.42 years (min = 30 years, max = 75 years), meanwhile the mean age of male patients was 48.87 years (min = 27 years, max = 86 years). Regarding the sex incidence, female patients are leaders in CVT (70%, $n = 7/10$), due to their post-partum and post abortion condition.

4. Discussion

CVT is a special type of cerebro-vascular pathology. The clinical signs are frequently the consequence of increased intracranial pressure and/or focal brain injury determined by venous infarction or hemorrhage. Venous territories are served by an extensive and widespread network. This is the reason venous territories are less demarcated compared to the arterial territories. CVT can also alter the absorption of the cerebro-spinal fluid (CSF) thru the arachnoid villi. As a result, intracranial pressure increases (with or without cerebral damage), usually in association with superior sagittal sinus (SSS) thrombosis. All these pathophysiological altered mechanisms lead to typical focal neurologic signs and symptoms, depending on the territory of the brain in which the venous drainage is altered, the rapidity of the thrombosis process (immediately or gradually), and the magnitude of brain damage. Superior sagittal sinus (62–80%) and lateral sinus (38–86%) are the most frequently involved sites for thrombosis [3].

Regarding the focal neurologic deficits, specific clinical symptomatology and neurological signs can suggest which area of the brain is damaged. However, the topographic clinical diagnosis of CVT is not as well-defined as in arterial occlusion, frequently being misleading. This characteristic is the consequence of concomitant multiple cerebral veins and dural sinuses thrombosis (more than two-thirds of cases), the numerous anatomic variants of some dural sinuses and some cerebral veins, and the existence of venous collateral circulation [16,25].

When aphasic syndromes are the consequence of dural sinus/sinuses thrombosis or cerebral veins thrombosis, establishing the exact site of lesions might be a challenge. However, the clinical aspects of aphasic syndromes may vary depending on the concomitant occlusion of other dural sinuses or cerebral veins.

1. **Superior Sagittal Sinus (SSS) Thrombosis**

   In SSS thrombosis, aphasia is the result of left fronto-parietal hemispheric lesions, secondary to progression of thrombosis to the tributaries bilateral cortical veins [3,16,25,26]. The specific types of aphasias are represented by nonfluent Broca's aphasia (secondary to left frontal cortical veins thrombosis) and mixed aphasias. Analyzing our results, isolated SSS thrombosis was not found in any of these case-studies. This result strengthens the hypothesis that aphasia is not the result of isolated SSS thrombosis but the consequence of extension of thrombosis to tributaries fronto-parietal cortical veins.

2. **Lateral Sinus (LS) Thrombosis**

   Lateral sinus contains two parts: the transverse sinus and the sigmoid sinus, respectively. Regarding the left transverse sinus thrombosis, it is well known that the association of adjacent temporal veins occlusion is the one that produces fluent Wernicke aphasia (40%) [16,25].

   Another specific characteristic of this dural sinuses is that the left LS is often hypoplasic; due to this characteristic, after right LS thrombosis, a pseudotumor syndrome is installed, causing bilateral venous drainage deficiency, affecting contralateral structures, especially the inferior part of temporal lobe and cerebellum [25].

   In many cases, thrombosis of lateral sinus spreads to other sinuses (especially to SSS) and veins [3,13,26,27]. Analyzing our data, only two case-report studies described aphasic syndromes (one case of non-fluent aphasia and the other one of fluent aphasia) in patients with isolated left LS–transverse part–thrombosis. The other cases of LS thrombosis were accompanied by other sinuses or cerebral veins thrombosis ($n = 7/10$).

3. **Isolated Cortical Veins Thrombosis**

Without association with dural sinus thrombosis, isolated thrombosis of cortical veins is considered a rare affection (2%) [16,25]. A plausible explanation would be that it is frequently underdiagnosed, due to imaging barriers, being identified with difficulty using the traditional MRI sequences and MRV [16,25]. The most common localization of occlusion is at the levels of the superior cortical veins, producing nonfluent Broca's aphasia or mixed aphasias [25]. From our collected data, there is only one case of isolated left cortical veins thrombosis.

4. **Deep Cerebral Veins Thrombosis**

Deep venous system thrombosis can be suspected in patients with altered state of consciousness (diffuse encephalopathy or even coma) and motor deficits (bilateral or fluctuating alternating paresis) [3,26]. Deep cerebral veins thrombosis (vein of Galen, basal veins of Rosenthal, internal cerebral veins, straight sinus) produces damages into the caudate nucleus and thalami, being present in almost 18% of patients diagnosed with CVT [16]. In rare situations, benign cases of thrombosis of the deep cerebral veins were noted producing left thalamic lesions with mixed transcortical aphasia [16].

Over the last few years, several case reports have brought to attention the small incidence of aphasia in the clinical picture of CVT. Unfortunately, few of those studies made a precise evaluation of the aphasic syndrome and a clinical-imagistic correlation.

Alexander Engelmann and his collaborators [20] published in 2021 an interesting case-report of an 86-year-old right-handed male with a complex oncological and neurosurgical pathology (history of colon adenocarcinoma, surgically treated, and recent surgery for right sphenoid wing meningioma), which presented in their emergency department with several transient episodes of fluent aphasia, during at most 10 min, being accompanied by one episode of involuntary right-handed grip, being initially considered as a TIA, taking into consideration that the symptomatology completely remitted. Although the Non-contrast head CT, CT Angiography head and neck, and perfusion CT did not highlight any sign of arterial occlusion or perfusion defects, they revealed the absence of opacification of the left transverse and sigmoid sinuses. They continued the investigations, and after performing the brain MRI with gadolinium, they found a new left transverse sinus thrombus. After 13 days of anticoagulation (LMWH) the patient did not experience any of the previous symptoms.

Giovana Ennis and her team [18] brought to attention another interesting and also a complex case of a 76-year-old woman (history of immune thrombocytopenic purpura, treated at that time with prednisolone, arterial hypertension, atrial fibrillation, hypothyroidism and pulmonary embolism), which presented in the emergency department complaining of amnesia and lethargy that had started a week earlier and were becoming more frequent, multiple episodes of transient right hemiparesis in the last two days, with a duration of 1–2 h. At the admission, the neurological examination revealed a 2/5 MRC right sided hemiparesis and global aphasia. The patient underwent cerebral computed tomography (CT) that excluded ischemic or hemorrhagic vascular event or any space-occupying process. After these examinations, the patient was re-examined, and, surprisingly, aphasia had disappeared, but a slight (4/5) right hemiparesis remained. Five hours later, her clinical status deteriorated, again presenting global aphasia and 3/5 MRC right hemiparesis. They decided to perform a CT angiography, which did not bring any pathological signs, excluding intracranial arterial occlusion or stenosis. On the first day after the admission in the Stroke Unit, the patient suffered three tonic-clonic seizures, with involuntary movements in the right limbs. Twelve hours later, a new cerebral CT was performed and revealed a vascular lesion situated in the left Rolandic cortico-subcortical region, with a hemorrhagic component and reduced amplitude of the regional sulci. Taking into consideration the high density of the medial third of the superior longitudinal sinus (SSS), cerebral veno-CT was immediately performed, which confirmed the lack of opacification of the superior longitudinal sinus and the right lateral sinus. The presence of the left fronto-parietal intraparenchymatous lesion was evocative for a venous infarct. She was also treated with LMWH, adjusted to the hematological pathology.

Another recent study conducted by Ayele et al. [15], reported the case of a 30-year-old right-handed Ethiopian female patient, who gave birth to a stillborn fetus 2 months previously, which presented with resistant to usual medications headache, accompanied by word-finding difficulty, nausea, and blurred vision, with a 2-week onset. At the neurological examination there were no focal deficits or cranial nerves signs. The language assessment showed normal fluency, compression, repetition, and reading. At the naming probe (assessed using a word generating test of 60 s), she has been found with difficulties, indicating anomia. The examination of fundus showed bilaterally papilledema. Brain MRI showed left temporo-parietal ischemia. MR venography showed thrombosis of the left transverse, sigmoid sinus, and corresponding cortical veins. During their research, they found only two similar cases, described by Kuan et al. (2014) [23], which symptoms were the consequence of left transverse sinus, sigmoid sinus and internal jugular vein thrombosis, with parenchymal hemorrhages in the left temporo-parietal region with effacement of the left cerebral sulci, and Sarma et al. (2004) [15], which symptoms were the consequence of superior, inferior, straight sinuses and also vein of Galen thrombosis.

In 2014, Tuncel and his collaborators [24] reported the case of a young patient (a 27-year-old male), diagnosed with advanced-stage small cell lung cancer two months previously, which presented to the Department of Medical Oncology, with Broca's aphasia and general seizures. The MRI of the brain did not show any pathological features. After initiating the chemotherapy, on day six of the second cycle, the patient presented in the emergency department 4 h succeeding the onset of a stroke. Using the MRI scan, they revealed a left transverse sinus, as well as a left sigmoid sinus thrombosis, accompanied by acute left parietal venous infarction.

In 2021, Jianu et al. [16], handled a case, that was both difficult and interesting, of a 38-year-old woman with pre-existing hypertension, on her 18th postpartum day, which was presented in the emergency department accusing sudden onset of severe headache for 2 days, accompanied by moderate right hemiparesis (4/5 MRC) and language disturbances (she was unable to speak or to understand orders properly, although the repetition of words and sentences was possible–mixed transcortical aphasia). All of these symptoms can be explained by the localization of the left cerebral deep venous infarcts (affecting the caudate, putamen, left thalamus, and periventricular white matter-internal capsule) that she presented [16].

Searching into the specialized literature, we observed a small number of observational studies which followed the clinical features of aphasic patience with CVT. The VENOST study [28] is the latest and the largest retrospective, prospective, multicenter, hospital-based, observational study that followed the records of 1144 patients with CVT, collected between 2000 and 2013 from patients' medical files. Between 2013 and 2015 the patients were included prospectively. Statistical data showed that the percentage of aphasia or dysarthria among all those patients who suffered from CVT was only 1.2% [28].

Analyzing all this data, we can easily observe that it is hard to make a statistically significant hypothesis regarding the incidence of different types of aphasic syndromes in CVT, taking into consideration that the diagnosis of a certain type of aphasia requires specific assessments, using approved tests, while the patient is cooperating (patients frequently have reduced arousal). However, some conclusions are clear from this study:

- aphasia is commonly the consequence of concomitant left transverse sinus thrombosis with left cortical temporal veins, followed by the superior sagittal sinus thrombosis with extension into tributary fronto-parietal cortical veins;
- depending on the site and the size of the brain damage (cerebral vasogenic/cytotoxic edema, venous infarction, intracranial hypertension), the most frequent types of aphasias are: non-fluent aphasias-Broca's aphasia and anomic plus aphasia (if the lesions are situated in the anterior language areas), fluent aphasias-Wernicke's aphasia, transcortical sensory aphasia (if the lesions are situated in the posterior language areas), mixed or global aphasias (in the cases of larger lesions);

- in LS sinus thrombosis (the transversal portion) associated with left cortical temporal veins thrombosis, the most common type of aphasia is Wernicke's aphasia (40%) [16];
- in many cases, the LS thrombosis spreads to the SSS, symptoms and signs of SSS thrombosis depending on the involvement of cerebral veins and other dural sinuses. The most often involved are the superior cerebral veins (Rolandic, parieto-occipital and posterior temporal) which empty into the SSS. If the thrombosis spreads to the deep veins system, altering the Ascending Reticular Activating System (ARAS), awakening alteration may occur;
- the clinical picture depends on the location and the dimensions of cerebral lesion: extensive lesions can determine global aphasia, or mixed transcortical aphasias; meanwhile smaller lesions might determine Wernicke's aphasia, transcortical sensory aphasia, Broca aphasia or anomic aphasia.

Our small study managed to highlight the small amount of information that has been gathered until now regarding the characteristics of aphasic syndromes in CVT, and this might be considered a great limitation. Unfortunately, the small number of cases described in the literature made difficult our intention to demonstrate a certain pattern of language disturbances, using the localization of the CVT. Mostly, the greatest impediment was the fact that few authors focused their attention on the clinical characteristics of aphasic syndromes, analyzing and describing the clinical aspects of language disturbances in an incomplete manner. However, this might be the beginning of a new research theme in this rare and underdiagnosed condition. We aim to continue our study and to gather further information over the next years to support us in outlining a clinical template that will guide clinicians in establishing the diagnosis of CVT much faster, more easily, and more accurately.

5. Conclusions

In conclusion, the early identification of aphasia in CVT can help us to provide a better prognosis of patients and the site of the lesion and guide us in the differential diagnosis of this cerebro-vascular pathology. Although aphasia is a rare syndrome in a rare disease (CVT), we should look toward new clinical data regarding this issue, insisting over the examination of the patients' language and trying to determine whether, the presence of aphasia might be a severity marker as it is considered in stroke. We should carefully look after patients with associated conditions that have fully demonstrated their potentially prothrombotic characteristic, especially in young women (postpartum/post abortion) and patients with inherited thrombophilia.

What is worth underlying is that aphasic syndromes are not the consequence of thrombosis of a specific, isolated dural sinus, but the result of thrombosis extension to cortical veins or other dural sinuses (especially the left LS and the SSS). Venous infarction in strategic language areas is also the main determining cause of aphasic syndromes.

Author Contributions: Conceptualization, G.M. and D.C.J.; methodology, G.M. and D.C.J.; software, G.M. and T.F.D.; validation, G.M., A.G.M.M., T.F.D., A.E.G. and D.C.J.; formal analysis, G.M. and D.C.J.; investigation, G.M., A.G.M.M., T.F.D., A.E.G. and D.C.J.; resources, G.M. and D.C.J.; data curation, G.M. and D.C.J.; writing—original draft preparation, G.M. and D.C.J.; writing—review and editing, G.M. and D.C.J.; visualization, G.M., A.G.M.M., T.F.D., A.E.G. and D.C.J.; supervision, G.M. and D.C.J.; project administration, G.M. and D.C.J. All authors have read and agreed to the published version of the manuscript.

Funding: This research received no external funding.

Institutional Review Board Statement: Not applicable.

Informed Consent Statement: Not applicable.

Data Availability Statement: Not applicable.

Conflicts of Interest: The authors declare no conflict of interest.

References

1. Ferro, J.M.; Canhaão, P.; Stam, J.; Bousser, M.-G.; Barinagarrementeria, F. Prognosis of cerebral vein and dural sinus thrombosis: Results of the International Study on Cerebral Vein and Dural Sinus Thrombosis (ISCVT). *Stroke* **2004**, *35*, 664–670. [CrossRef]
2. Sparaco, M.; Feleppa, M.; Bigal, M.E. Cerebral Venous Thrombosis and Headache-A Case-Series. *Headache* **2015**, *55*, 806–814. [CrossRef] [PubMed]
3. Jianu, D.C.; Jianu, S.N.; Munteanu, G.; Dan, F.T.; Bârsan, C. Cerebral Vein and Dural Sinus Thrombosis. In *Ischemic Stroke of Brain*; Intech Open: London, UK, 2018; Chapter 3. [CrossRef]
4. Bousser, M.-G.; Ferro, J.M. Cerebral venous thrombosis: An update. *Lancet Neurol.* **2007**, *6*, 162–170. [CrossRef]
5. Devasagayam, S.; Wyatt, B.; Leyden, J.; Kleinig, T. Cerebral Venous Sinus Thrombosis Incidence Is Higher Than Previously Thought: A retrospective population-based study. *Stroke* **2016**, *47*, 2180–2182. [CrossRef] [PubMed]
6. Damak, M.; Crassard, I.; Wolff, V.; Bousser, M.-G. Isolated Lateral Sinus Thrombosis: A series of 62 patients. *Stroke* **2009**, *40*, 476–481. [CrossRef]
7. Ferro, J.; Lopes, M.G.; Rosas, M.; Ferro, M.; Fontes, J. Long-Term Prognosis of Cerebral Vein and Dural Sinus Thrombosis: Results of the VENOPORT study. *Cerebrovasc. Dis.* **2002**, *13*, 272–278. [CrossRef]
8. Jianu, D.C.; Jianu, S.N.; Petrica, L.; Dan, T.F.; Munteanu, G. Vascular Aphasias. In *Ischemic Stroke*; Sanchetee, P., Ed.; Intech Open: London, UK, 2021; Chapter 3; pp. 37–59.
9. Abou Zeki, D.; Hillis, A. Acquired Disorders of Language and Speech. In *Oxford Textbook of Cognitive Neurology and Dementia*; Masud, H., Schott, J.M., Eds.; Oxford University Press: Oxford, UK, 2016; Chapter 12; pp. 123–133.
10. Croquelois, A.; Godefroy, O. Vascular Aphasias. In *The Behavioral and Cognitive Neurology of Stroke*, 2nd ed.; Godefroy, O., Ed.; Cambridge University Press: Cambridge, UK, 2013; Chapter 7; pp. 65–75/.
11. Goodglass, H.; Kaplan, E. (Eds.) *The Assessment of Aphasia and Related Disorder*, 2nd ed.; Lea and Febiger: Philadelphia, PA, USA, 1983.
12. Swanberg, M.M.; Nasreddine, Z.S.; Mendez, M.F.; Cummings, J.L. Speech and Language. In *Goetz, Textbook of Clinical Neurology*, 3rd ed.; Christopher, G., Ed.; W.B. Saunders: Philadelphia, PA, USA, 2007; pp. 79–98. Available online: https://www.sciencedirect.com/science/article/pii/B9781416036180100062 (accessed on 1 April 2022)ISBN 9781416036180. [CrossRef]
13. Ferro, J.M.; Canhão, P. Cerebral Venous Thrombosis. In *Stroke (Pathophysiology, Diagnosis, and Management)*, 6th ed.; Grotta, J.C., Albers, G.W., Broderick, J.P., Kasner, S.E., Lo, E.H., Mendelow, A.D., Sacco, R.L., Wong, L.K.S., Eds.; Elsevier: Beijing, China, 2016; Chapter 45; pp. 716–730.
14. Einhäupl, K.; Bousser, M.G.; de Bruijn, S.F.; Ferro, M.; Martinelli, I.; Masuhr, F.; Stam, J. FEFNS guideline on the treatment of cerebral venous sinus thrombosis. *Eur. J. Neurol.* **2006**, *13*, 553–559. [CrossRef] [PubMed]
15. Ayele, B.A.; Abdella, R.I.; Wachamo, L.Z. Reversible anomia and cerebral venous thrombosis: A case report and review of the literature. *J. Med. Case Rep.* **2022**, *16*, 56. [CrossRef] [PubMed]
16. Jianu, D.; Jianu, S.; Dan, T.; Iacob, N.; Munteanu, G.; Motoc, A.; Băloi, A.; Hodorogea, D.; Axelerad, A.; Pleș, H.; et al. Diagnosis and Management of Mixed Transcortical Aphasia Due to Multiple Predisposing Factors, including Postpartum and Severe Inherited Thrombophilia, Affecting Multiple Cerebral Venous and Dural Sinus Thrombosis: Case Report and Literature Review. *Diagnostics* **2021**, *11*, 1425. [CrossRef]
17. Das, S.; Dubey, S.; Pandit, A.; Ray, B.K. Bilateral thalamic lesion presenting as Broca's type subcortical aphasia in cerebral venous thrombosis: Index case report. *BMJ Case Rep.* **2021**, *14*, e240196. [CrossRef] [PubMed]
18. Ennis, G.; Domingues, N.; Marques, J.S.; Ribeiro, P.; Andrade, C. Cerebral Venous Thrombosis and Its Clinical Diversity. *Cureus* **2021**, *13*, e14750. [CrossRef]
19. Hwang, S.R.; Wang, Y.; Weil, E.L.; Padmanabhan, A.; Warkentin, T.E.; Pruthi, R.K. Cerebral venous sinus thrombosis associated with spontaneous heparin-induced thrombocytopenia syndrome after total knee arthroplasty. *Platelets* **2021**, *32*, 936–940. [CrossRef] [PubMed]
20. Engelmann, A.; DiPastina, K.; Liu, T. The ugly duckling of aphasia: Cerebral venous sinus thrombosis as a mimic of TIA and stroke. *J. Community Hosp. Intern. Med. Perspect.* **2021**, *11*, 156–157. [CrossRef] [PubMed]
21. Lan, R.; Ma, Y.Z.; Shen, X.M.; Wu, J.T.; Gu, C.Q.; Zhang, Y. Bilateral corpus callosum and corona radiata infarction due to cerebral venous sinus thrombosis presenting as headache and acute reversible aphasia: A rare case report. *BMC Neurol.* **2020**, *20*, 249. [CrossRef] [PubMed]
22. Croci, D.M.; Michael, D.; Kahles, T.; Fathi, A.R.; Fandino, J.; Marbacher, S. Ipsilateral Dural Thickening and Enhancement: A Sign of Isolated Cortical Vein Thrombosis? A Case Report and Review of the Literature. *World Neurosurg.* **2016**, *90*, 706.e11–706.e14. [CrossRef] [PubMed]
23. Kuan, W.S. Anomia and Mild Headache: A Subtle Presentation of Cerebral Venous Thrombosis. *Hong Kong J. Emerg. Med.* **2014**, *21*, 172–175. [CrossRef]
24. Tuncel, T.; Ozgun, A.; Emirzeoğlu, L.; Celiïk, S.; Demiïr, S.; Bilgi, O.; Karagoz, B. Broca's aphasia due to cerebral venous sinus thrombosis following chemotherapy for small cell lung cancer: A case report and review of literature. *Oncol. Lett.* **2014**, *9*, 937–939. [CrossRef]
25. Jianu, D.C.; Jianu, S.N.; Dan, T.F.; Munteanu, G.; Copil, A.; Birdac, C.D.; Motoc, A.G.M.; Axelerad, A.D.; Petrica, L.; Arnautu, S.F.; et al. An Integrated Approach on the Diagnosis of Cerebral Veins and Dural Sinuses Thrombosis (a Narrative Review). *Life* **2022**, *12*, 717. [CrossRef]

26. Ulivi, L.; Squitieri, M.; Cohen, H.; Cowley, P.; Werring, D.J. Cerebral venous thrombosis: A practical guide. *Pract. Neurol.* **2020**, *20*, 356–367. [CrossRef]
27. Bousser, M.G.; Barnett, H.J.M. Cerebral Venous Thrombosis. In *Stroke (Pathophysiology, Diagnosis, and Management)*, 4th ed.; Mohr, J.P., Choi, D.W., Grotta, J.C., Weir, B., Wolf, P.A., Eds.; Churchill Livingstone: Philadelphia, PA, USA, 2004; Chapter 12; pp. 301–325.
28. Duman, T.; Uluduz, D.; Midi, I.; Bektas, H.; Kablan, Y.; Goksel, B.K.; Milanlioglu, A.; Orken, D.N.; Aluclu, U.; Colakoglu, S.; et al. A Multicenter Study of 1144 Patients with Cerebral Venous Thrombosis: The VENOST Study. *J. Stroke Cerebrovasc. Dis.* **2017**, *26*, 1848–1857. [CrossRef] [PubMed]

Review

Cerebral Venous Outflow Implications in Idiopathic Intracranial Hypertension—From Physiopathology to Treatment

Sorin Tuță [1,2]

1. Department of Neurology, "Carol Davila" University of Medicine and Pharmacy, 050471 Bucharest, Romania; sorin.tuta@umfcd.ro
2. Department of Neurology, National Institute of Neurology and Neurovascular Diseases, 041914 Bucharest, Romania

Abstract: In this review, we provide an update on the pathogenesis, diagnosis, and management of adults with idiopathic intracranial hypertension (IIH) and implications of the cerebral venous system, highlighting the progress made during the past decade with regard to mechanisms of the venous outflow pathway and its connection with the cerebral glymphatic and lymphatic network in genesis of IIH. Early diagnosis and treatment are crucial for favorable visual outcomes and to avoid vision loss, but there is also a risk of overdiagnosis and misdiagnosis in many patients with IIH. We also present details about treatment of intracranial hypertension, which is possible in most cases with a combination of weight loss and drug treatments, but also in selected cases with surgical interventions such as optic nerve sheath fenestration, cerebral spinal fluid (CSF) diversion, or dural venous sinus stenting for some patients with cerebral venous sinus stenosis, after careful analysis of mechanisms of intracranial hypertension, patient clinical profile, and method risks.

Keywords: idiopathic intracranial hypertension; pseudotumor cerebri; cerebral venous sinus stenosis; magnetic resonance venography; cerebral venous sinus stenting; optical nerve sheath fenestration

1. Introduction

Idiopathic intracranial hypertension (IIH) is considered a relatively rare disorder characterized by elevated intracranial pressure (ICP) without a clear cause, remaining a diagnosis of exclusion, after other known situations associated with raised ICP have been evaluated. Several approaches have proposed different names of this entity according to the knowledge and understanding at that point in time. In 1904, 'pseudotumor cerebri' was proposed by Nonne, and in 1937 Walter Dandy [1] described it under the name 'intracranial pressure without brain tumor'; later, in the 1950s, it was named benign intracranial hypertension. Unfortunately, if left untreated, the disorder can lead to prolonged headache, pulsatile tinnitus, reactive depression with reduced quality of life, but also substantial visual morbidity, including complete blindness. All these reasons changed the opinion on benign intracranial hypertension, and the actual term of IIH is the most used. Pseudotumor cerebri is still used for the secondary forms of intracranial hypertension, after cerebral magnetic resonance imaging (MRI) excludes an intracranial mass lesion. Exclusion of a secondary cause of intracranial hypertension is part of the IIH diagnosis workflow, and from this point of view the cerebral venous and sinus thrombosis is a much better known and accepted cause of intracranial hypertension: 10% of patients with cerebral venous thrombosis developed chronic intracranial hypertension during follow-up in one study [2] and dural sinus thrombosis was identified in 26% of patients with initial IIH, but in the last two decades, more evidence has emerged toward a similar role of dural venous sinus stenosis without thrombosis [3].

Although early diagnosis and treatment are crucial for favorable visual outcomes in IIH patients, there is also a risk of overdiagnosis and misdiagnosis in as many as 40% of patients initially diagnosed with IIH [4]. Patients with a secondary cause of intracranial hypertension (with the exception of those with a cerebral mass lesion) belong to the category of pseudotumor cerebri, but on the other hand, in 355 patients analyzed with CT angiography in a recent study [5], the prevalence of unilateral transverse sinus stenosis or hypoplasia in the general population was up to 33%, 5% for bilateral transverse sinus stenosis, and 1% for unilateral stenosis with contralateral hypoplasia. Therefore, a diagnosis of cerebral sinus stenosis is important, but to prove there is a causal link with intracranial hypertension is sometimes challenging and requires measurement of the pressure gradient at the level of the stenosis with all other plausible causes to be excluded. This is the reason why in the present review the venous sinus stenosis is often discussed in relation to idiopathic intracranial hypertension and not considered a priori to belong to the pseudotumor cerebri category.

The process of collection and selection of published papers for this review started with a search of the PubMed and Cochrane Libraries for all peer-reviewed articles from 2002 to date with a combination of key words, including "idiopathic intracranial hypertension," "pseudotumor cerebri", and "benign intracranial hypertension", and after that a second search was started for more narrow and detailed information about "cerebral glymphatic ", "cerebral lymphatic", "cerebral venous sinus stenosis", "cerebral venous sinus stenosis stenting", "lumboperitoneal shunts and intracranial hypertension", and "optical nerve sheath fenestration". Other references from the articles that were identified in the initial search and important data for clinical studies of IIH treatment were also selected and reviewed for extraction of additional information or points of view.

In this synthetic review of the literature, we provide the latest information and points of view with respect to the pathogenesis, diagnosis, and management of adult idiopathic intracranial hypertension, and we highlight the progress made during the past decade regarding the mechanisms of venous outflow pathway obstruction, emphasizing the role of cerebral venous sinus stenosis, but also of its connection with the cerebral glymphatic and lymphatic network in genesis of IIH. We present details about treatment of intracranial hypertension related to venous sinus stenosis and IIH, which is possible in most cases using a combination of weight loss and drug treatments, but also surgical interventions such as optic nerve sheath fenestration, cerebral spinal fluid (CSF) diversion, and dural venous sinus stenting in selected cases of cerebral sinus stenosis, after careful analysis of mechanisms of intracranial hypertension, patient clinical profile, and risks.

2. Physiopathology of Idiopathic Intracranial Hypertension—A Connection between CSF, Cerebral Glymphatic, Lymphatic, and Venous Drainage

Starting with the historical hypothesis of Monro and Kelly, later completed by Magendie and Burrows, the skull was described as a rigid structure containing incompressible brain, and it was stated that the sum of the volume of brain, blood, and cerebrospinal fluid (CSF) is constant: an increase in one causes a decrease in one or both of the remaining two, but once the period of compliance due to the displacement of CSF or blood runs out, there is an exponential curve of a rise in intracranial pressure. An increased volume of the brain parenchyma is classically associated with cerebral edema (such as in large ischemic strokes, encephalitis, traumatic brain injury, and malignant tumors), or intraparenchymal expanding lesions such as hematomas or tumors, but this is not the main objective of this review [6,7].

The epithelial cells of the choroid plexus are the main source of CSF secretion, with a rate of 0.3–0.4 mL/min, while a secondary source is the interstitial fluid of the brain resulting from filtration through the blood–brain barrier, which is estimated to be of a much lower importance, but the overall volume of CSF is about 150–160 mL [6]. The difference in hydrostatic pressure between choroid plexus capillaries, epithelial cells, and ventricles also depends on blood pressure and represents an important factor for the net filtration process resulting in CSF production [7].

Both osmotic and hydrostatic pressure gradients contribute to CSF formation. As alterations to osmolarity modify water flux across the choroid plexus, the transport of ions across the blood–CSF barrier is important in the secretion process. In this process, ions are transported from circulating blood into the CSF via their respective transporters in the choroid cells' walls, while water is likely transported by a combination of a transcellular process against an osmotic gradient by cotransporters and via tight junctions [6].

Although osmotic and hydrostatic pressure gradients between choroid plexus cells and ventricles could play a role for CSF secretion in some instances, this role is minor, and some cotransporter proteins may have a significant role. While aquaporin-1 (AQP1)-dependent water channels have an important role at the apical membrane of choroid cells, the water permeability at the basolateral membrane is dependent on other proteins, such as the glucose carrier GLUT1. At the same time, paracellular water transport through the tight junctions toward lateral spaces between epithelial cells is determined by proteins from the claudin family (most often claudin-1, -2, and -3, but also -9, -19, and -20) [7,8].

Water enters from interstitial space and the capillary pole into the choroid cells through the basolateral membrane and participates in CSF formation at the apical membrane of choroid plexus, with both processes mediated by aquaporin-1, and it can be upregulated by retinoids and glucocorticoids, which explains the implication of some medications in IIH [6,8].

The cotransporter proteins act at the basolateral membrane of epithelial cells (interstitial space border) and the apical membrane (CSF border of the epithelial cells), facilitating the movement of some ions with importance in CSF production, the Na^+ gradient driving HCO_3^- and Cl^- into the epithelial cells. The Na^+–K^+-ATPase pump and Na^+–K^+–$2Cl^-$ cotransporter (NKCC1) are very important to these processes, but also the Na^+–HCO_3 cotransporter, with accumulation of HCO_3^- and H^+ from carbonic anhydrase activity. This derives the role of acetazolamide inhibition of carbonic anhydrase and the further reduction of CSF production by almost 50%, as well as the same effect of the NKCC1 inhibitor bumetanide [6,8–10].

The secretion and resorption of CSF must be balanced to maintain a constant volume of CSF of around 150–160 mL, whereby an excess amount will produce a rise in intracranial pressure through an increase of the total fluid content of the brain. There are several possibilities for CSF's contribution to raised intracranial pressure. First, it could be an increased production with insufficient outflow, such as in tumors of the choroid plexus, where sometimes hydrocephalus can occur, whereas in idiopathic intracranial hypertension the ventricles remain a normal size. Another mechanism is the case of obstructive hydrocephalus that could result secondary to an obstruction along the CSF pathway, in contrast with non-obstructive hydrocephalus, where a decreased resorption is the cause of accumulation of CSF. Classically, the arachnoid granulations have the main role in CSF clearance. Absorption of CSF depends on the pressure gradient between the venous sinus and the subarachnoid space, so a rise in venous pressure needs a concomitant increase in CSF pressure to maintain absorption rates. There are instances such as subarachnoid hemorrhage or meningitis where a blockage of the arachnoid granulation and lymphatics by blood cells or fibrosis is produced, where reduced absorption of CSF could result in intracranial hypertension and communicating hydrocephalus, but in IIH such development is not visible [10,11].

Through a similar mechanism, both CSF hypercellularity, as seen in malignant meningitis, and high CSF protein in Guillian–Barré syndrome, can elevate ICP. Vitamin A deficiency can also lead to elevated ICP, with evidence of thickening of the extracellular matrix in the arachnoid villi [10,11].

Interstitial fluid of the brain is produced by fluid secretion and filtration at the blood–brain barrier level, being distributed between neurons, glial cells, and capillary cells within the parenchyma, while CSF fills the ventricles and subarachnoid space. There is an interaction between interstitial fluid and cerebrospinal fluid that takes place in the perivascular spaces surrounding the small penetrating vessels in the brain parenchyma, where a slow convective flow takes place through the glymphatic system [10,11].

From the subarachnoid spaces, the CSF enters the periarterial spaces, traveling from the cortex toward the deep white matter along the courses of the pial and the perforator arteries in a centripetal distribution [12]. This process of slow flow is passively driven by pressure gradients, including the difference in pressure during respiration, but actively by the arterial pulsations pump. It looks as though this process is more active during nighttime sleep. Another fraction of interstitial fluid derives from trans ependymal passing of CSF from cerebral ventricles and from the periventricular area, reaching periarterial spaces in a centrifugal fashion, a process mediated by aquaporin-4 (AQP4), expressed in the astrocytic end-feet from the structure of the blood–brain barrier. AQP4, which occupies ~50% of the surface area of capillary-facing end-feet, constitutes a low-resistance pathway for water movement between these compartments. AQP4 localized to astroglial end-feet around the microvasculature also has a role in draining the interstitial fluid (water and accompanying solute) efflux into the paravenous compartment [13–15].

This slow flow of CSF into the brain parenchyma induces a convective flow of interstitial fluid toward the perivenous spaces surrounding the large-caliber draining veins [13]. The drainage of the CSF from periarachnoid spaces and intraparenchymal perivenular spaces (together with interstitial fluid) will follow two pathways: the lymphatic outflow and the venous outflow pathways. The interstitial cerebral fluid forms the glymphatic network, and finally drains in the sinus-associated lymphatics, but a fraction of the subarachnoid CSF also arrives in the dural sinus lymphatics [13,16].

The lymphatic system of the brain was described as a dural network extending from the dural sinuses to both eyes, the cribriform plate via the olfactory bulbs and following the dural arteries and veins into the dura mater, penetrating the skull base with the adjacent vessels through the anatomical foramina, and the transported CSF is discharged into the sheaths of the cranial nerves, finally joining the deep cervical lymph nodes [11]. Therefore, the cranial nerve sheaths represent a common CSF and interstitial fluid outflow pathway from the glymphatic system through the lymphatic dural vessels and from the subarachnoid space (through the dural lymphatic vessels and direct anatomical communications between the cranial nerve sheaths and the subarachnoid space) [13–16].

Traditionally, it was considered that the arachnoid villi (invaginations of the arachnoid across the dura mater into the lumen of the venous sinus) represent the main pathway of resorption of the CSF from the subarachnoid spaces. Some authors [13] consider that functionally, these arachnoid granulations could be described as "vascular", centered by a small cortical vein entering the venous sinus, and they are preferentially located in the wall of the transverse sinus, in the area where the Labbé vein joins the sinus, and the rest are the "nonvascular" arachnoid granulations. It was hypothesized that these "vascular" arachnoid granulations represent continuation of the perivenous space of the large-caliber draining veins and receive a part of the CSF and cerebral interstitial fluid from the glymphatic system into the venous blood of the dural sinuses, with another part draining into the dural lymphatics and from there into the general lymphatic circulation [13,16]. The CSF from subarachnoid spaces is drained directly through "nonvascular" arachnoid granulation in large venous sinuses, and from there in the jugular vein and general venous circulation. The proportion of the CSF and interstitial fluid draining through these pathways is not constant, and if one subsystem is not functioning properly (the lymphatic chain or the venous system), the other one will have an increased flow to compensate. From these observations, a combined model of CSF drainage was derived, in which cervical lymphatic exit is the primary site of drainage with the recruitment of arachnoid venous projections under excessive CSF pressure gradients [11,17].

There are medical hypotheses linking the CSF and interstitial fluid with the glymphatic, lymphatic, and venous pathways of drainage and idiopathic intracranial hypertension. First, it was observed (with 3D volumetric MRI measurements) that IIH patients have an excess of cerebral interstitial fluid and CSF in subarachnoid spaces, suggesting a congestion of the glymphatic system [13]. A second observation derives from imaging in cases with IIH, with an excess of CSF observed along the sheaths of the cranial nerves, more frequently described as being the optic nerve sheath dilatation, scleral flattening, and optic nerve tortuosity, that can be explained by the overflow of the lymphatic CSF outflow pathway [18]. The third possibility is related to a stenosis of the transverse sinus, especially at the junction with the Labbé vein, with a backward increase of central venous pressure and inefficient glymphatic venous drainage leading to an excess of cerebral interstitial fluid and overload of the lymphatic CSF outflow pathway [13].

In more than half of the population, the cerebral venous drainage is asymmetric, with predominance of the right side in most cases. An obstruction of the dominant transverse sinus will have a more deleterious effect than of the non-dominant one.

There is a debate as to whether a collapsed wall of the intracranial venous sinus is the cause of intracranial hypertension, or the result of it, but at some point, a cycle of venous hypertension, cerebral swelling, further venous compression, and therefore augmented intracranial hypertension occurs, and this could be a mechanism of worsening. There is a close connection between intracranial pressure and cortical venous pressure, with cortical venous pressure being ~2–5 mmHg higher than intracranial pressure, so there will be a venous flow as long as the ICP does not exceed the inflow venous pressure [19].

The lack of valves in the cranio-vertebral venous system leads the vena cava pressure to be reflected in the CSF pressure, revealing the fact that the venous side of cerebral circulation has much more impact for ICP than the arterial resistance side, but also explaining why an obstacle in venous outflow could be located not only in the intracranial region but also in cervical, thoracal, or abdominal regions.

In case of intracranial obstruction of venous outflow generating an increase of intracranial pressure, the cause of the obstacle could be a focal external venous compression (depressed skull fracture compressing a large venous sinus, periosteal hematoma, tumors), an internal obstruction (most often a sagittal or transverse sinus thrombosis), or a local venous sinus stenosis with idiopathic anatomical local changes; however, sometimes the sinus stenosis could be functional, due to a large volume of arterial blood flowing into the sinus, such as in arteriovenous malformations (AVM) and dural arteriovenous fistulas (DAF) [12]. In these situations of AVM and DAF, the increased venous flow initially produces a maximum distension of the draining vein, but after it reaches the limit of distension, an increased intradural venous pressure will follow (with possible local venous wall changes such as thickening, but also possible thinning and distention producing a local aneurysm), as well as impairment of the mechanisms of CSF absorption with a possible further increase of intracranial pressure until a new level of equilibrium is attained with or without a hydrocephalus development [12,20].

Except for the direct connection between dural venous sinuses of the posterior cranial fossa and sigmoid–jugular venous system, the lateral, posterior, and anterior condylar veins and the mastoid and occipital emissary veins were found to represent another venous connection between the posterior cranial fossa venous sinuses and the vertebral venous systems. All these structures were shown by MR venography. In upright positions, venous drainage preferentially occurs via the spinal venous system, while it is the anterior jugular system in the lying position [21].

An obstruction or difficulty of the venous outflow at the cervical level is possible in particular positions of the neck, such as persistent flexion with lateral rotation, in tight cervical collars, local tumors, and very rarely in jugular compression due to a long styloid process, especially when the opposite venous sigmoid sinus is hypoplastic [22].

Intrathoracic and abdominal causes of venous mechanisms of increased intracranial pressure were associated with positive pressure ventilation in the treatment of chest infection and adult respiratory distress syndrome (ARDS), that can severely raise intrathoracic pressure, severe obesity, and abdominal compartment syndrome with raised intraabdominal pressure [12].

Severe obesity is indeed frequently encountered in IIH patients, and the hypothesis that it produces a retrograde increase of venous pressure, and further intracranial transmitted, only partly explained the IIH since most of the obese persons with IIH were women, but men with an even higher body mass index (BMI) did not have intracranial hypertension. In some trials, a decrease in BMI was clearly associated with a reduction of headache, papilledema, and CSF opening pressure. The mechanism by which weight loss improves idiopathic intracranial hypertension is not known. The effect of weight in terms of mass alone is not a complete explanation, because BMI and lumbar puncture opening pressure have a non-significant correlation [23]. Obesity is increasingly perceived as an inflammatory disorder, and it is supposed that some cytokines (IL-1β, IL-8, and TNF-α) seem to be associated with IIH pathogenesis [24]. The role of adipokines is not consistently related to IIH in all studies.

3. Clinical Manifestations and Diagnosis Criteria of Idiopathic Intracranial Hypertension

The vast majority of patients with IIH are obese (BMI > 30 kg/m^2) women of fertile age, developing some classical signs of intracranial hypertension dominated by headache and visual disturbances (including papilledema).

The most frequent manifestations associated with idiopathic intracranial hypertension are headache 75–94%, nausea with or without vomiting 72–75%, photophobia, phonophobia, or both 42–73%, transient visual obscurations 68–72%, and pulsatile tinnitus in 52–60% of cases [25].

3.1. Headache

Idiopathic intracranial hypertension-associated headaches are of significance to severe intensity, holocranial, frontal, or retro-orbital headaches, but one quarter have moderate and persistent headaches [25,26].

Almost half of the patients have migraine-like headaches, with associated throbbing quality, nausea, photophobia, and phonophobia. There are sometimes some helpful features to raise questions about the diagnosis of "migraine", such as back-, neck-, or radicular-associated pain, increased severity with Valsalva-type maneuvers, or being worse in the morning and when lying flat [26].

In the Idiopathic Intracranial Hypertension Treatment Trial [27], for the assessment of clinical profiles at baseline for the 165 included patients, the average (SD) headache severity on a scale of 0 to 10 was 6.3, with 5.4% of patients reporting a severity of 10. In 51% of those reporting headache, the headache was either constant or daily (median number of days per month with headache was 12), and 41% reported a premorbid history of migraine (17% had migraine with aura).

There are patients with chronic daily headache-like manifestation, frequently associated with analgesic abuse, but almost two-thirds of IIH patients complain of persisting chronic headache despite a normalization of ICP [28].

A potential risk for missing or delaying the diagnosis are the patients without papilledema, when a long-time refractory headache and resultant neurological disability is in fact due to idiopathic intracranial hypertension. One study found, in evaluating patients with IIH, that about 6% of patients with chronically high ICP have no papilledema [29]. Local anatomical anomalies within the optic nerve sheath might prevent the development of papilledema in IIH patients, since sometimes papilledema could be unilateral, or the moment of the ophthalmology evaluation was before the development of the papilledema. The threshold of CSF pressure required to develop papilledema may depend on individual patient characteristics, and it is possible that those without papilledema have a higher threshold than others, but also the moment of measurement of the CSF opening pressure could find different values of ICP at different moments in the same patient. The opposite situation is encountered when some patients can have higher CSF opening pressures than some with papilledema, but normal cerebral MRI findings, and may simply have chronic daily headaches with coincident elevated intracranial pressure (ICP) at that moment [29]. Due to this particular situation, there are specific diagnosis criteria for pseudotumor cerebri syndrome without papilledema, recommended by Friedman et al. [30] When the usual clinical signs and symptoms of intracranial hypertension are present, the neurological examination is without pathological signs (except for possible 6th nerve palsy), but ophthalmoscopy reveals papilledema, the following steps for a diagnosis of pseudotumor cerebri syndrome are MRI neuroimaging (to rule out intracranial expansive mass, hydrocephalus, cerebral veins or sinus thrombosis, or pathologic meningeal enhancement after gadolinium), a normal CSF composition, but elevated CSF opening pressure at lumbar puncture ($\geq$250 mm CSF in adults and $\geq$280 mm CSF in children). In the situation of a patient fulfilling the above criteria but without papilledema, he has to present instead of a unilateral or bilateral abducens nerve palsy. If abducens nerve palsy is not present, MRI supportive arguments are required for a probable diagnosis (at least three from empty sella, posterior optic globe flattening, distension of the optical nerve sheath, eventually with tortuosity of the optic nerve, or transverse sinus stenosis).

3.2. Visual Features of IIH

Anamnesis should assess the eventual episodes of transient visual obscurations and diplopia and ophthalmology examination should test the visual acuity (each eye separately for the best-corrected distance visual acuity with glasses), color vision with Ishihara's plates, pupil examination, and visual fields (either a Humphrey's or Goldmann's automated perimetry, as confrontational visual fields detect only major defects). The visual field evaluation is considered more sensitive than the decrease of visual acuity in patients with IIH, so it should be carefully assessed at each visit. Dilated fundus examination for optic nerve head and retina is the first very important step to rule out or to confirm a papilledema, which if present should be graded by severity and exclude other ocular causes for disc swelling.

Transient visual obscurations (TVOs) refer to sudden loss or shadowy, fogginess, black, white, or grey vision in one or both eyes, lasting for a minute or less than 30 s, sometimes related to a change of position of the body. Increased pressure in liquid from surrounding optic nerve sheaths could compress the thin vascular small arteries and veins at this level, producing a transient ischemia of the optic nerve head [31]. While not specific for raised ICP, the daily occurrence of these symptoms without other explanation (e.g., ischemic amaurosis fugax) is much more frequently encountered in IIH patients.

Diplopia in patients with IIH is due in most cases to a sixth nerve palsy, with this nerve being particularly vulnerable to increased intracranial pressure. Diplopia is horizontal, binocular, and if associated with significant abducens nerve palsy, there is a limited abduction of the eye and strabismus. Third and fourth cranial nerve palsies have been described in patients with IIH but are much less frequently encountered.

Papilledema is encountered in a vast majority (~95%) of patients with IIH, and because of that it is one of the most important elements of the diagnosis criteria and should be assessed in all patients suspected of having this condition. Sometimes, papilledema may be asymmetrical, with 7% of patients having a difference of 2 Frisen grades or more between the two eyes [27]. In chronic untreated cases, optic disc edema can be followed by optic atrophy due to damage to the retinal ganglion cells. Optic nerve pallor suggests that permanent injury to the optic nerve has occurred. The presence of spontaneous venous pulsations has been considered to exclude the possibility of raised ICP, however the evidence from some studies [32] proved that there are patients with lumbar puncture pressure > 30 cm H_2O presenting spontaneous venous pulsation, so this situation does not rule out raised intracranial pressure [31].

Sometimes, distinguishing pseudo-papilledema from papilledema requires clinical experience. Pseudo-papilledema may be due to congenitally anomalous discs, optic nerve head drusen, titled myopic discs, inflammation associated with a juxtapapillary optical neuritis, or malignant arterial hypertension. Ophthalmic ultrasound scanning is a useful method to more precisely detect the drusen of the optic nerve head. Optic nerve head drusen was responsible for 6% of misdiagnoses of IIH. B-scan ultrasound is considered diagnostic if there is an area of hyperreflectivity present at the nerve head or if acoustic shadowing of posterior structures of the optic nerve head is detected [33].

Optical coherence tomography (OCT) generates non-invasive, high-resolution cross-sectional images of the retina using a near-infrared light source through undilated pupils. OCT is a useful tool to identify and quantify papilledema, along with some details such as an increase of peripapillary retinal nerve fiber layer thickness and peripapillary choroidal and/or retinal folds, proving a true papilledema [34]. The optic nerve contour, longitudinal assessment of optic nerve swelling, the shape of the back of the eye, and the shape of the scleral opening around the optic nerve are more precisely measurable using OCT. Quantification of the thickness of the retinal ganglion cell layers in the macula is important to alert the clinician that a decrease can reflect irreversible injury to the optic nerve and that the patient is at risk of permanent vision loss [26].

Visual loss in IIH could associate a loss in the visual field with a loss of visual acuity. An enlarged blind spot is well-recognized as a common early visual field defect in raised ICP. In the baseline patient group from the Idiopathic Intracranial Hypertension Treatment Clinical Trial, the co-existence of visual field defects with a loss of visual acuity manifesting as an enlarged blind spot and inferior partial arcuate defects were described as the most frequent pathological changes, even in patients with mild disease [27]. Loss of visual acuity is generally accepted to be a feature of advanced disease, but clinicians should be aware that in some cases, we can witness a rapid development of a severe visual loss within the first four weeks from symptoms' onset in severe cases of intracranial hypertension, prompting surgical intervention to prevent permanent visual deficits [31].

Pulsatile tinnitus [27,31] is another common feature of idiopathic intracranial hypertension (in more than half of patients), with two-thirds presenting bilaterally. It consists of hearing a whooshing, whistling, humming, or marching noise, continuously or synchronously with the heartbeats (pulsatile is much more frequent) and is thought to represent an auditory perception of turbulent pulsatile flow in intracranial vessels, or in case of intracranial hypertension, probably secondary to a turbulent flow in transverse venous sinus stenosis [26,31]. It is not specific for intracranial hypertension and also occurs due to other underlying vascular abnormalities (including arteriovenous malformations, arterial stenoses), eustachian tube dysfunction, and other benign causes, but in most cases, remains idiopathic.

4. Neuroimaging, Ultrasound, and Lumbar Puncture in Intracranial Hypertension

4.1. Neuroimaging

The primary role of brain imaging in idiopathic intracranial hypertension (IIH) is to exclude other pathologies causing intracranial hypertension, but also to sustain the diagnosis with evidence of subtle radiologic findings suggestive of IIH.

Some visible modifications derive from bony erosion from IIH, such as empty sella, meningocele, and foramen ovale widening, while others are due to mechanical deformation from IIH (posterior ocular globe flattening, vertical tortuosity of the optic nerve, transverse sinus venous stenosis), or a limitation of normal flow of fluids in the optic nerve sheath with optic nerve head protrusion and distention of the optic nerve sheath [35,36] (Figure 1).

In a meta-analysis [35] of MRI modification associated with intracranial hypertension, the empty sella had a pooled sensitivity of 62.2% and a pooled specificity of 90.7%, with absolute pituitary area <151 mm^2 being the most sensitive modification (95.5%). Posterior globe flattening had a sensitivity of 56.3% and specificity of 95.3%, optic nerve head protrusion had a sensitivity of 29.1% and specificity of 97.0%, and optic nerve sheath distension had a pooled sensitivity and specificity of 68.6% and 86.1%, respectively, with individual sensitivity of 78.8% and specificity of 94.2% for a maximum optic nerve sheath diameter > 5.60 mm.

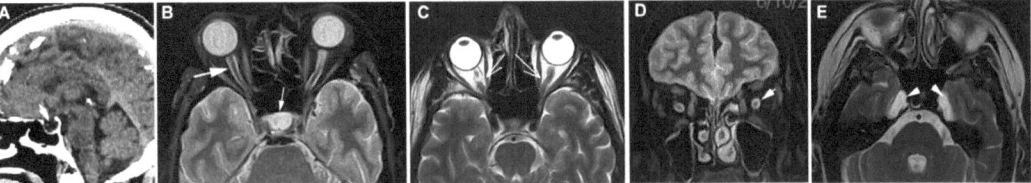

Figure 1. MRI changes in patients with IIH. (**A**) Partial empty sella, T1 weighted MRI. (**B**) Distention of the optic nerve sheath with enlarged cerebrospinal fluid (CSF) spaces surrounding the optic nerve in T2 weighted MRI with fat suppressed sequence (arrow), empty sella also visible (hyperintense signal). (**C**) Noncontrast axial T2 scan reveals that the right optic nerve cannot be entirely displayed along a single plane because the signal of orbital fat obscures the mid-portion of the nerve ("smear sign"). (**D**) Coronal T2 weighted MRI—distention of the optic nerve sheath with enlarged hyperintense CSF ring. (**E**) Axial T2 scan reveals meningoceles involving both of Meckel caves (arrowheads).

4.1.1. Empty Sella

Empty sella is the most commonly reported imaging finding in patients with IIH, with a sensibility up to 80%, but it is also encountered in the general population. When using the definition based on the cross-sectional area of the sella, the pooled specificity is estimated as 83% (95% CI: 76–90) [18]. When the pituitary gland is not visible on T1 mid-sagittal MRI, being replaced by CSF, without any other lesions, we can assign the case as primary empty sella, while in secondary empty sella, the size of the pituitary gland is decreased compared to the size of sella due to other pathologies, such as pituitary tumor, radiotherapy, drug therapy, head trauma, surgery, or rarely, Sheehan syndrome. Primary empty sella associated with increased intracranial pressure is believed to be related to an intrasellar herniation of arachnoid mater and CSF, which flattens the pituitary gland and remodels the sella turcica, a very slow process which take years.

4.1.2. Changes in the Optic Nerve: Protrusion, Tortuosity, and Sheath Distension

Optic nerve protrusion is defined by a focal hyperintensity at the optic nerve head, protruding in the eye, visible on MRI with contrast, and is a representation of papilledema due to increased CSF pressure in the optic nerve sheath and correlates with optic nerve edema seen on OCT as well as the papilledema grade. The detection of contrast enhancement has a smaller sensitivity due to the small dimension of the nerve head and could also be produced in some inflammatory lesions of the optic nerve [36]. In a comparison of neuroimaging findings in patients with idiopathic intracranial hypertension and others with cerebral venous thrombosis, optic nerve head protrusion was present only in patients with IIH, and none in the cerebral venous thrombosis group [37].

Posterior ocular globe flattening can be seen on axial MRI at the bulbar insertion of the optic nerve, and is probably produced by increased pressure in posterior juxtabulbar perioptic CSF, compared with the pressure inside the ocular globe. However, this pressure gradient could also be encountered in situations with decreased intraocular pressure and normal ICP, such as ocular hypotony, with similar posterior globe flattening on MRI appearance, an aspect that explains why this sign is not of absolute specificity in IIH. The sensitivity of MRI-detected posterior globe flattening in IIH ranges from 43% to 85% but is still important to be recognized because in some cases, it may precede the installation of papilledema [18].

Distension of the optical nerve sheaths is possibly correlated with high CSF pressure in the optic nerve sheath and can be seen on MRI imaging (best in coronal T2 sequences) as a widened ring of CSF surrounding an optic nerve. Definitions for distention of the optical nerve sheaths vary, but a diameter of the CSF ring of more than 2 mm is commonly used [36].

Tortuosity of the optic nerve occurs due the fixation of the nerve at proximal and distal points and increased CSF pressure in the optic nerve sheath enlarging the nerve and forcing it to be "kinked". Detection of tortuosity depends on the MRI slice thickness and orientation, with horizontal tortuosity being less common but more specific for increased ICP than vertical tortuosity [38].

In a dedicated comparison of before and after treatment of patients with IIH with papilledema, in the group with resolution of papilledema, all patients showed improvement in two or more of the MRI characteristics of IIH (height of the midsagittal pituitary gland and optic nerve sheath thickness). Sella configuration, ocular globe configuration, and horizontal orbital optic nerve tortuosity were different between the IIH pretreatment group and controls, but not between controls and the IIH post-treatment group [39].

4.1.3. Slit-like Lateral Ventricles

Narrowing or collapse of the walls of the lateral ventricles, referred to as slit-like ventricles, are very rarely described in association with IIH compared to other causes of intracranial hypertension with associated cerebral edema.

4.1.4. Changes in the Cerebral Venous Sinuses: Transverse Venous Sinus Stenosis

Multiple studies have found that severe bilateral transverse sinus stenosis is present on magnetic resonance venography (MRV) in almost 100% of people with IIH, depending on the definition of transverse sinus stenosis, but as was detailed in pathogenesis, whether transverse sinus stenosis is a primary cause or a consequence of IIH is still under debate. A pathological cycle of stenosis of the sinus contributing to intracranial hypertension with further collapsing of the sinus is possible. This could explain both the reversibility of stenosis with treatment of the increased ICP and the success of the stenting procedure of transverse sinus stenosis in people with IIH. Bilateral transverse sinus stenosis greater than 50% has been found to be a very sensitive imaging marker of IIH [18].

Transverse sinus diameter has been demonstrated to correlate with invasive measured venous pressure gradients in patients with IIH. The degree of stenosis of 30–35%, predictive of a clinically significant pressure gradient in the venous sinuses, was considerably lower than the arterial stenosis at which pathologic hemodynamic alterations occur with a significant pressure gradient. For every 10% increase in the degree of venous stenosis, an approximate increase in the pressure gradient of 3.5 mmHg was seen [40].

In another published study [41], a significant stenosis of both transverse sinuses was found before lumbar puncture in IIH patients, with an average diameter of 1.77 mm of the right transverse sinus and 1.57 mm of the left transverse sinus. After the lumbar puncture, there was a significant increase in all venous sinus diameters, but no correlation between the changes in diameter of the venous sinuses after lumbar puncture and measured CSF opening pressure, or the body mass index. This is to be considered when measurements of sinus diameter are planned a short time after a lumbar puncture.

Accurate assessment of transverse sinus diameter is important to diagnose IIH, but also for treatment decisions and follow-up. MR venography (MRV) can be performed by gadolinium-enhanced or by non-enhanced (including time-of-flight and phase-contrast) techniques. Non-enhanced MRV may be susceptible to effects related to slow or turbulent flow with a risk of underestimating the degree of stenosis, while Gadolinium-enhanced MRV may overestimate the lumen of the transverse sinus, because the dural lining also enhances. In a prospective evaluation, the dural venous sinus diameters were measured in an IIH patient population on two-dimensional time-of-flight MRV and three-dimensional contrast-enhanced (3D-CE), and thereafter MRV were compared with real-time endoluminal measurements with intravascular ultrasound (IVUS) as the reference. The CE-MRV significantly overestimated the cerebral venous sinuses compared to TOF-MRV, while the TOF-MRV sinus measurements were in good agreement with the IVUS measurements [42].

Finally, it is better to use MRV (or CT venography) as a screening tool in case of indication of endoluminal stenting, and if the degree of venous stenosis is significant, the catheter venography will be used for further analysis and measurement of the pressure inside the transverse sinus, before and after the stenosis area, so one can make sure of whether there is a significant pressure gradient or not.

In some, but not all, of these patients, the diameter of optic nerve sheaths decreased after lumbar puncture, and maybe this could be a useful sign for selection of patients for methods of treatment such as CSF diversion, while a close follow-up of visual acuity and visual field for the non-responders and selection of other methods of treatment could be helpful. Mean values of optic nerve diameters were around 2.4–2.7 mm, while mean optic disc elevation in IIH patients was 1.2 ± 0.3 mm in both eyes, and neither were influenced by lumbar puncture CSF removal [42].

In a retrospective study, MRI findings of patients with migraine and IIH (including patients with migraine-like headache) were significantly different, where decreased pituitary gland height, optic nerve sheath distention, and flattened posterior globe were found to be statistically significant ($p < 0.001$) in IIH patients. Bilateral transverse sinus stenosis was also more common in IIH patients than in the control group and the migraine group ($p = 0.02$) [43].

Overall, in a meta-analysis, the bilateral > 50% transverse sinus stenosis with MRI diagnosis had a sensibility of 93.0% and a specificity of 96.4% [35].

4.2. The Ultrasound Assessment of Orbital Region

The ultrasound assessment of the orbital region could provide important information for IIH patients in an accessible manner, especially about the mean optic disk elevation as a result of papilledema, the diameter of the optic nerve, and the optic nerve sheaths measured 3 mm behind the papilla. In a published study [44], the mean sheath diameter was 5.4 ± 0.5 mm bilaterally in controls, but with significantly higher values among individuals with IIH, with a mean diameter of 6.4 ± 0.6 mm bilaterally. A cut-off value of a 5.8 mm mean optic nerve sheath diameter for patients with raised intracranial pressure was proposed.

4.3. Lumbar Puncture (LP) to Confirm Intracranial Hypertension

LP is mandatory for the diagnosis of IIH but checking for a normal CSF composition should also exclude meningitis or meningeal carcinomatosis. Reference values of ICP and lumbar pressure of CSF were evaluated in a recent meta-analysis [45] which included 9 studies for ICP and 27 studies for lumbar CSF pressure. The measured values for intracranial pressure were −5.9 to 8.3 mmHg in the upright position and 0.9 to 16.3 mmHg in the supine position, while lumbar CSF pressure values were dependent on position, with 7.2 to 16.8 and 5.7 to 15.5 mmHg in the lateral recumbent position and supine position, respectively.

All patients with papilledema and MRI examination without an expanding intracerebral lesion should have a lumbar puncture to measure the CSF pressure [46].

The diagnostic criteria of pseudotumor cerebri [30] require that opening pressure (which should be measured in the lateral decubitus position with stretched legs and without sedative medications, with a manometer zero positioned level with the foramen magnum regardless of patient positioning), should be above 25 cm H_2O in adults and 28 cm H_2O in children. However, it is important to note that these cut-offs are not of absolute value, with 2.5% of normal adults having ICP above 25 cm H_2O in some populational studies and 10% of patients with acute pseudotumor cerebri having ICP less than 25 cm H_2O [23,47].

Since increased values of ICP may occur intermittently, especially in IIH patients without papilledema, in the presence of suspected intracranial hypertension syndrome with classical clinical presentation and suggestive MRI findings for intracranial hypertension, a second lumbar puncture should be performed if the first lumbar puncture revealed an opening pressure of CSF within the normal range [28].

5. Management of IIH

The main principles of management of IIH are targeting the underlying disease if diagnosed, the protection of vision, and to reduce the headache morbidity. During the last decades, a combination of lifestyle measures, drug treatments, and in selected cases different surgical and endovascular interventional therapies were developed. Before deciding the treatment strategy of an IIH patient, the first step is to check if other known factors associated with increased intracranial hypertension are present, and if identified, they should be addressed. According to Friedman [30], the most frequent causes of pseudotumor cerebri are cerebral venous abnormalities (cerebral venous sinus thrombosis, arteriovenous fistulas, venous decreased CSF absorption from previous intracranial infection or subarachnoid hemorrhage, bilateral jugular vein thrombosis or surgical ligation, increased right heart pressure, superior vena cava syndrome, and the risk factors for cerebral venous and sinus thrombosis, such as middle ear or mastoid infection, hypercoagulable states). Exposure to specific medication and abuse of some substances is another possible cause (tetracycline, minocycline, doxycycline, nalidixic acid, vitamin A excess and retinoids, isotretinoin, lithium, chlordecone), but also some endocrine dysfunction (related to human growth hormone, thyroxine—in children, Addison disease, hypoparathyroidism, anabolic steroids, but also withdrawal from chronic steroid treatment). Obesity is frequently associated with hypercapnic status due to sleep apnea or Pickwickian syndrome. Finally, other diseases such as anemia, renal failure, and Turner and Down syndrome are sometimes associated with high ICP values.

5.1. Weight Reduction

A large majority of patients with pseudotumor cerebri are overweight, but especially obese (90–95%), with 90% of them being women of fertile age. In the year preceding a diagnosis of IIH, many patients had a weight gain of about 5–15%, but in a cohort study, a weight loss of 15% was associated with a significant reduction of ICP (mean 8 cm H_2O), headache, and papilledema, although a correlation between the amount of obesity and CSF pressure was not always found [46,47].

Considering the association between weight gain and IIH recurrence, a weight management plan should be a long-term, sustainable target. Once definite IIH is diagnosed, all patients with a BMI > 30 kg/m^2 should be counselled about weight management with a low-energy diet [48] and integrated in community weight management programs. For those without significant results from community management programs, bariatric surgery is another option and has an increasing role. A comparison between these two options is now available, following the results of a recent randomized study [49] in these obese patients. In this randomized clinical trial of 66 women with idiopathic intracranial hypertension and a body mass index of 35 or higher, bariatric surgery was superior to a community weight management intervention in decreasing intracranial pressure at 12 and 24 months (mean difference 6 and 8.2 cm, respectively, in CSF opening pressure between groups), with weight loss being more significant in the bariatric surgery group (mean 21.4 kg at 12 months and 26.6 kg at 24 months).

5.2. Drug Treatments

Acetazolamide is considered the drug of choice for IIH patients. The mechanism of acetazolamide's effect in reducing the CSF production is thought to be related to inhibition of carbonic anhydrase that causes a reduction in the transport of sodium ions across the choroid plexus epithelium. It has been shown to reduce CSF production by 6% to 50% using a relatively high dosage in humans.

Two double-blind, randomized trials with acetazolamide in patients with IIH were analyzed in a 2015 Cochrane review [50]. The first one was a pilot study with 25 patients per arm [51] and the second one was The Idiopathic Intracranial Hypertension Treatment Trial (IIHTT) [52] with 165 participants (86 patients in the acetazolamide group and 79 in the placebo control). Both trials' participants had a mild form of disease, meaning that evidence for the use of acetazolamide in participants with moderate to severe visual loss is lacking. In the IIHTT, compared with the placebo, the treatment with acetazolamide demonstrated an improvement in visual perimetric mean deviation, papilledema grade, visual related quality of life, and CSF opening pressure at 6 months, but it did not find a benefit in visual acuity or symptomatic headache relief. The IIHTT used a maximal dose of 4 g daily (but only 44% of participants achieved 4 g/day, with the majority tolerating 1 g/day). The usual starting dose of acetazolamide is 250–500 mg twice a day, and a slow dose increase thereafter within the limits of tolerance. The most frequent adverse effects of acetazolamide include increased risk of diarrhea, dysgeusia, fatigue, nausea, paresthesia, tinnitus, vomiting, depression, and rarely, renal stones. Overall, the Cochrane review considered the two studies too small and not representative for the whole population of patients with IIH, and they did not allow quantification of either relative or absolute benefit of treatment, so there is still a need for a large RCT that can provide this information.

A possible alternative to acetazolamide is topiramate, which theoretically could have some advantages: it is also a weak carbonic anhydrase inhibitor, has some migraine preventive effects (and some IIH patients have a migraine-type headache or a previous migraine), and induces appetite suppression, leading to potential weight loss.

An open-label study of 40 patients with idiopathic intracranial hypertension compared topiramate (100–150 mg per day) and acetazolamide (1000–1500 mg per day) [53]. The main outcome was the visual field-graded deficit, which at the 3-month, 6-month, and 12-month visits, improved without a significant difference in the 2 groups. The topiramate group had the advantage of an associated significant weight loss. A prominent relief in headache was reported after a mean treatment period of 3.75 months in the topiramate and 3.3 months in the acetazolamide group, while papilledema grades began to regress after the second month with a mean treatment period of 5.5 months for the topiramate and 5.1 months for the acetazolamide group, but the difference did not reach a significance level. Patients need to be cautioned about potential side effects of topiramate, such as depression, cognitive slowing, reduction of the efficacy of oral contraceptives, and some potential for teratogenic effects.

For patient with previous migraine overlapping with an increased intracranial pressure syndrome, some classical drugs used for migraine attack treatment are still useful (triptan acute therapy used in combination with NSAID or paracetamol and antiemetics), avoiding long-term abuse of analgesics. Topiramate could be used for the prevention of migraine attacks, but in some cases for patients with associated depression, venlafaxine could also play a positive role, avoiding the risk of weight gain seen with betablockers, tricyclic antidepressants, or sodium valproate.

5.3. Surgical and Interventional Therapeutic Methods

5.3.1. CSF Diversion Methods

CSF divergence can be the logical step to reduce the disturbed balance between secretion and drainage of CSF, with an increase in total intracranial fluid content, to compensate for other possible links such as intracerebral venous and glymphatic system compression secondary to intracranial hypertension, but also large venous sinus compression with extrinsic stenosis. This secondary venous sinus stenosis can lead to a further increase in ICP, which creates a vicious cycle where the increase in ICP produces a worsened secondary sinus stenosis and higher venous pressure [51,54]. There is evidence that drainage of CSF with a reduction of ICP can also reverse the transverse sinus collapse in patients with idiopathic intracranial hypertension [54,55].

In patients with a high risk for visual loss, CSF divergence can be sight-saving. If the surgical procedure is likely to be delayed for 24–48 h, it is possible to insert a lumbar drain at the time of the lumbar puncture. Other methods are a lumbo-peritoneal shunt, where a catheter is inserted into the subarachnoid space at the lumbar spine and the distal part enters the peritoneum, but this method is not appropriate in the case of patients with low-lying cerebellar tonsils, as there is an increased risk of tonsillar herniation following the shunt. A ventriculoperitoneal shunt diverts CSF from the lateral ventricle to the peritoneum, and a ventriculoatrial shunt diverts CSF from the lateral ventricle to the atrium of the heart, while a ventriculopleural shunt diverts it to the pleural cavity, but the last two techniques are less used. The surgical risks include shunt malfunction, infection, and over-drainage. Due to the lower reported rate of shunt revisions per patient, the ventriculoperitoneal route should be the preferred CSF diversion procedure for visual deterioration in IIH [46].

The results of CSF drainage methods were evaluated through some retrospective case series and a meta-analysis of them. In a retrospective study [56] with 53 cases of CSF diversion (in most cases, lumbo-peritoneal shunt), significantly fewer patients experienced declining vision and a visual acuity improvement at 6 and 12 months, although headache continued at 6, 12, and 24 months (68%, 77%, and 79%, respectively). Additionally, post-operative low-pressure headache occurred in 28%. Shunt revision occurred in 51% of patients, with 30% requiring multiple revisions.

In a meta-analysis of 17 studies with a CSF diversion including 435 patients [57], the headache improved in 80% of patients, papilledema in 70%, and visual acuity in 54%, but 43% needed another additional surgical procedure, and most of them were related to revision of the shunt for shunt obstruction or failure, malposition, valve dysfunction, or low-pressure headache. The other complications were subdural hematoma, tonsillar herniation, radicular pain, and CSF fistula. The rate of major complications was 7.6% (shunt infection, tonsillar herniation, subdural hematoma, and CSF fistula) [57].

Overall, different methods of CSF shunting have benefits in reducing CSF pressure, in improving visual deficits, and in preventing visual loss, but this is not the procedure of choice for intracranial hypertension headache prevention or treatment.

5.3.2. Venous Sinus Stenting

Stenosis, as previously defined by Marmarou et al. [58], is an acute reduction in the caliber of the venous vessel by at least 40%, while a hypoplastic sinus is decreased in diameter on average by 40% compared to the dominant venous sinus. There is an increased prevalence of right transverse sinus (RTS) dominance, being larger on average than left transverse sinus (LTS).

The DSA estimated pattern of venous drainage in a cohort of patients showed that a right-side dominance is the most prevalent pattern of drainage (49%), while codominance occurs in 43% and left-side dominance in 8%. A complete unilateral drainage is seen in 19% (right) and 1% (left) of patients [59].

Dural sinus stenosis is generally described as intrinsic or extrinsic, although some patients may have both. An intrinsic obstruction pattern is a focal filling defect secondary to arachnoid granulation (often round/oval touching a dural sinus wall), whereas an extrinsic stenosis may be related to local hypertrophic scarring or related to elevated intracranial hypertension, which itself compresses the wall of the sinus (in this situation, the stenosis appears often as a long, tapered, and smooth narrowing) [60].

The arachnoid granulations were present in the superior sagittal sinus in 50% of patients, with a 7% incidence of sinus stenosis. Most of the stenosis in the sinuses was due to the arachnoid granulations (77% on LTS and 71% on RTS) [60]. Overall, only 6% had decreased flow through both sinuses, either by bilateral transverse sinus stenosis or unilateral stenosis with contralateral hypoplastic sinus. Contrary to non-IIH patients, bilateral transverse sinus stenosis is prevalent in 90% of IIH patients [60,61].

The hypothesis linking the dural venous sinus stenosis and IIH leads to the conclusion that solving the stenosis using angioplasty and placement of a stent could serve as another method for treatment of the disease, especially in patients who are unresponsive to medical therapy. Research evaluating this therapy began with Higgins and colleagues, in 2003, who demonstrated a clinical improvement in 7 of 12 medically refractory IIH patients treated with venous sinus stenting, 5 of whom experienced complete resolution of symptoms [62].

Recently, a new proposal emerged [63] for changing the name of idiopathic intracranial hypertension to chronic intracranial venous hypertension syndrome (CIVHS) and to change the diagnostic criteria with a new, combined criteria which requires opening pressure on lumbar puncture or intracranial pressure > 25 cm H_2O and elevated superior sagittal sinus pressures (>18 mmHg) in the absence of an intracranial mass lesion. Based on central venous pressure and the presence of significant venous sinus stenosis, four subtypes of CIVHS were proposed: (1) Central-type patients have elevated central venous pressure without concomitant venous sinus stenosis, whereby morbid obesity or cardiorespiratory disease result in significant central venous pressure elevations with subsequent elevations in intracranial venous pressures. These patients account for about 25% of patients with IIH, are not candidates for venous sinus stents, and tend to respond to weight loss or furosemide to reduce central venous volume and therefore central venous pressure. (2) Craniocervical-type patients demonstrate pathologic venous sinus stenosis with low–moderate CVP, wherein the venous outflow obstruction at the venous stenosis manifests as the primary driver of elevated intracranial venous pressure. These patients are often excellent candidates for venous sinus stents. (3) Mixed-type patients are the largest subset of patients and demonstrate both pathologic venous sinus stenosis as well as moderate to high venous sinus stents, wherein both are independent and additive drivers of high intracranial venous pressure. (4) Post-thrombotic patients demonstrate impaired intracranial venous outflow due to chronic venous sinus thrombosis, and are the rarest [63,64].

Evaluation of venous cerebral circulation should especially detail the location, extension, and degree of stenosis of dural venous sinuses, if possible, with noninvasive imaging such as CT venography, or contrast-enhanced magnetic resonance venography, which can also demonstrate intrinsic/extrinsic stenoses. A direct retrograde catheter venography with venous manometry is required to determine whether a venous pressure gradient exists across the stenotic segment. Pressures are measured from the segments of the superior sagittal sinus, bilateral transverse sinuses, sigmoid sinus, jugular bulb, and cervical internal jugular. A stenosis is considered clinically significant if a trans-stenotic gradient above a certain level is found between the proximal and distal segments of the evaluated venous stenosis. Normal gradients between the superior sagittal sinus and the jugular bulb range between 0 and 3 mmHg in healthy patients. A universally recognized cut-off value for the trans-stenotic gradient to determine which patients are appropriate candidates for stenting has not been established, although most practitioners prefer 8 mmHg for the selection of patients for stenting, and the maximum values are frequently more than 10 mmHg [65].

The likelihood for a cerebral venous pressure gradient is almost 5 times higher (OR 4.97, 95% CI 1.71–14.47) in patients diagnosed with IIH, but very low in patients with a preexisting shunt (OR 0.09, 95% CI 0.02–0.44) and absent in those with normal ICP [66].

There are opinions that the trans-stenotic venous gradient should be measured before and after lumbar puncture, and confirmation of indication for stenting of the venous stenosis remains in patients without significant post-puncture improvement of the gradient. Secondary venous sinus stenosis due to external compression within an intracranial hypertension syndrome may respond to a decrease of ICP after lumbar puncture, while gradient pressure due to intrinsic stenosis is thought to be less responsive to a post-lumbar puncture decrease of ICP [65]. However, the secondary extrinsic venous sinus stenosis can lead to a further increase in ICP, which creates a vicious cycle, a proven fact that, together with case series demonstrating the efficacy of stenting in reducing ICP in patients with extrinsic stenosis, supports the consideration of the procedure in both extrinsic and intrinsic venous sinus stenosis. The cerebrospinal fluid opening pressure and trans-stenotic pressure gradient were significantly decreased post-intervention. The stent reinforces the walls of the transverse sinus and increases its resistance to extramural compression, restoring a more physiologic gradient of venous outflow. This helps with lowering the ICP by preventing the development of upstream venous congestion [64,65].

In a meta-analysis of 32 eligible studies, a total of 186 patients were included for predicting outcome values of pressure gradients [67]. Patients who had favorable outcomes had higher mean pressure gradients (22.8 ± 11.5 mmHg vs. 17.4 ± 8.0 mmHg, $p = 0.033$) and higher changes in pressure gradients after stent placement (19.4 ± 10.0 mmHg vs. 12.0 ± 6.0 mmHg, $p = 0.006$) compared with those with unfavorable outcomes. In a multivariate stepwise logistic regression controlling for multiple factors, the change in pressure gradient with stent placement was found to be an independent predictor of favorable outcome ($p = 0.028$). Using a pressure gradient of 21 mmHg as a cut-off, 94.2% of patients with a gradient > 21 mmHg achieved favorable outcomes, compared with 82.0% of patients with a gradient $\leq$ 21 mmHg ($p = 0.022$), but the high percentage (82%) of patients with favorable outcome with pressure gradient $\leq$ 21 mmHg made it difficult to choose this value as a definitive indication for intervention [67].

Ultimately, venous manometry is the most important parameter to select a venous stent indication as a treatment after diagnosis of significant intracranial hypertension with progressive symptoms/vision loss and an obstructive venous outflow pattern (isolated sigmoid sinus stenosis, bilateral transverse/sigmoid sinus stenosis, or ipsilateral transverse/sigmoid sinus stenosis with contralateral transverse/sigmoid sinus hypoplasia or absence of sinus), without a response to weight loss and maximal medical therapy, after careful comparison of other alternative surgical methods and patient particularities.

Prior to stent placement, patients are provided with seven days of aspirin 75 mg and clopidogrel 75 mg daily or loading doses of aspirin 325 mg and clopidogrel 600 mg. Trans-stenotic maximal venous pressures and pressure gradients are reconfirmed prior to placement of the venous stent. For venous sinus stenosis, the stents need to be self-expanding with adequate radial force to overcome any external stenosis from elevated ICP and long constructs to ensure they extend >10 mm pre- and post-stenosis [68].

Post-stenting venograms are performed to look at the drainage patterns. A CT scan is performed to rule out an intracranial hemorrhage. Patients will be on dual-antiplatelet therapy for one month and single-antiplatelet therapy for at least 3–6 months [46,69]. An array of stents are used for this purpose, such as Zilver 518 of 10 mm-diameter (Cook Medical), the SMART 10 mm-diameter stent (Cordis), Protégé Everflex (Covidien), Precise (Cordis), and Wallstent (Boston Scientific), but the list is continuously expanding [68]. An ongoing study (estimated study completion date January 2024), "Operative Procedures vs. Endovascular Neurosurgery for Untreated Pseudotumor Trial OPEN-UP", which compares venous sinus stenting versus ventriculoperitoneal shunt placement, uses the Zilver stent (ClinicalTrials.gov identifier NCT number NCT02513914).

There are no studies specifically reporting on synchronous bilateral transverse sinus stenting for patients with IIH. The vast majority of published studies performed unilateral stenting of the most stenotic transverse sinus, with good procedural outcomes [69].

The clinical outcomes of dural sinus stenting are related to headache, but especially improvement of visual parameters (visual acuity, papilledema), and as a secondary achievement, the improvement or disappearance of the tinnitus. In the published meta-analysis and retrospective reviews of case series (Table 1), there was a consistent benefit with respect to these parameters: headache subsided or was significantly improved in 73–93% of patients, papilledema in 68–100%, visual acuity and visual field improvement in 70.3–86.5%, and tinnitus in 84.5–100% of patients [57,61,65,70–73].

Table 1. Improvement of clinical outcomes after dural venous sinus stenting.

Authors/Parameter	Headache	Papilledema	Visual Performance	Tinnitus
Satti S.R. et al., 2015 [57]	83%	97%	78%	-
Leishangthem, L et al., 2018 [61]	82%	92%	78%	-
Dinkin M. et al., 2019 [65]	73%	68%	74%	85.1%
Ahmed R.M. et al., 2011 [70]	93%	100%	-	100%
Starke R.M.et al., 2015 [71]	78.3%	94.4%	86.5%	92.9%
Saber H.et al., 2018 [72]	77.6%	85.8%	70.3%	84.5%
Liu X. et al., 2019 [73]	-	-	84.2%	-

In a dedicated meta-analysis of 395 patients [72] with available follow-up data on stenting outcome (mean of 18.9 months), the stent survival and stent-adjacent stenosis rates were 84% (95% confidence interval (CI): 79–87%) and 14% (95% CI 11–18%), respectively. In a retrospective case series [74], overall, 25.9% of patients underwent further surgical intervention following venous sinus stenting, including 6.2% of the total number of patients who repeated a venous sinus stenting procedure and 22.2% who underwent cerebrospinal fluid shunting. Except for restenosis, adjacent stent stenosis or stent thrombosis represent other parts of the treatment failure. The opposite-side venous sinus stenosis is explained by unexpected development of contralateral transverse sinus stenosis after previous stenting of the culprit stenotic sinus. It is assumed that the post-stenting reduction of internal pressure in the opposite transverse sinus—after a large part of venous flow is again directed through the stented dilated sinus—will favor shrinking of the non-stented sinus, and in the most extreme situation, even an occlusion, with re-initiation of a negative vicious cycle of increasing intracranial hypertension and venous collapsing.

The rate of major complication of the procedure (intracranial hemorrhage, subdural hematoma, and subarachnoid hemorrhage, permanent neurological disability) varied from 0% to 1.5–2.9% [57,61,74]. Some minor complications in 3.4–5.4% of cases [57,61,68] were most often related to angiography, or were transient and described as retroperitoneal hemorrhage, retroperitoneal hematoma, femoral artery pseudo-aneurysms, femoral vein thrombosis, neck hematoma, transient hearing losses, transient headache, urinary tract infection, syncope, and post-stenting headache. The mechanism of cerebral venous sinus stenting headache (clinically different than that produced by IIH) remains unknown. Suggestions have included: mechanical stimulation of the venous sinus wall during the procedure, local toxicity, a chemical reaction to the dye, or inflammatory changes, a lower pain threshold, variation in the locations of the hypersensitive pressure receptors of the venous vessel walls, or changes in the pain threshold in the context of physical and psychological stress related to the procedure [75]. According to ICHD-3 criteria [76], cerebral venous sinus stenting headache is defined as any new headache or previous headache that has significantly worsened within one week after jugular or cranial venous stenting has been performed, is ipsilateral to the stenting, or bilateral, and is not better accounted for by another diagnosis. In a dedicated analysis of post-cerebral venous stent headache of 48 patients [75], the headache was present in 29%, of which 92.9% were on the same side as the stent, mild and moderate, in most cases occipital-located, persisted for less than 3 days in 42.8%, for 3 days to 3 months in 28.6%, and for longer than 3 months in 28.6%.

Compared with the other interventional/surgical procedures for IIH, the rate of improvement of the associated tinnitus is higher with stenting of venous sinus stenosis. Pulsatile tinnitus in the majority of patients with IIH is described as a whooshing sound synchronous with their pulse. This has been attributed to turbulent venous flow through a stenotic segment, and compression of the ipsilateral jugular vein may result in its cessation. A 3 T/four-dimensional (4D) flow magnetic resonance imaging with fast-field echo study [77] proved that on the tinnitus side, all patients had sigmoid sinus wall dehiscence, and patients with transverse sinus stenosis showed significantly higher maximum flow velocities than those without transverse sinus stenosis. A jet-like flow in the stenosis and downstream of the stenosis was observed in all patients with transverse sinus stenosis. Since increased prevalence of sigmoid sinus diverticulum/dehiscence and transverse sinus stenosis in idiopathic intracranial hypertension did not correlate with the presence of pulsatile tinnitus in another study [78], there are probably other hemodynamic factors such as intra-stenotic maximum velocity dependent on the local trans-stenotic pressure gradient and complex flow patterns, such as vortex flow, turbulent flow, and helical flow, that are better correlated with pulsatile tinnitus [79].

5.3.3. Optical Nerve Sheath Fenestration (ONSF)

There are very few dedicated studies on ONSF in IIH patients, and in general, they are retrospective case series. The mechanisms through which ONSF reduces the optic nerve consequences of high ICP are not clear. The MRI-proven increase of optic sheath thickness and increased tortuosity of the optical nerve could lead to the idea that the ONSF exerts its action by local fistula formation between the nerve sheath and dura, with slow drainage and resorption of the excess of fluid in the orbital tissue, or a local hypertrophic scarring in the first segment of the optic nerve with a further limitation of transmission of increased pressure in the distal optic nerve and papilla [31].

ONSF was more often considered in patients with asymmetrical papilledema and mainly in patients where headache is not significant, because of the more modest improvement rate compared to the other treatment methods, or in a situation when CSF diversion surgery is considered to carry a high risk or is contraindicated.

The meta-analysis of Satti et al. of optic nerve sheath fenestration included 712 patients. Post-procedure, there was an improvement of vision in 59%, headache in 44%, and papilledema in 80%, and 14.8% of patients required a repeated procedure with major and minor complication rates of 1.5% and 16.4%, respectively [57]. The major complications following ONSF included retinal artery occlusions, retrobulbar hemorrhage, traumatic optic neuropathy, orbital apex syndrome, orbital cellulitis, and manifest strabismus, while minor complications included transient double vision, anisocoria, conjunctival problems/cysts, and optic nerve hemorrhages [46,57].

Unilateral ONSF in a case series of 62 patients [80] significantly decreased the grade of papilledema in both ipsilateral (operated) and contralateral (unoperated) eyes. The reduction of the papilledema and the stability of the visual field in the contralateral (not operated) eye suggest that bilateral ONSF may not always be necessary in patients with bilateral visual loss and papilledema due to IIH, and probably that the cerebrospinal fluid that filters through the dural opening fistula into the orbit produces a subsequent decrease of subarachnoid CSF pressure, and this could explain the therapeutic effect. Unilateral superomedial transconjunctival ONSF was the single treatment method in another small retrospective case series of patients with IIH [81]. Visual acuity, perimetric mean deviation, papilledema grade, and optic nerve head elevation were significantly improved after 6 months in both the operated and non-operated eye. Optic nerve head elevation and visual field testing with automated perimetry could be viable biomarkers for assessing early treatment efficacy after ONSF.

6. Conclusions

The accurate diagnosis of idiopathic intracranial hypertension is essential as visual deterioration due to papilledema may be irreversible. An increase in incidence is expected in the future because of the rising levels of obesity. Although the mechanisms of this heterogeneous syndrome are complex and not all of them are fully elucidated, there are advances in the understanding of idiopathic intracranial hypertension and improvements in diagnosis, based on current available criteria, including specific CSF pressure levels. The therapeutic options include reducing weight strategies (low-calorie diet and bariatric surgery), medication (especially acetazolamide and topiramate), and in selected severe cases, some interventional therapies such as ventriculoperitoneal shunts, optical nerve sheath fenestration, and intracranial venous sinus stenosis stenting, with a possibility to adapt them to the patient's clinical profile for the best results.

Funding: This research received no external funding.

Institutional Review Board Statement: Not applicable.

Informed Consent Statement: Not applicable.

Conflicts of Interest: The author declares no conflict of interest.

References

1. Dandy, W.E. Intracranial pressure without brain tumor. *Ann. Surg.* **1937**, *106*, 492–513. [CrossRef] [PubMed]
2. Geisbüsch, C.; Herweh, C.; Gumbinger, C.; Ringleb, P.A.; Möhlenbruch, M.A.; Nagel, S. Chronic Intracranial Hypertension after Cerebral Venous and Sinus Thrombosis—Frequency and Risk Factors. *Neurol. Res. Pract.* **2021**, *3*, 28. [CrossRef] [PubMed]
3. Leker, R.R.; Steiner, I. Features of Dural Sinus Thrombosis Simulating Pseudotumor Cerebri. *Eur. J. Neurol.* **1999**, *6*, 601–604. [CrossRef] [PubMed]
4. Fisayo, A.; Bruce, B.B.; Newman, N.J.; Biousse, V. Overdiagnosis of Idiopathic Intracranial Hypertension. *Neurology* **2016**, *86*, 341–350. [CrossRef]
5. Durst, C.R.; Ornan, D.A.; Reardon, M.A.; Mehndiratta, P.; Mukherjee, S.; Starke, R.M.; Wintermark, M.; Evans, A.; Jensen, M.E.; Crowley, R.W.; et al. Prevalence of Dural Venous Sinus Stenosis and Hypoplasia in a Generalized Population. *J. NeuroInterv. Surg.* **2016**, *8*, 1173–1177. [CrossRef]
6. Brinker, T.; Stopa, E.; Morrison, J.; Klinge, P. A New Look at Cerebrospinal Fluid Circulation. *Fluids Barriers CNS* **2014**, *11*, 10. [CrossRef]
7. Johanson, C.E.; Duncan, J.A.; Klinge, P.M.; Brinker, T.; Stopa, E.G.; Silverberg, G.D. Multiplicity of Cerebrospinal Fluid Functions: New Challenges in Health and Disease. *Cereb. Fluid Res.* **2008**, *5*, 10. [CrossRef]
8. MacAulay, N.; Zeuthen, T. Water Transport between CNS Compartments: Contributions of Aquaporins and Cotransporters. *Neuroscience* **2010**, *168*, 941–956. [CrossRef]
9. Hladky, S.B.; Barrand, M.A. Fluid and ion transfer across the blood-brain and blood-cerebrospinal fluid barriers; a comparative account of mechanisms and roles. *BioMed Cent.* **2016**, *13*, 19. [CrossRef]
10. Mollan, S.P.; Ali, F.; Hassan-Smith, G.; Botfield, H.; Friedman, D.I.; Sinclair, A.J. Evolving Evidence in Adult Idiopathic Intracranial Hypertension: Pathophysiology and Management. *J. Neurol. Neurosurg. Psychiatry* **2016**, *87*, 982–992. [CrossRef]
11. Bothwell, S.W.; Janigro, D.; Patabendige, A. Cerebrospinal Fluid Dynamics and Intracranial Pressure Elevation in Neurological Diseases. *Fluids Barriers CNS* **2019**, *16*, 9. [CrossRef]
12. Wilson, M.H. Monro-Kellie 2.0: The Dynamic Vascular and Venous Pathophysiological Components of Intracranial Pressure. *J. Cereb. Blood Flow Metab.* **2016**, *36*, 1338–1350. [CrossRef]
13. Lenck, S.; Radovanovic, I.; Nicholson, P.; Hodaie, M.; Krings, T.; Mendes-Pereira, V. Idiopathic Intracranial Hypertension The Veno Glymphatic Connections. *Neurology* **2018**, *91*, 515–522. [CrossRef]
14. Benveniste, H.; Lee, H.; Volkow, N.D. The Glymphatic Pathway: Waste Removal from the CNS via Cerebrospinal Fluid Transport. *Neuroscientist* **2017**, *23*, 454–465. [CrossRef]
15. Iliff, J.J.; Wang, M.; Liao, Y.; Plogg, B.A.; Peng, W.; Gundersen, G.A.; Benveniste, H.; Vates, G.E.; Deane, R.; Goldman, S.A.; et al. A Paravascular Pathway Facilitates CSF Flow through the Brain Parenchyma and the Clearance of Interstitial Solutes, Including Amyloid β. *Sci. Transl. Med.* **2012**, *4*, 147ra111. [CrossRef]
16. Aspelund, A.; Antila, S.; Proulx, S.T.; Karlsen, T.V.; Karaman, S.; Detmar, M.; Wiig, H.; Alitalo, K. A Dural Lymphatic Vascular System That Drains Brain Interstitial Fluid and Macromolecules. *J. Exp. Med.* **2015**, *212*, 991–999. [CrossRef]
17. Zakharov, A.; Papaiconomou, C.; Koh, L.; Djenic, J.; Bozanovic-Sosic, R.; Johnston, M. Integrating the Roles of Extracranial Lymphatics and Intracranial Veins in Cerebrospinal Fluid Absorption in Sheep. *Microvasc. Res.* **2004**, *67*, 96–104. [CrossRef]
18. Bidot, S.; Saindane, A.M.; Peragallo, J.H.; Bruce, B.B.; Newman, N.J.; Biousse, V. Brain Imaging in Idiopathic Intracranial Hypertension. *J. Neuro-Ophthalmol.* **2015**, *35*, 400–411. [CrossRef]
19. Schaller, B. Physiology of Cerebral Venous Blood Flow: From Experimental Data in Animals to Normal Function in Humans. *Brain Res. Rev.* **2004**, *46*, 243–260. [CrossRef]
20. Rossitti, S. Pathophysiology of Increased Cerebrospinal Fluid Pressure Associated to Brain Arteriovenous Malformations: The Hydraulic Hypothesis. *Surg. Neurol. Int.* **2013**, *4*, 42. [CrossRef]
21. Rúiz, D.S.M.; Gailloud, P.; Rüfenacht, D.A.; Delavelle, J.; Henry, F.; Fasel, J.H.D. The Craniocervical Venous System in Relation to Cerebral Venous Drainage. *Am. J. Neuroradiol.* **2002**, *23*, 1500–1508.
22. Li, M.; Sun, Y.; Chan, C.C.; Fan, C.; Ji, X.; Meng, R. Internal Jugular Vein Stenosis Associated with Elongated Styloid Process: Five Case Reports and Literature Review. *BMC Neurol.* **2019**, *19*, 112. [CrossRef]
23. Whiteley, W.; Al-Shahi, R.; Warlow, C.P.; Zeidler, M.; Lueck, C.J. CSF Opening Pressure: Reference Interval and the Effect of Body Mass Index. *Neurology* **2006**, *67*, 1690–1691. [CrossRef]
24. Samancl, B.; Samancl, Y.; Tüzün, E.; Altlokka-Uzun, G.; Ekizoglu, E.; Içöz, S.; Sahin, E.; Küçükali, C.I.; Baykan, B. Evidence for Potential Involvement of Pro-Inflammatory Adipokines in the Pathogenesis of Idiopathic Intracranial Hypertension. *Cephalalgia* **2017**, *37*, 525–531. [CrossRef]
25. Markey, K.A.; Mollan, S.P.; Jensen, R.H.; Sinclair, A.J. Understanding Idiopathic Intracranial Hypertension: Mechanisms, Management, and Future Directions. *Lancet Neurol.* **2016**, *15*, 78–91. [CrossRef]
26. Ahmad, S.R.; Moss, H.E. Update on the Diagnosis and Treatment of Idiopathic Intracranial Hypertension. *Semin. Neurol.* **2019**, *39*, 682–691. [CrossRef]
27. Wall, M.; Kupersmith, M.J.; Kieburtz, K.D.; Corbett, J.J.; Feldon, S.E.; Friedman, D.I.; Katz, D.M.; Keltner, J.L.; Schron, E.B.; McDermott, M.P. The Idiopathic Intracranial Hypertension Treatment Trial Clinical Profile at Baseline. *JAMA Neurol.* **2014**, *71*, 693–701. [CrossRef]

28. Hoffmann, J.; Mollan, S.P.; Paemeleire, K.; Lampl, C.; Jensen, R.H.; Sinclair, A.J. European Headache Federation Guideline on Idiopathic Intracranial Hypertension. *J. Headache Pain* **2018**, *19*, 93. [CrossRef] [PubMed]
29. Mathew, N.T.; Ravishankar, K.; Sanin, L.C. Coexistence of Migraine and Idiopathic Intracranial Hypertension without Papilledema. *Neurology* **1996**, *46*, 1226–1230. [CrossRef] [PubMed]
30. Friedman, D.I.; Liu, G.T.; Digre, K.B. Revised Diagnostic Criteria for the Pseudotumor Cerebri Syndrome in Adults and Children. *Neurology* **2013**, *81*, 1159–1165. [CrossRef] [PubMed]
31. Raoof, N.; Hoffmann, J. Diagnosis and Treatment of Idiopathic Intracranial Hypertension. *Cephalalgia* **2021**, *41*, 472–478. [CrossRef]
32. Wong, S.H.; White, R.P. The Clinical Validity of the Spontaneous Retinal Venous Pulsation. *J. Neuro-Ophthalmol.* **2013**, *33*, 17–20. [CrossRef]
33. Bakola, E.; Alonistiotis, D.; Arvaniti, C.; Salakou, S.; Nana, N.; Foska, A.; Kotsali-Peteinelli, V.; Voumvourakis, K.; Tsivgoulis, G. Optic disc drusen mimicking Idiopathic Intracranial Hypertension (IIH): Rely on ultrasound. *Neurol. Res. Pract.* **2021**, *3*, 33. [CrossRef]
34. Jensen, R.; Vukovic-Cvetkovic, V.; Korsbaek, J.; Wegener, M.; Hamann, S.; Beier, D. Awareness, Diagnosis and Management of Idiopathic Intracranial Hypertension. *Life* **2021**, *11*, 718. [CrossRef]
35. Kwee, R.M.; Kwee, T.C. Systematic Review and Meta-Analysis of MRI Signs for Diagnosis of Idiopathic Intracranial Hypertension. *Eur. J. Radiol.* **2019**, *116*, 106–115. [CrossRef]
36. Barkatullah, A.; Lakshmi, L.; Moss, H.E. MRI Findings as Markers of Idiopathic Intracranial Hypertension. *Curr. Opin. Neurol.* **2021**, *34*, 75–83. [CrossRef]
37. Onder, H.; Kisbet, T. Neuroimaging Findings in Patients with Idiopathic Intracranial Hypertension and Cerebral Venous Thrombosis, and Their Association with Clinical Features. *Neurol. Res.* **2020**, *42*, 141–147. [CrossRef]
38. Passi, N.; Degnan, A.J.; Levy, L.M. MR Imaging of Papilledema and Visual Pathways: Effects of Increased Intracranial Pressure and Pathophysiologic Mechanisms. *Am. J. Neuroradiol.* **2013**, *34*, 919–924. [CrossRef]
39. Batur Caglayan, H.Z.; Ucar, M.; Hasanreisoglu, M.; Nazliel, B.; Tokgoz, N. Magnetic Resonance Imaging of Idiopathic Intracranial Hypertension: Before and after Treatment. *J. Neuro-Ophthalmol.* **2019**, *39*, 324–329. [CrossRef]
40. West, J.L.; Greeneway, G.P.; Garner, R.M.; Aschenbrenner, C.A.; Singh, J.; Wolfe, S.Q.; Fargen, K.M. Correlation between Angiographic Stenosis and Physiologic Venous Sinus Outflow Obstruction in Idiopathic Intracranial Hypertension. *J. NeuroInterv. Surg.* **2019**, *11*, 90–94. [CrossRef]
41. Horev, A.; Hallevy, H.; Plakht, Y.; Shorer, Z.; Wirguin, I.; Shelef, I. Changes in Cerebral Venous Sinuses Diameter after Lumbar Puncture in Idiopathic Intracranial Hypertension: A Prospective MRI Study. *J. Neuroimaging* **2013**, *23*, 375–378. [CrossRef]
42. Boddu, S.R.; Gobin, P.; Oliveira, C.; Dinkin, M.; Patsalides, A. Anatomic Measurements of Cerebral Venous Sinuses in Idiopathic Intracranial Hypertension Patients. *PLoS ONE* **2018**, *13*, 25–30. [CrossRef]
43. Guliyeva, A.; Apaydin, M.; Beckmann, Y.; Sezgin, G.; Gelal, F. Migraine or Idiopathic Intracranial Hypertension: Magnetic Resonance Venography and Magnetic Resonance Imaging Findings. *Neuroradiol. J.* **2020**, *33*, 244–251. [CrossRef]
44. Bäuerle, J.; Nedelmann, M. Sonographic assessment of the optic nerve sheath in idiopathic intracranial hypertension. *J. Neurol.* **2011**, *258*, 2014–2019. [CrossRef]
45. Norager, N.H.; Olsen, M.H.; Pedersen, S.H.; Riedel, C.S.; Czosnyka, M.; Juhler, M. Reference Values for Intracranial Pressure and Lumbar Cerebrospinal Fluid Pressure: A Systematic Review. *Fluids Barriers CNS* **2021**, *18*, 19. [CrossRef]
46. Mollan, S.P.; Davies, B.; Silver, N.C.; Shaw, S.; Mallucci, C.L.; Wakerley, B.R.; Krishnan, A.; Chavda, S.V.; Ramalingam, S.; Edwards, J.; et al. Idiopathic intracranial hypertension: Consensus guidelines on management. *J. Neurol. Neurosurg. Psychiatry* **2018**, *89*, 1088–1100. [CrossRef]
47. Corbett, J.J.; Mehta, M.P. Cerebrospinal Fluid Pressure in Normal Obese Subjects and Patients with Pseudotumor Cerebri. *Neurology* **1983**, *33*, 1386. [CrossRef]
48. Sinclair, A.J.; Burdon, M.A.; Nightingale, P.G.; Ball, A.K.; Good, P.; Matthews, T.D.; Jacks, A.; Lawden, M.; Clarke, C.E.; Stewart, P.M.; et al. Low Energy Diet and Intracranial Pressure in Women with Idiopathic Intracranial Hypertension: Prospective Cohort Study. *BMJ* **2010**, *341*, 138. [CrossRef]
49. Mollan, S.P.; Mitchell, J.L.; Ottridge, R.S.; Aguiar, M.; Yiangou, A.; Alimajstorovic, Z.; Cartwright, D.M.; Grech, O.; Lavery, G.G.; Westgate, C.S.J.; et al. Effectiveness of Bariatric Surgery vs Community Weight Management Intervention for the Treatment of Idiopathic Intracranial Hypertension: A Randomized Clinical Trial. *JAMA Neurol.* **2021**, *78*, 678–686. [CrossRef]
50. Piper, R.J.; Kalyvas, A.V.; Young, A.M.H.; Hughes, M.A.; Jamjoom, A.A.B.; Fouyas, I.P. Interventions for Idiopathic Intracranial Hypertension. *Cochrane Database Syst. Rev.* **2015**, *2015*, CD003434. [CrossRef]
51. Ball, A.K.; Howman, A.; Wheatley, K.; Burdon, M.A.; Matthews, T.; Jacks, A.S.; Lawden, M.; Sivaguru, A.; Furmston, A.; Howell, S.; et al. A Randomised Controlled Trial of Treatment for Idiopathic Intracranial Hypertension. *J. Neurol.* **2011**, *258*, 874–881. [CrossRef] [PubMed]
52. Wall, M.; McDermott, M.P.; Kieburtz, K.D.; Corbett, J.J.; Feldon, S.E.; Friedman, D.I.; Katz, D.M.; Keltner, J.L.; Schron, E.B.; Kupersmith, M.J. Effect of Acetazolamide on Visual Function in Patients with Idiopathic Intracranial Hypertension and Mild Visual Loss: The Idiopathic Intracranial Hypertension Treatment Trial. *JAMA—J. Am. Med. Assoc.* **2014**, *311*, 1641–1651. [CrossRef] [PubMed]
53. Çelebisoy, N.; Gökçay, F.; Şirin, H.; Akyürekli, Ö. Treatment of Idiopathic Intracranial Hypertension: Topiramate vs Acetazolamide, an Open-Label Study. *Acta Neurol. Scand.* **2007**, *116*, 322–327. [CrossRef] [PubMed]

54. Buell, T.; Ding, D.; Raper, D.; Chen, C.J.; Aljuboori, Z.; Taylor, D.; Wang, T.; Ironside, N.; Starke, R.; Liu, K. Resolution of Venous Pressure Gradient in a Patient with Idiopathic Intracranial Hypertension after Ventriculoperitoneal Shunt Placement: A Proof of Secondary Cerebral Sinovenous Stenosis. *Surg. Neurol. Int.* **2021**, *12*, 14. [CrossRef]
55. Onder, H.; Gocmen, R.; Gursoy-Ozdemir, Y. Reversible Transverse Sinus Collapse in a Patient with Idiopathic Intracranial Hypertension. *BMJ Case Rep.* **2015**, *2015*, 3–6. [CrossRef]
56. Sinclair, A.J.; Kuruvath, S.; Sen, D.; Nightingale, P.G.; Burdon, M.A.; Flint, G. Is Cerebrospinal Fluid Shunting in Idiopathic Intracranial Hypertension Worthwhile? A 10-Year Review. *Cephalalgia* **2011**, *31*, 1627–1633. [CrossRef]
57. Satti, S.R.; Leishangthem, L.; Chaudry, M.I. Meta-Analysis of Csf Diversion Procedures and Dural Venous Sinus Stenting in the Setting of Medically Refractory Idiopathic Intracranial Hypertension. *Am. J. Neuroradiol.* **2015**, *36*, 1899–1904. [CrossRef]
58. Marmarou, A.; Shulman, K.; Rosende, R.M. A Nonlinear Analysis of the Cerebrospinal Fluid System and Intracranial Pressure Dynamics. *J. Neurosurg.* **1978**, *48*, 332–344. [CrossRef]
59. Cheng, Y.; Li, W.A.; Fan, X.; Li, X.; Chen, J.; Wu, Y.; Meng, R.; Ji, X. Normal Anatomy and Variations in the Confluence of Sinuses Using Digital Subtraction Angiography. *Neurol. Res.* **2017**, *39*, 509–515. [CrossRef]
60. Farb, R.I.; Vanek, I.; Scott, J.N.; Mikulis, D.J.; Willinsky, R.A.; Tomlinson, G.; terBrugge, K.G. Idiopathic Intracranial Hypertension: The Presence and Morphology of Sinovenous Stenosis. *Neurology* **2003**, *60*, 1418–1424. [CrossRef]
61. Leishangthem, L.; SirDeshpande, P.; Dua, D.; Satti, S.R. Dural Venous Sinus Stenting for Idiopathic Intracranial Hypertension: An Updated Review. *J. Neuroradiol.* **2019**, *46*, 148–154. [CrossRef]
62. Higgins, J.N.P.; Cousins, C.; Owler, B.K.; Sarkies, N.; Pickard, J.D. Idiopathic Intracranial Hypertension: 12 Cases Treated by Venous Sinus Stenting. *J. Neurol. Neurosurg. Psychiatry* **2003**, *74*, 1662–1666. [CrossRef]
63. Fargen, K.M. Idiopathic Intracranial Hypertension Is Not Idiopathic: Proposal for a New Nomenclature and Patient Classification. *J. NeuroInterv. Surg.* **2020**, *12*, 110–114. [CrossRef]
64. Townsend, R.K.; Fargen, K.M. Intracranial Venous Hypertension and Venous Sinus Stenting in the Modern Management of Idiopathic Intracranial Hypertension. *Life* **2021**, *11*, 508. [CrossRef]
65. Dinkin, M.; Oliveira, C. Men Are from Mars, Idiopathic Intracranial Hypertension Is from Venous: The Role of Venous Sinus Stenosis and Stenting in Idiopathic Intracranial Hypertension. *Semin. Neurol.* **2019**, *39*, 692–703. [CrossRef]
66. Levitt, M.R.; Hlubek, R.J.; Moon, K.; Kalani, M.Y.S.; Nakaji, P.; Smith, K.A.; Little, A.S.; Knievel, K.; Chan, J.W.; McDougall, C.G.; et al. Incidence and Predictors of Dural Venous Sinus Pressure Gradient in Idiopathic Intracranial Hypertension and Non-Idiopathic Intracranial Hypertension Headache Patients: Results from 164 Cerebral Venograms. *J. Neurosurg.* **2017**, *126*, 347–353. [CrossRef]
67. McDougall, C.M.; Ban, V.S.; Beecher, J.; Pride, L.; Welch, B.G. Fifty Shades of Gradients: Does the Pressure Gradient in Venous Sinus Stenting for Idiopathic Intracranial Hypertension Matter? A Systematic Review. *J. Neurosurg.* **2019**, *130*, 999–1005. [CrossRef]
68. Daggubati, L.C.; Liu, K.C. Intracranial Venous Sinus Stenting: A Review of Idiopathic Intracranial Hypertension and Expanding Indications. *Cureus* **2019**, *11*, e4008. [CrossRef]
69. Fargen, K.M.; Liu, K.; Garner, R.M.; Greeneway, G.P.; Wolfe, S.Q.; Crowley, R.W. Recommendations for the Selection and Treatment of Patients with Idiopathic Intracranial Hypertension for Venous Sinus Stenting. *J. NeuroInterv. Surg.* **2018**, *10*, 1203–1208. [CrossRef]
70. Ahmed, R.M.; Wilkinson, M.; Parker, G.D.; Thurtell, M.J.; Macdonald, J.; McCluskey, P.J.; Allan, R.; Dunne, V.; Hanlon, M.; Owler, B.K.; et al. Transverse Sinus Stenting for Idiopathic Intracranial Hypertension: A Review of 52 Patients and of Model Predictions. *Am. J. Neuroradiol.* **2011**, *32*, 1408–1414. [CrossRef]
71. Starke, R.M.; Wang, T.; Ding, D.; Durst, C.R.; Crowley, R.W.; Chalouhi, N.; Hasan, D.M.; Dumont, A.S.; Jabbour, P.; Liu, K.C. Endovascular Treatment of Venous Sinus Stenosis in Idiopathic Intracranial Hypertension: Complications, Neurological Outcomes, and Radiographic Results. *Sci. World J.* **2015**, *2015*, 140408. [CrossRef]
72. Saber, H.; Lewis, W.; Sadeghi, M.; Rajah, G.; Narayanan, S. Stent Survival and Stent-Adjacent Stenosis Rates Following Venous Sinus Stenting for Idiopathic Intracranial Hypertension: A Systematic Review and Meta-Analysis. *Interv. Neurol.* **2018**, *7*, 490–500. [CrossRef]
73. Liu, X.; Di, H.; Wang, J.; Cao, X.; Du, Z.; Zhang, R.; Yu, S.; Li, B. Endovascular Stenting for Idiopathic Intracranial Hypertension with Venous Sinus Stenosis. *Brain Behav.* **2019**, *9*, 3–9. [CrossRef]
74. Garner, R.M.; Aldridge, J.B.; Wolfe, S.Q.; Fargen, K.M. Quality of Life, Need for Retreatment, and the Re-Equilibration Phenomenon after Venous Sinus Stenting for Idiopathic Intracranial Hypertension. *J. NeuroInterv. Surg.* **2021**, *13*, 79–85. [CrossRef]
75. Su, H.; Li, B.; Wang, J.; Tian, C.; Cao, X.; Du, Z.; Liu, X.; Liu, R.; Yu, S. Headache Attributed to Cranial Venous Sinus Stenting: A Case Series and Literature Review. *Cephalalgia* **2019**, *39*, 1277–1283. [CrossRef]
76. Olesen, J. Headache Classification Committee of the International Headache Society (IHS): The International Classification of Headache Disorders, 3rd Edition. *Cephalalgia* **2018**, *38*, 1–211. [CrossRef]
77. Li, X.; Qiu, X.; Ding, H.; Lv, H.; Zhao, P.; Yang, Z.; Gong, S.; Wang, Z. Effects of Different Morphologic Abnormalities on Hemodynamics in Patients with Venous Pulsatile Tinnitus: A Four-Dimensional Flow Magnetic Resonance Imaging Study. *J. Magn. Reson. Imaging* **2021**, *53*, 1744–1751. [CrossRef]
78. Lansley, J.A.; Tucker, W.; Eriksen, M.R.; Riordan-Eva, P.; Connor, S.E.J. Sigmoid Sinus Diverticulum, Dehiscence, and Venous Sinus Stenosis: Potential Causes of Pulsatile Tinnitus in Patients with Idiopathic Intracranial Hypertension? *Am. J. Neuroradiol.* **2017**, *38*, 1783–1788. [CrossRef]

79. Ding, H.; Zhao, P.; Lv, H.; Li, X.; Qiu, X.; Zeng, R.; Wang, G.; Yang, Z.; Gong, S.; Jin, L.; et al. Correlation between Trans-Stenotic Blood Flow Velocity Differences and the Cerebral Venous Pressure Gradient in Transverse Sinus Stenosis: A Prospective 4-Dimensional Flow Magnetic Resonance Imaging Study. *Neurosurgery* **2021**, *89*, 549–556. [CrossRef] [PubMed]
80. Alsuhaibani, A.H.; Carter, K.D.; Nerad, J.A.; Lee, A.G. Effect of Optic Nerve Sheath Fenestration on Papilledema of the Operated and the Contralateral Nonoperated Eyes in Idiopathic Intracranial Hypertension. *Ophthalmology* **2011**, *118*, 412–414. [CrossRef]
81. Hagen, S.M.; Wegener, M.; Toft, P.B.; Fugleholm, K.; Jensen, R.H.; Hamann, S. Unilateral Optic Nerve Sheath Fenestration in Idiopathic Intracranial Hypertension: A 6-Month Follow-up Study on Visual Outcome and Prognostic Markers. *Life* **2021**, *11*, 778. [CrossRef] [PubMed]

Case Report

Case Reports of Pregnancy-Related Cerebral Venous Thrombosis in the Neurology Department of the Emergency Clinical Hospital in Constanta

Any Docu Axelerad [1], Lavinia Alexandra Zlotea [2], Carmen Adella Sirbu [3], Alina Zorina Stroe [1,*], Silviu Docu Axelerad [4], Simona Claudia Cambrea [5,6] and Lavinia Florenta Muja [1]

1. Department of Neurology, General Medicine Faculty, Ovidius University, 900470 Constanta, Romania; axelerad.docu@365.univ-ovidius.ro (A.D.A.); laviniamuja@gmail.com (L.F.M.)
2. Radiology-Medical Imaging, Sf Apostol Andrei Emergency County Clinical Hospital, 900591 Constanta, Romania; laviniazlotea23@gmail.com
3. Department of Neurology, Titu Maiorescu University, 040441 Bucharest, Romania; carmen.sirbu@prof.utm.ro
4. Faculty of General Medicine, 'Vasile Goldis' University, 317046 Arad, Romania; docu.silviu@yahoo.com
5. Infectious Diseases Clinic, Clinical Infectious Diseases Hospital, 900708 Constanta, Romania; claudia.cambrea@univ-ovidius.ro
6. Department of Infectious Diseases, General Medicine Faculty, Ovidius University, 900470 Constanta, Romania
* Correspondence: alina.stroe@365.univ-ovidius.ro or zorina.stroe@yahoo.com; Tel.: +40-727-987-950

Abstract: Cerebral venous thrombosis accounts for 0.5–1% of all cerebrovascular events and is one type of stroke that affects the veins and cerebral sinuses. Females are more affected than males, as they may have risk factors, such as pregnancy, first period after pregnancy, treatment with oral contraceptives treatment with hormonal replacement, or hereditary thrombophilia. This neurological pathology may endanger a patient's life. However, it must be suspected in its acute phase, when it presents with variable clinical characteristics, so that special treatment can be initiated to achieve a favorable outcome with partial or complete functional recovery. The case study describes the data and the treatment of two patients with confirmed cerebral venous thrombosis with various localizations and associated risk factors, who were admitted to the neurology department of the Sf. Apostol Andrei Emergency Hospital in Constanta. The first patient was 40 years old and affected by sigmoid sinus and right lateral sinus thrombosis, inferior sagittal sinus, and right sinus thrombosis, associated with right temporal subacute cortical and subcortical hemorrhage, which appeared following a voluntary abortion. The second case was a patient aged 25 who was affected by left parietal cortical vein thrombosis, associated with ipsilateral superior parietal subcortical venous infarction, which appeared following labor. The data are strictly observational and offer a perspective on clinical manifestations and clinical and paraclinical investigations, including the treatment of young patients who had been diagnosed with cerebral venous thrombosis and admitted to the neurology department.

Keywords: cerebral venous thrombosis; pregnancy; puerperium; voluntary abortion

1. Introduction

Cerebral venous thrombosis (CVT) is an uncommon type of neurological pathology. It is an embedded cerebrovascular disease, may appear regardless of age, and corresponds to 0.5–1% of all cerebral and vascular strokes [1]. It presents a remarkable range of symptoms and signs, the most frequent being cephalalgia, convulsions, focal neurological deficits, papillary edema, and alternating general health status and consciousness [2].

Around 20% of CVST-related strokes have been documented in young Asian females [3]. Bano et al. found that, in 68.8% of patients, the gender-specific pathogenesis of CVST was related to pregnancy and the postpartum [4]. CVT occurs in 2–57% of pregnancy-related strokes, with the majority of instances occurring during the postpartum period [5].

In Bajko et al.'s [6] research, females comprised around 60% of the study group, and a significant proportion of the female patient population was in the puerperium (17.2%).

Modifications of the cerebral parenchyma appear in cerebral venous thrombosis due to an obstruction in the venous system and intracranial sinuses. The primary locations of flow blockages appear to be at the intersections of cerebral veins and major cerebral sinuses, with a preference for the superior sagittal and transverse sinuses [7,8].

In patients with this neurological pathology, extremely diverse symptomatology may be encountered, both at the beginning and during its evolution, and younger patients can suffer from it. Female patients are particularly affected when they have risk factors such as pregnancy, puerperium, use of oral contraceptives or hormonal replacement therapy; patients with hereditary thrombophilia may also be affected [9].

Pregnancy-related stroke develops in 30.0 out of every 100,000 pregnancies; hemorrhagic and ischemic strokes happen in two thirds of cases, and CVST occurs in one third [10]. The first postpartum month, the perinatal period and the third trimester of pregnancy are the most strongly associated with the etiology of CVST, although just a few instances of CVST have been documented in early pregnancy. Our patients had pregnancy-related situations: the first patient had an abortion via curettage and the second patient was in the sixth day of puerperium after a caesarian delivery.

As a rare high-risk disease, cerebral venous thrombosis must be suspected in cases accompanied by cephalalgia and other focal neurological deficits, altered consciousness, and convulsions, even in the acute phase when the disease has variable symptoms [11].

The diagnosis of CVST should be confirmed by clinical and paraclinical manifestations, the associated risk factors, and a neurological examination. The imaging investigations are extremely important for confirming the diagnosis and the most reliable imaging type is nuclear magnetic resonance (NMR).

The most useful methods for establishing a diagnosis of CVT are imaging investigations, and the most precise method involves a combination of magnetic resonance imaging and angiography. All patients suspected of having CVT should undergo screening for prothrombotic states, along with an evaluation of the levels of antithrombin III, levels of S and C proteins, homocysteine levels, mutations of prothrombin levels, and levels of antiphospholipid antibodies [12].

The thrombophilia test is useful for people with CVST-associated risk factors who have a history of thromboembolism. In particular, it is beneficial and essential for pregnant women with another associated risk factor.

Treatment aims to halt the progression of a thrombus through the elimination of obstacles in the sinus lumen and the affected veins, thereby improving the prothrombotic status with the purpose of preventing venous thrombotic events, and at the same time, preventing the occurrence of relapses. Moreover, treatment also aims to optimize functional recovery. Drug treatments may consist of blood thinners or thrombolytic medications; the latter are suggested for destroying the blood clots that have formed if the thrombosis is serious.

In this article, we present the cases of two patients with neurological pathology who were admitted to the neurology department of Sf. Apostol Andrei Emergency Hospital of Constanta and who progressed favorably under special treatment. The Ethics Committee for Clinical Studies at the Constanta County Emergency Clinical Hospital (registration number 30/1.11.2021) approved the study, which was conducted in accordance with the Declaration of Helsinki. All subjects gave written informed permission before of the enrolment.

The first patient presented with sigmoid sinus and right lateral sinus thrombosis and inferior sagittal sinus, and right sinus thrombosis, associated with right temporal subacute cortical and subcortical hemorrhage, a pathology that appeared following a voluntary abortion. The second patient was affected by left parietal cortical vein thrombosis associated with an ipsilateral superior parietal subcortical venous infarction that appeared following labor and delivery by a caesarian operation.

2. Results

2.1. Case 1

The first case was a female patient aged 40, known to be affected by laparoscopic cholecystectomy and abortion by curettage in ambulatory surgery. The patient was admitted to the neurology department for a period of 11 days due to a decrease in muscular strength in the right hemibody and a speech disorder that onset during the same day.

At the emergency ward, the patient underwent a native and contrast-enhanced CT scan, which highlighted the following: the right temporal surface was most probably compatible, in terms of imaging, with encephalitis; a cranial cerebral MRI examination and a pulmonary radiography (X-ray), which did not reveal pleuro-pulmonary evolutive lesions, were recommended.

When admitted to the neurology department, during the neurological objective examination, the patient was conscious, barely cooperative, had expressive aphasia, had no stiffness in the back of the head, had normal ocular motricity, and had no nystagmus; further, the patient presented with right hemiparesis 3/5 equally distributed, and a cutaneous plantar reflex with bilateral flexion.

On the first day of hospitalization, the patient underwent a cerebral native and contrast-enhanced MRI and angiography, and a CT venography, which highlighted sigmoid sinus and right lateral sinus thrombosis, and inferior sagittal sinus and right sinus thrombosis, associated with right temporal cortical and subcortical subacute hemorrhage, supratentorial recent subacute synchronous lacunar infarct, (cytotoxic and vasogenic) thalamic–lenticular–caudal oedema, and supratentorial non-specific demyelinating lesions.

On the first day of hospitalization, biological material was collected in order to create the hereditary thrombosis profile, which was transmitted to the Clinical Service of Pathological Anatomy and tested to identify the mutations associated with cardiovascular disease and thrombophilia.

The following genotypes were identified: heterozygous for V factor mutation *H1299R* (R2) and heterozygous for mutation *4G* of *PAI-1*. Moreover, the *A1/A1* haplotype of *EPCR* was identified.

On the second day of admission, the patient underwent native thoracic CT and angiography for pulmonary arteries, without any images suggesting pulmonary thromboembolism.

On the same day (the second day of admission), the patient underwent a gynecological exam. The diagnosis of incomplete abortion was confirmed, and the patient was recommended to perform beta-human chorionic gonadotropin (hCG) after 48 h. The patient was recommended to take antibiotics (2 g intravenous ampicillin every 12 h and 80 g intravenous gentamicin every 12 h), and a nonsteroidal anti-inflammatory drug (75 mg diclofenac, one 0.2 mg tablet every 12 h) and to undergo reevaluation according to the results of the tests. Uterine curettage was recommended to be performed after neurological rebalancing of the patient.

During admission, on the fifth day of hospitalization, the patient underwent a cardiac assessment. She also had a blood pressure of 105/60 mmHg, a heart rate of 64 beats per minute, a normal electrocardiogram (ECG) with sinus rhythm, and angiography of the pulmonary arteries that infirmed pulmonary thromboembolism.

On the seventh day of admission, a gynecological reassessment was requested for the result of beta-hCG testing, and the investigation indicated a decrease in its value. Following a consultation, the patient was advised to continue therapy with antibiotics and to repeat the beta-hCG test after 7 days for a reassessment of the results.

On the ninth day, the gynecological reassessment indicated a paraclinical decrease in beta-hCG and the patient was recommended to repeat this test on a weekly basis until negative results were obtained and to have a gynecological assessment in ambulatory after 1 week. A hematological assessment was also requested on the ninth day of admission, which confirmed that the mutations detected in the hereditary thrombophilia profile fell into the low-risk class. It was recommended that the screening test for thrombophilia be intensified for C and S proteins, AT III, the dosage of serum homocysteine, and lupus anticoagulant in the ambulatory. The details of treating the patient and the findings can be seen in Figure 1.

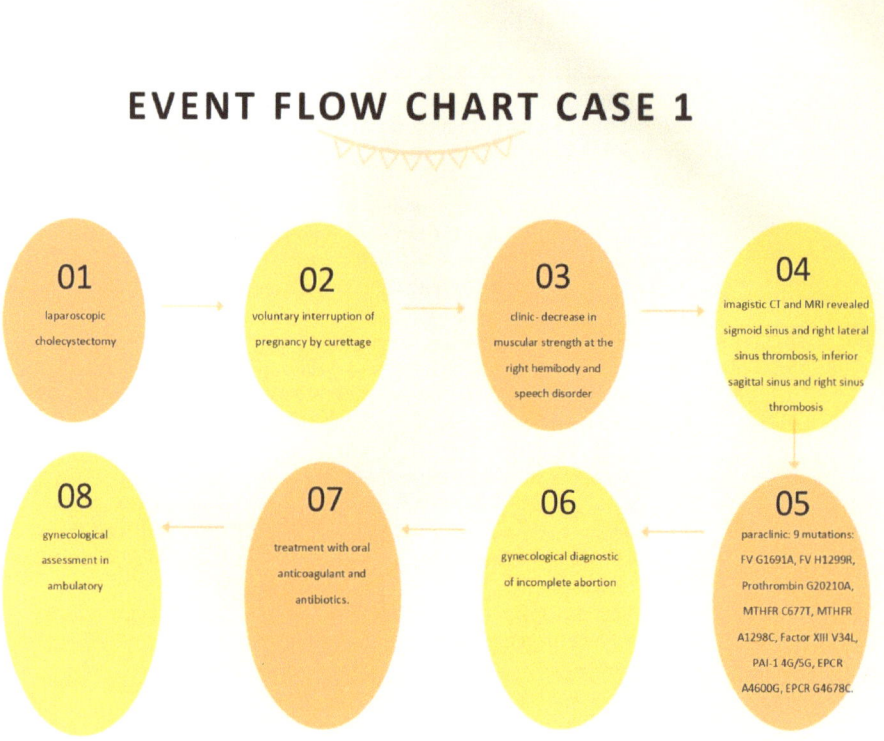

Figure 1. Event flow chart case 1.

During her admission, the patient received brain depletive medication (20% mannitol, 250 mL every 12 h, for 5 days), hydro-electrolytic rebalancing (500 mL of normal saline solution every 12 h), heparin with a small molecular weight (0.4 mL enoxaparin sodium, one ampoule per day during the entire period of admission), cortico-steroid anti-inflammatory drugs (one ampoule of intravenous dexamethasone every 12 h for the first 2 days of admission), benzodiazepine (one ampoule of diazepam in 10 mL of a normal intravenous saline solution, given slowly in case of convulsive spasm), antibiotics (2 g intravenous ampicillin every 12 h, 80 mg intravenous gentamicin every 12 h), a non-steroidal anti-inflammatory (one ampoule of ketoprofen per day), a gastric protector (one 40 mg pantoprazole tablet per day), a probiotic enhancer (one 250 mg enterolum tablet twice a day, 2 h after the antibiotic), and an oral anticoagulant (4 mg acenocoumarol) as follows: 1/4 tablet on the seventh day of admission; 1/2 tablet per day on days 8 and 9; 3/4 tablet per day on days 10 and 11, with international normalized ratio (INR) control performed on a daily basis, in order to adjust the dose according to the INR. The patient recovered well.

At discharge, the patient continued the treatment with the oral anticoagulant (4 mg acenocoumarol as follows: 3/4 tablet alternating with 1 tablet per day, according to the INR dosage every 7, 14, and 21 days, then, on a monthly basis), to which a pain-killer was added (one tablet metamizole, if necessary), along with a brain trophic (one 400 mg Actovegin tablet, three times per day) and a dietary supplement with alpha-lipoic acid and a complex of vitamins.

Upon discharge, the neurological examination indicated that the patient was conscious, cooperative, oriented in time and space, without stiffness in the back of the head, no nystagmus, with normal ocular motricity, denial of diplopia, possible deglutition for liquid and solid food, normal speech, no movement deficits, no sensitivity or coordination disorders, and a cutaneous plantar reflex with bilateral flexion. The images of the MRI can be seen below in Figure 2.

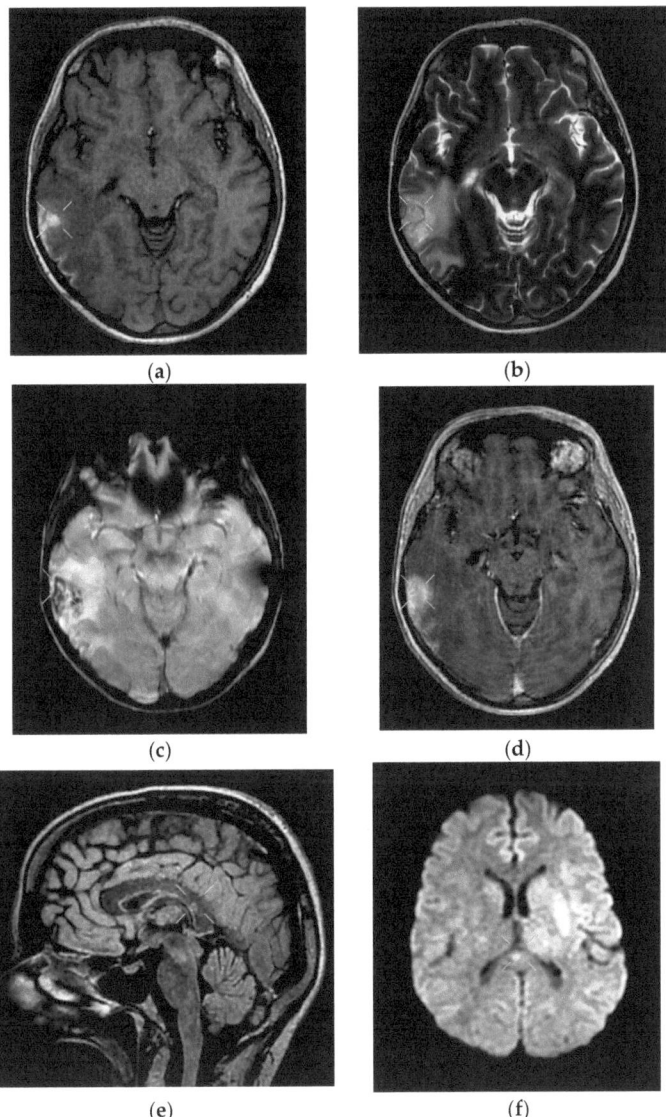

Figure 2. Cont.

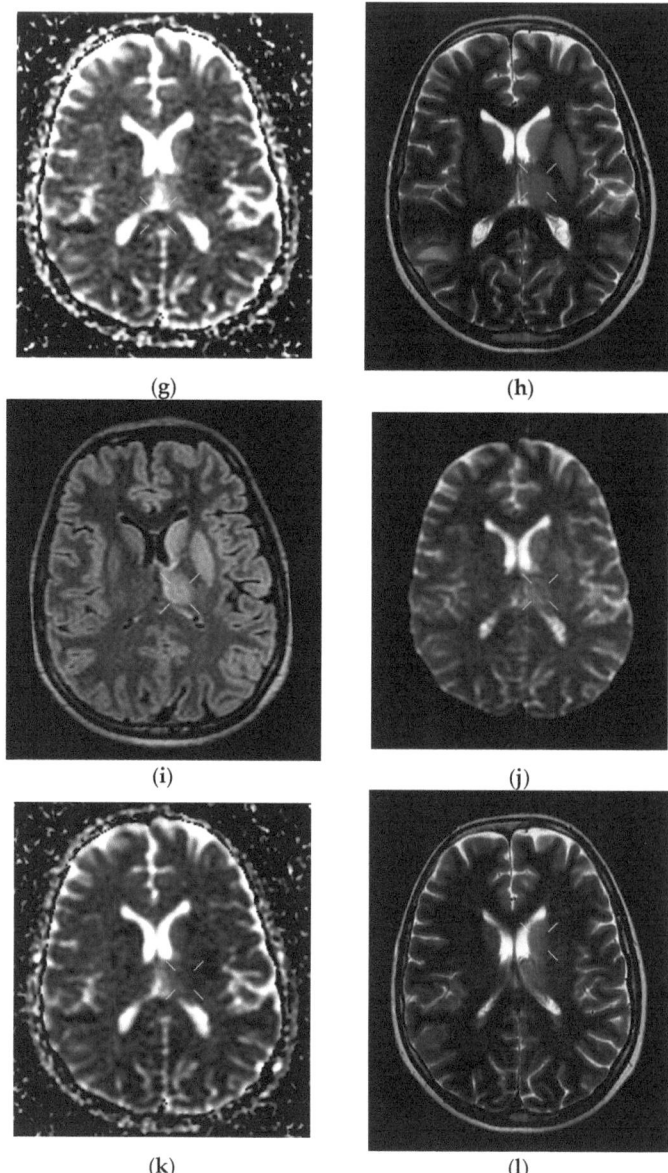

Figure 2. Cont.

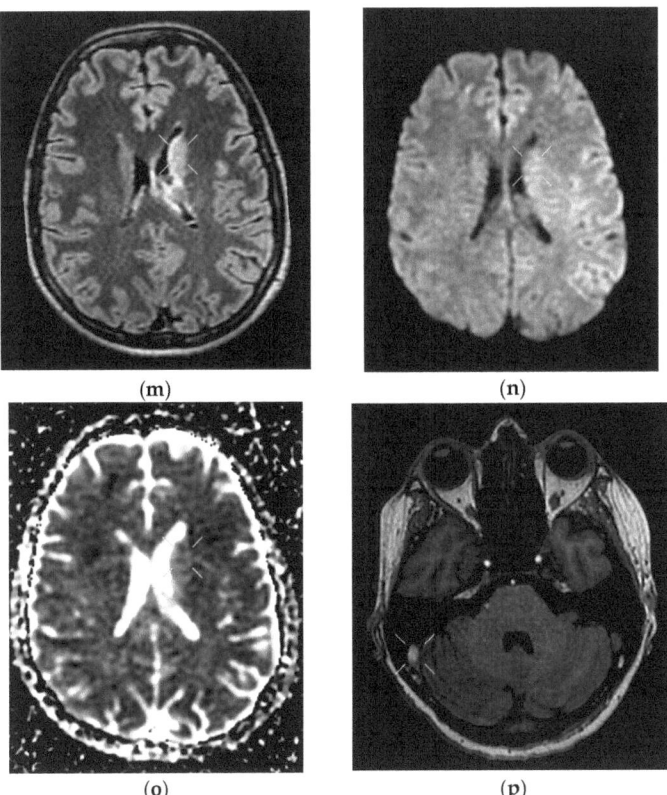

Figure 2. Cerebral native and contrast-enhanced MRI and angiography, and CT cerebral venography highlighting the sigmoid sinus and right lateral sinus thrombosis and the inferior sagittal sinus and right sinus thrombosis, associated with right temporal cortical and subcortical subacute hemorrhage, supratentorial recent subacute synchronous lacunar infarct, (cytotoxic and vasogenic) thalamic–lenticular–caudal edema, and supratentorial non-specific demyelinating lesions. Magnetic resonance imaging shows cortico-subcortical subacute hemorrhage in the right temporal lobe (**a,b**) T1 and T2 hyperintensities. (**c**) methemoglobin signal. (**d**) heterogeneous contrast enhancement. (**e**) supratentorial recent subacute lacunar infarction in a millimeter lesion in hypersignal FLAIR, restrictive in diffusion coefficient. (**f,g**) supratentorial recent subacute lacunar infarction located in the corpus callosum. (**h,i,j,k**) cytotoxic and vasogenic edema in diffuse T2 and FLAIR high signal and moderate restriction in diffusion coefficient in the left thalamus. (**l,m,n,o**) cytotoxic and vasogenic edema in left lenticular-caudate nucleus. (**p**) right sigmoid and lateral sinuses thrombosis—T1 and T2 hyperintense material, without contrast enhancement. The intravenous post-contrast and native cranio-cerebral MRI examination highlights are as follows: oval globular formations with a non-homogeneous central portion and a periphery with a methemoglobin signal, hyper-intense T1–T2, axial dimensions of 11/10 mm maximally and heterogeneous contrast outlet, along with right temporal cortical and subcortical conglomerates, with extended moderate perilesional oedema; FLAIR hyper-intense millimeter lesions, intense and homogeneous restriction in diffusion and no-contrast outlets in the semioval centers, in the corpus callosum and in the middle temporal gyrus; diffuse signal T2–FLAIR increased in the left and left lenticular–caudal thalamus,

with minimum diffusion restriction and no detectable contrast outlets; a few T2–FLAIR hypersignal millimeter outbreaks, with no diffusion restriction and no corresponding T1, located in the white matter in the periventricular hemisphere and bilateral frontal–parietal subcortical area; normal supra- and infratentorial pericerebral liquid spaces; a symmetric ventricular system, with normal dimensions; structures of the median line in normal position; orbits and orbital content without anomalies; and paranasal sinuses with normal development and pneumatization. Magnetic resonance (MR) cerebral arteriography and venography indicated the following: internal carotid arteries symmetrically disposed, with a normal trajectory and caliber; anterior cerebral arteries and normal average bilaterally detached from the internal carotid, with no areas of stenosis or circumscribed dilation, with a homogeneous intralumenal signal; vertebral arteries, basilar artery, upper cerebral arteries and communicating arteries with a normal trajectory and caliber; hyperintense T1–T2 material, with a no-contrast outlet, which transversely occupied the sinuses and sigmoid on the right side; and a lesion with the same signal characteristics situated along the right sinus and extended towards the inferior sagittal sinus; the rest of the dural sinuses had no detectable lesions in the sequences observed.

2.2. Case 2

The second case we present was a 25-year-old female patient, with no pathological personal history, in the sixth day of puerperium after caesarian delivery, who came to the Emergency Unit of the Sf. Apostol Andrei Clinical Hospital in Constanta. The patient presented with cephalalgia, paresthesia of the right hemibody, a decrease in muscular strength in the right upper limb, and tonic–clonic convulsive spasms.

Following medical history, clinical examination and clinical and paraclinical investigations, it was decided that the patient should be admitted to the obstetrics and gynecology department, with the following diagnostics: 6-day puerperium after caesarian delivery, a mild form of secondary anemia and convulsion spasms to be investigated. She was oriented in time and space, was afebrile, had normally colored skin, had post-caesarian operation soft plaque in the process of healing (sutures removed), had a weak muscular system, was hypokinetic in the right upper and lower limbs, had a soft abdomen, and had a contracted uterus, had serosanguinous leaking, had supple breasts, was lactating, had a movement deficit in the right upper limb, with a lingual trauma mark.

The native cerebral CT scan highlighted a normality, with no detectable cranio-cerebral pathological modifications. The patient also underwent a native thorax CT and angiography for the pulmonary arteries, which did not indicate images suggestive of pulmonary thromboembolism.

A neurological consultation was requested when she was admitted to the gynecology department. When consulted, the patient was conscious, cooperative, oriented in time and space, had symmetrical pupils, was reactive on the median line, with a bitten tongue, showed right hemiparesis (upper limb 3/5 and lower limb 4/5) and had a bilaterally traced plantar cutaneous reflex. The diagnosis of tonic–clonic generalized convulsive spasm with tongue biting, and a post-critical status was given.

A cerebral and angiography MRI with venous time and reevaluation of the result was recommended, along with treatment with antiepileptic drugs (200 mg carbamazepine, 1/2 tablet per day; one intravenous ampoule of phenytoin 250 mg/5 mL, diluted in case of convulsive spasm), and a platelet antiaggregatory agent (one 75 mg aspenter tablet per day). Another neurological examination was requested on the same day, as the patient presented involuntary movements of the right lower limb. She received treatment with antiepileptic drugs (the dose was increased to one 200 mg carbamazepine tablet three times per day, plus one ampoule of intravenous phenytoin 250 mg/5 mL in 20 mL of normal saline solution), a cerebral depletive (20% mannitol, one 250 mL ampoule twice a day), a corticosteroid anti-inflammatory (one dexamethasone ampoule twice a day), a gastric protector (one 40 mg pantoprazole tablet per day), and heparin with a small molecular weight (one 0.6 mL enoxaparin sodium ampoule per day). The use of the steroid anti-inflammatory drugs in cerebral venous thrombosis was the choice of the treating physician.

On the second day of hospitalization, the patient underwent a native and contrast-enhanced cerebral MRI and angiography with arterial and venous sequence. The examination was suggestive of the left parietal cortical vein associated with ipsilateral superior parietal subcortical venous infarction and demyelinating lesions organized in the crown radiated and parietal on the right side, most probably with an ischemic vascular sublayer. This was the reason why the patient was transferred to the neurology department on the same day.

When admitted to the neurology department, on the second day of hospitalization, the patient was objectively examined and presented a good general health: a Glasgow Coma Scale (GCS) of 15 points, afebrile, conscious, cooperative, oriented in time and space, no deficit of the cranial nerves, a tongue with a traumatic trace, right hemiparesis 4/5 (predominantly brachial), right tactile hypesthesia; she denied any lost pregnancies, thrombophilia, or eclampsia.

On the third day of admission, biological material was drawn for the purpose of examining the hereditary thromboliphilia profile and was sent to the Clinical Service of Pathological Anatomy to be tested to identify mutations associated with cardiovascular disease and thrombophilia.

The test indicated the following genetic variants: heterozygous double genotype for the *C677T* and *A1298C* alleles in the *MTHFR* gene, mutant homozygous for the *V34L* allele in the *factor XIII* gene, wild type homozygous genotype *5G/5G* of the *PAI-1* gene and haplotype *A2/A2 (H2/H2)* of *EPCR*. The findings about and treatment of the patient can be seen in Figure 3.

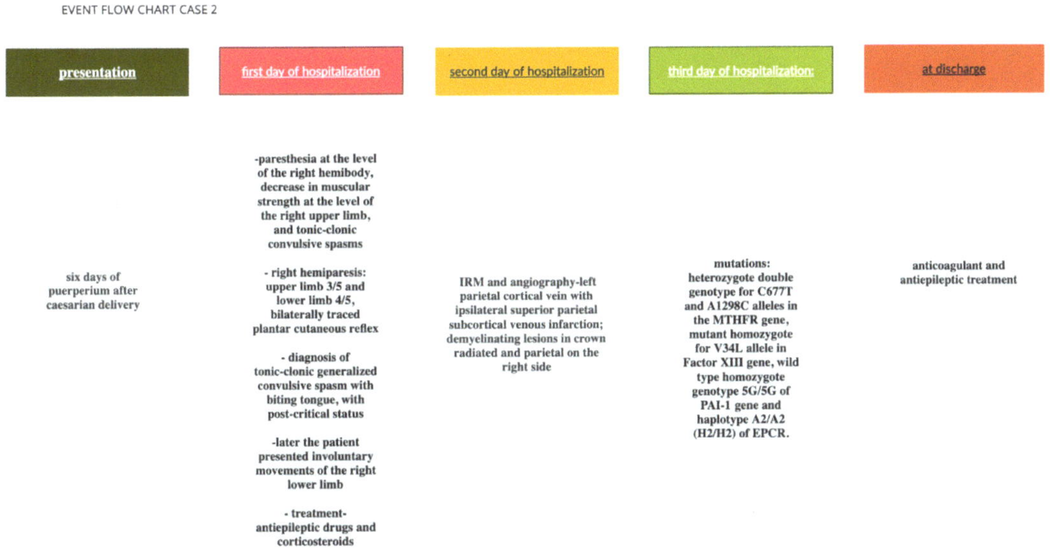

EVENT FLOW CHART CASE 2

presentation	first day of hospitalization	second day of hospitalization	third day of hospitalization:	at discharge
six days of puerperium after caesarian delivery	-paresthesia at the level of the right hemibody, decrease in muscular strength at the level of the right upper limb, and tonic-clonic convulsive spasms - right hemiparesis: upper limb 3/5 and lower limb 4/5, bilaterally traced plantar cutaneous reflex - diagnosis of tonic-clonic generalized convulsive spasm with biting tongue, with post-critical status -later the patient presented involuntary movements of the right lower limb - treatment- antiepileptic drugs and corticosteroids	IRM and angiography-left parietal cortical vein with ipsilateral superior parietal subcortical venous infarction; demyelinating lesions in crown radiated and parietal on the right side	mutations: heterozygote double genotype for C677T and A1298C alleles in the MTHFR gene, mutant homozygote for V34L allele in Factor XIII gene, wild type homozygote genotype 5G/5G of PAI-1 gene and haplotype A2/A2 (H2/H2) of EPCR.	anticoagulant and antiepileptic treatment

Figure 3. Event flow chart: Case 2.

During admission to the neurology department, the patient was treated with a cerebral depletive (20% mannitol, 250 mL every 12 h for 5 days), hydro-electrolytic rebalancing (500 mL normal saline solution two times a day), heparin with low molecular weight (one 0.6 mL enoxaparin sodium ampoule every 12 h), painkillers (one metamizole ampoule every 12 h), antiepileptic medicines (one 200 mg carbamazepine tablet three times a day), a corticosteroid anti-inflammatory (dexamethasone, 1/2 ampoule every 12 h), benzodiazepine (one ampoule of intravenous diazepam slowly in 10 mL of normal saline solution, in case of convulsive spasm), a gastric protector (one 40 mg pantoprazole tablet per day), an oral anticoagulant (4 mg acenocoumarol, 1/2 tablet, according to the INR dosage; the patient was administered this medicine on the seventh day of admission). She recovered well.

When discharged, the patient continued to take oral anticoagulants (4 mg acenocoumarol, 1/2 tablet per day, according to the INR dosage on days 7 and 14, and on a monthly basis thereafter), antiepileptic medicines (200 mg carbamazepine, 1/2 tablet three times a day), and painkillers (one metamizole tablet if necessary).

When discharged, the patient was conscious, cooperative, oriented in time and space, without stiffness in the back of the head, had no nystagmus, showed normal ocular motricity, denied diplopia, had possible deglutition for liquid and solid food, displayed symmetric facies, had no movement deficits, had no superficial tactile sensitivity or coordination disorders and showed a cutaneous plantar reflex with bilateral flexion. The images of the MRI can be seen below in Figure 4.

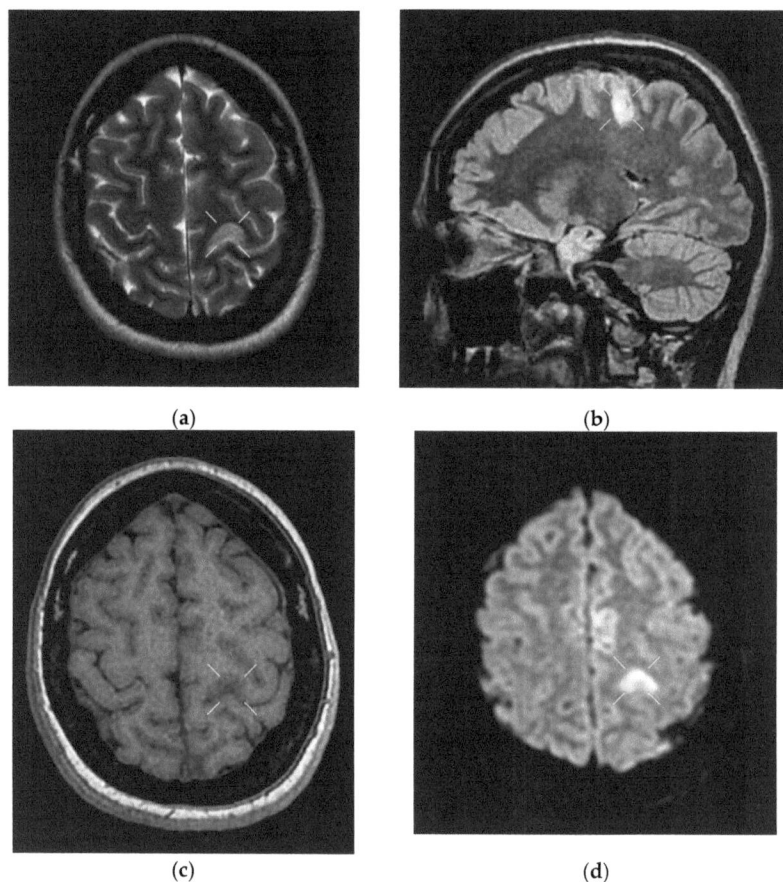

Figure 4. *Cont.*

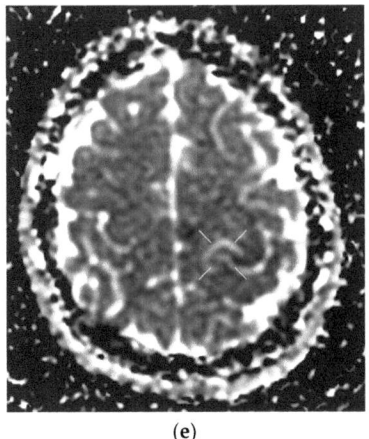
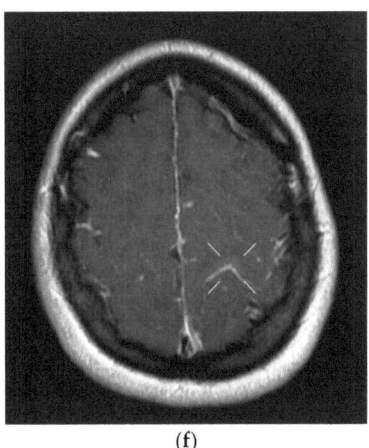

(e) (f)

Figure 4. Native and contrast-enhanced cerebral MRI and angiography with arterial and venous sequencing, performed on the second day of hospitalization. The scan indicates thrombosis of the left parietal cortical vein associated with ipsilateral superior parietal subcortical venous infarction—(**a**) band in T2 and FLAIR hypersignal. (**b**) band in T2 and FLAIR hypersignal. (**c**) T1 hyposignal. (**d**) restrictive in diffusion coefficient. (**e**) restrictive in diffusion coefficient. (**f**) restrictive in diffusion coefficient with weak contrast enhancement. Demyelinating lesions are organized in the crown, radiated and parietal on the right side, most probably with an ischemic vascular sublayer. The native cranio-cerebral and post-contrast MRI examination with arterial and venous angiographic sequencing highlighted the following: normal pericerebral liquid spaces; a symmetric ventricular system, with normal dimensions; an area in the hypersignal band T2, and a FLAIR/iso-hypo signal T1, with restricted diffusion weighing, weak gadolinophilia, axial dimensions of about 9/16 mm, located subcortically and parietally on the upper left side; two millimeter focal points of the T2 and FLAIR hypersignal, with no diffusion restrictions or detectable contrast outlet organized in the crown, radiated and parietal subcortical on the right side, in the area adjacent to the dorsal horn of the VL; structures of the median line in the right position; orbits and orbital content without anomalies; paranasal sinuses with normal development and pneumatization; the absence of images evoking hemorrhagic accumulations or masses with a tumor sublayer; symmetrically disposed internal carotid arteries with normal trajectories and caliber; a normal bilateral carotid siphon with no position or extrinsic compression anomalies, with homogeneous intensity of the intralumenal signal; anterior and middle cerebral arteries that were normally detached from the internal carotid on both sides, without any areas of inferior longitudinal stenosis with an aspect within the normal limits; transverse and symmetric sigmoid sinuses, without lesions; the rest of the patient's evaluable venous segments did not present any defect in the lumen signal.

3. Discussion

The diagnoses of the cases presented herein were based on the clinical manifestations, neurological objective examinations, imaging investigations, and biological profiles.

The first case described was a 40-year-old female patient, who had and a voluntary abortion. Following the imaging investigations, the diagnosis of sigmoid sinus and right lateral sinus thrombosis of the lower sagittal sinus and right sinus was confirmed, associated with right temporal cortical–subcortical subacute hemorrhage. The following genotypes were identified for the identification of the hereditary thrombophilia profile: heterozygous for V factor mutation *H1299R* (R2), heterozygous for mutation *4G* of *PAI-1*, and haplotype *A1/A2* of *EPCR*.

The second case was a young female patient, on day 6 of the puerperium after caesarian delivery. As the diagnosis was confirmed after the imaging investigations, namely, thrombosis of the left parietal cortical vein associated with ipsilateral superior parietal subcortical venous infarction. The hereditary thrombophilia test indicated the following genetic variants: heterozygous double genotype for the *C677T* and *A1298C* alleles in the *MTHFR* gene, mutant homozygous for the *V34L* allele in *factor XIII* gene, wild type homozygous genotype 5G/5G of *PAI-1*, and haplotype A2/A2 (H2/H2) of *EPCR*. According to the literature, CVST appeared 13 times more often during the puerperium than throughout pregnancy [12].

The patient also had generalized tonic–clonic convulsions. This case demonstrates the critical nature of a wide differential diagnosis in women with postpartum seizures. While eclampsia is the most frequent source of these instances, additional uncommon illnesses can develop throughout the puerperium which necessitate markedly different care strategies. MRI has considerable sensitivity for detecting the existence of cerebral venous thrombosis; therefore, it should be used, if feasible, to aid in diagnosis. In summary, women's healthcare practitioners can enhance postpartum patient care by evaluating etiologies other than eclampsia and seeking diagnostics that can differentiate them.

During admission, the progression of the two patients presented herein rapidly became favorable, even though both of them presented with intracerebral hemorrhage.

The uniqueness of our cases consisted first of the neurological symptomatology of the patient in the first case, which was significant, as she presented with motor deficits and aphasia. The first patient also presented with subacute cerebral hemorrhage and thrombosis of several sinus areas. In this patient, we also observed mutations associated with cardiovascular disease and thrombophilia. Furthermore, the second patient presented with sensory and motor impairments, and tonic–clonic convulsive spasms and mutations associated with cardiovascular disease and thrombophilia. Imaging showed that the left parietal cortical vein was associated with ipsilateral superior parietal subcortical venous infarction.

Although both patients had procoagulant changes due to genetic mutations in their coagulation gene profiles, neither patient had a pathological episode until the hospitalizations reported on, which shows the extreme importance of pregnancy in the development of cerebral venous thrombosis, and in the case of the first patient, the even greater importance of genital infection and incomplete abortion in the development of cerebral venous thrombosis.

In these two cases, pregnancy-related cerebral venous thrombosis increased the risk of stroke and led to cerebral hemorrhage. Hemorrhagic infarctions are independent indicators of poor prognosis; therefore, early detection and treatment are critical. As the postpartum and post-abortion situations have distinct hemodynamic properties, we hypothesized that cerebral venous thrombosis would appear differently in these phases, as it did in our patients, but the prognosis and outcome were both favorable.

The prognosis of the two patients was favorable, with complete functional recovery. Even though venous cerebral thrombosis has a severe clinical presentation that may endanger the patient's life, the application of adequate therapeutic measures in due time leads to recovery.

Physiological changes occur throughout pregnancy that encourage the appearance of venous thromboembolism. Increased coagulation factor production and decreased fibrinolytic activity lead to a physiological hypercoagulant state. Additionally, the pressure exerted by the larger uterus decreases blood flow and may potentially induce stasis. Additionally, acute blood loss after childbirth, postpartum infection and extended bed rest all significantly enhance the risk of venous thromboembolism, especially in patients with mutations associated with cardiovascular disease and thrombophilia. In our first patient, another CVT risk factor besides the pregnancy interruption and mutations was the infection for which the patient received treatment with antibiotics.

A solitary prothrombotic factor might not have been a substantial risk factor for CVT in our patients and may not be common. In physiological conditions associated with increased sensitivity to thrombosis, such as pregnancy, puerperium, and abortion, the occurrence of numerous prothrombotic states can turn the situation in favor of thrombosis. The identification of intrinsic prothrombotic conditions can have a considerable influence on the long-term treatment of puerperal CVT, particularly in terms of oral anticoagulant duration, future pregnancies, and the use of estrogen-containing oral contraceptives.

Cerebral venous thrombosis is a very uncommon disorder that may result in cerebral infarction by raising venous and capillary pressure, thereby impairing cerebral perfusion [13]. The condition is caused by a mismatch between the coagulation and anticoagulation systems, which results in venous outflow obstruction and metabolic disorders in brain cells. Increased capillary pressure facilitates hemorrhagic transition, which happens more often in this condition than in other ischemic states.

In the article of Piazza, a case of cerebral venous thrombosis is described, and it resembles the cases presented in this study. The patient was young and came to the hospital for severe headaches on the left side, nausea, photophobia, and phonophobia. Symptoms were reduced by the treatment; thus, the patient was discharged. However, after 12 h, she came back, reporting recurrent severe headaches. The venogram by magnetic resonance revealed thrombosis of the transverse sinus, left sigmoid and internal proximal jugular vein. The patient started the treatment with heparin of low molecular weight; then she took an oral anticoagulant, warfarin. For the hereditary thrombophilia profile, the test described heterozygosity for the mutation of the V Leiden factor [14].

4. Conclusions

The coexistence of risk factors in young patients increases the risk of developing cerebral venous thrombosis. Early diagnosis and treatment of cerebral venous thrombosis are critical for a positive outcome with no neurological deficits.

Maternal stroke, characterized as a stroke that occurs during pregnancy or the postpartum period, is becoming a more acknowledged cause of maternal death and disability. Individuals suffering cerebral venous thrombosis must be hospitalized in a stroke unit or neurology clinic, where they should receive triple therapy—antithrombotic therapy; symptomatic therapy; and when necessary, etiologic therapy. These therapies are used identically in young women with sex-specific risk factors and in all other patients with cerebral venous thrombosis.

Despite cerebral venous thrombosis being an uncommon complication of pregnancy, it must be evaluated in differential diagnoses, particularly when a pregnant woman or a woman who has had an abortion presents with an abrupt neurological impairment that raises suspicion of ischemic disease. Delayed diagnosis can be explained by a number of factors, including the disease's rareness, the disease's late presentation, the vague symptoms that are typically attributed to pregnancy, the multiple restrictions associated with examining a pregnant woman, avoidance of imaging examinations and the presumably reduced specificity of imaging studies.

While early detection and effective treatment are strongly related to a favorable outcome, the incidence and diversity of pregnancy-related CVT imply that clinicians seem to have little knowledge of its course and that diagnosis is often incorrect or delayed. The features of CVT vary according to the physiological characteristics of pregnant and postpartum women; a significant rate of cerebral infarction is seen in pregnant CVT patients. Neurological symptoms, including headaches and vision loss, along with motor and sensory impairments and seizures, during pregnancy, must alert clinicians to the possibility of CVT.

In summary, oral contraceptive use and pregnancy or puerperium coincide with a significant number of cerebral venous thrombosis cases in young women, often in conjunction with other prothrombotic risk factors, most notably congenital thrombophilia. Although the clinical manifestations, diagnostic testing, and treatment of these cerebral venous thrombosis cases are non-specific, the overall prognosis is favorable, with full recovery occurring in the majority of patients. Future pregnancies are not contraindicated; however, all estrogen-based contraception is permanently contraindicated.

Author Contributions: Conceptualization, A.D.A. and L.F.M.; methodology, A.D.A.; software, L.F.M.; validation, A.D.A., A.Z.S. and L.F.M.; formal analysis, A.D.A., A.Z.S. and L.F.M.; investigation, A.D.A., A.Z.S. and L.F.M.; resources, A.D.A., A.Z.S. and L.F.M.; data curation, A.D.A., A.Z.S. and L.F.M.; writing—original draft preparation, A.Z.S., L.A.Z. and C.A.S.; writing—review and editing, A.Z.S. and S.D.A.; visualization, S.C.C.; supervision, A.D.A. and L.F.M.; project administration, A.D.A. and L.F.M.; funding acquisition, A.D.A. and L.F.M. All authors have read and agreed to the published version of the manuscript.

Funding: This research received no external funding.

Institutional Review Board Statement: The study was conducted according to the guidelines of the Declaration of Helsinki and approved by the Ethics Committee of Sf Apostol Andrei Clinical County Hospital of Constanta (protocol code 30/1 November 2021).

Informed Consent Statement: Informed consent was obtained from all subjects involved in the study.

Data Availability Statement: Third-party data restrictions apply to the availability of these data. The data were obtained from Constanta's Sf Apostol Andrei County Emergency Clinical Hospital and are available from the authors with the permission of the Institutional Ethics Committee of Clinical Studies of the Constanta's Sf Apostol Andrei County Emergency Clinical Hospital.

Conflicts of Interest: The authors declare no conflict of interest.

References

1. Liang, Z.-W.; Gao, W.-L.; Feng, L.-M. Clinical characteristics and prognosis of cerebral venous thrombosis in Chinese women during pregnancy and puerperium. *Sci. Rep.* **2017**, *7*, 43866. [CrossRef] [PubMed]
2. Bousser, M.-G.; Ferro, J.M. Cerebral venous thrombosis: An update. *Lancet Neurol.* **2007**, *6*, 162–170. [CrossRef]
3. Mubarak, F.; Azeemuddin, M.; Anwar, S.; Nizamani, W.; Beg, M. In-hospital imaging prevalence, patterns of neurological involvement in cerebral venous sinus thrombosis: Analysis from Pakistan. *J. Adv. Med. Med. Res.* **2018**, *25*, 1–9. [CrossRef]
4. Bano, S.; Farooq, M.U.; Nazir, S.; Aslam, A.; Tariq, A.; Javed, M.A.; Rehman, H.; Numan, A. Structural imaging characteristic, clinical features and risk factors of cerebral venous sinus thrombosis: A prospective cross-sectional analysis from a tertiary care hospital in Pakistan. *Diagnostics* **2021**, *11*, 958. [CrossRef] [PubMed]
5. Lanska, D.J.; Kryscio, R.J. Risk factors for peripartum and postpartum stroke and intracranial venous thrombosis. *Stroke* **2000**, *31*, 1274–1282. [CrossRef] [PubMed]
6. Bajko, Z.; Motataianu, A.; Stoian, A.; Barcutean, L.; Andone, S.; Maier, S.; Drăghici, I.-A.; Cioban, A.; Balasa, R. Gender differences in risk factor profile and clinical characteristics in 89 consecutive cases of cerebral venous thrombosis. *J. Clin. Med.* **2021**, *10*, 1382. [CrossRef] [PubMed]
7. Ferro, J.M.; Crassard, I.; Coutinho, J.M.; Canhão, P.; Barinagarrementeria, F.; Cucchiara, B.; Derex, L.; Lichy, C.; Masjuan, J.; Massaro, A.; et al. Decompressive surgery in cerebrovenous thrombosis: A multicenter registry and a systematic review of individual patient data. *Stroke* **2011**, *42*, 2825–2831. [CrossRef] [PubMed]
8. Aaron, S.; Alexander, M.; Moorthy, R.K.; Mani, S.; Mathew, V.; Patil, A.K.B.; Sivadasan, A.; Nair, S.; Joseph, M.; Thomas, M.; et al. Decompressive craniectomy in cerebral venous thrombosis: A single centre experience. *J. Neurol. Neurosurg. Psychiatry* **2013**, *84*, 995–1000. [CrossRef] [PubMed]
9. Ferro, J.M.; Bousser, M.-G.; Canhão, P.; Coutinho, J.M.; Crassard, I.; Dentali, F.; di Minno, M.; Maino, A.; Martinelli, I.; Masuhr, F.; et al. European Stroke Organization guideline for the diagnosis and treatment of cerebral venous thrombosis—Endorsed by the European Academy of Neurology. *Eur. Stroke J.* **2017**, *2*, 195–221. [CrossRef] [PubMed]
10. Swartz, R.H.; Cayley, M.L.; Foley, N.; Ladhani, N.N.N.; Leffert, L.; Bushnell, C.; McClure, J.A.; Lindsay, M.P. The incidence of pregnancy-related stroke: A systematic review and meta-analysis. *Int. J. Stroke* **2017**, *12*, 687–697. [CrossRef] [PubMed]
11. Kristoffersen, E.S.; Harper, C.E.; Vetvik, K.G.; Faiz, K.W. Cerebral venous thrombosis-epidemiology, diagnosis and treatment. *Tidsskr. Den Nor. Legeforening* **2018**, *138*. [CrossRef]
12. Cantú, C.; Barinagarrementeria, F. Cerebral venous thrombosis associated with pregnancy and puerperium. *Stroke* **1993**, *24*, 1880–1884. [CrossRef] [PubMed]
13. Pizzi, M.A.; Alejos, D.A.; Siegel, J.L.; Kim, B.Y.S.; Miller, D.A.; Freeman, W.D. Cerebral venous thrombosis associated with intracranial hemorrhage and timing of anticoagulation after hemicraniectomy. *J. Stroke Cerebrovasc. Dis.* **2016**, *25*, 2312–2316. [CrossRef] [PubMed]
14. Piazza, G. Cerebral Venous Thrombosis. *Circulation* **2012**, *125*, 1704–1709. [CrossRef] [PubMed]

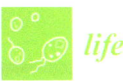

Case Report

Cerebral Venous Sinus Thrombosis Following an mRNA COVID-19 Vaccination and Recent Oral Contraceptive Use

Timothy C. Frommeyer [1,*], Tongfan Wu [1], Michael M. Gilbert [1], Garrett V. Brittain [1] and Stephen P. Fuqua [2]

1. Department of Pharmacology & Toxicology, Boonshoft School of Medicine, Wright State University, Dayton, OH 45435, USA
2. Department of Neurology, Boonshoft School of Medicine, Wright State University, Dayton, OH 45435, USA
* Correspondence: tcfrommeyer@gmail.com

Abstract: Rising concerns of cerebral venous sinus thrombosis (CVST) and other forms of venous thromboembolism have been associated with the SARS-CoV-2 vaccinations. Adverse effects with vector-based vaccines are well documented in the literature, while less is known about the mRNA vaccines. This report documents a case of CVST in a 32-year-old female patient who received her second Pfizer mRNA COVID-19 vaccination 16 days prior to hospital admission and had started oral combined contraceptives approximately 4 months beforehand. Clinicians should be cognizant of the possibility that mRNA vaccines, when combined with other risk factors like oral contraceptive pill use, may enhance one's hypercoagulable status.

Keywords: cerebral venous thrombosis; COVID-19; vaccination; oral contraception; mRNA

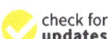

Citation: Frommeyer, T.C.; Wu, T.; Gilbert, M.M.; Brittain, G.V.; Fuqua, S.P. Cerebral Venous Sinus Thrombosis Following an mRNA COVID-19 Vaccination and Recent Oral Contraceptive Use. *Life* **2023**, *13*, 464. https://doi.org/10.3390/life13020464

Academic Editors: Morayma Reyes Gil, Jean Claude SADIK, Dafin Fior Mureşanu and Dragos Catalin Jianu

Received: 21 November 2022
Revised: 25 January 2023
Accepted: 1 February 2023
Published: 7 February 2023

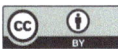

Copyright: © 2023 by the authors. Licensee MDPI, Basel, Switzerland. This article is an open access article distributed under the terms and conditions of the Creative Commons Attribution (CC BY) license (https://creativecommons.org/licenses/by/4.0/).

1. Introduction

Cerebral venous sinus thrombosis (CVST) is a rare and potentially fatal cause of stroke. It can present with a multitude of signs and symptoms, which make it difficult to differentiate from other neurological conditions. As such, it is frequently overlooked due to the vague nature of its clinical and radiological presentation, making CVST a challenging diagnosis. Early recognition of its presentation and associated symptoms with prompt treatment can improve overall health outcomes and prognosis in patients [1].

CVST accounts for 0.5–1% of all strokes and is estimated to occur more often in females, with a 3:1 female-to-male ratio [2,3]. This stroke subtype is a multifactorial disease with 85% of affected adults having at least one risk factor [4]. While the pathophysiology is not fully understood, the main risk factors include prothrombotic conditions such as factor V Leiden, antiphospholipid syndrome, protein C deficiency, and antithrombin III deficiency [1,5]. Additional risk factors include infections, mechanical trauma, vasculitis, intracranial defects, hematological conditions, systemic diseases, and medications such as oral contraceptives pills (OCPs) [1].

Combined OCPs containing ethinylestradiol and progestogen are associated with an increased risk of venous thromboembolism (VTE) in women of reproductive age [6,7]. This relationship is related to OCP-induced changes in coagulation and fibrinolysis, which alters the hemostatic balance towards a prothrombotic direction [8,9]. In fact, the use of OCPs has been shown to increase the odds of CVST by 5- to 22-fold [10]. Another known risk factor for VTE that has recently emerged is infection with the novel coronavirus, SARS-CoV-2 [11]. In patients with combined OCPs, infection with COVID-19 is thought to aggravate the risk of VTE and strokes [12]. While the VTE risks of OCPs and COVID-19 are well-known, less is known about the thromboembolic effects of mRNA COVID-19 vaccines, especially in combination with OCPs.

While COVID-19 vaccination administrations are being widely conducted to overcome the pandemic, an emerging concern about thromboembolic side effects has been realized. A case series of CVST and thrombocytopenia associated with virus vector COVID-19 vaccines

(Johnson & Johnson (New Brunswick, NJ, USA); AstraZeneca (Cambridge, UK)) has been reported [13–17]. This vaccine associated syndrome, called vaccine-induced immune thrombocytopenia (VITT), has a pathogenesis similar to heparin-induced thrombocytopenia via immune-mediated platelet activation. Now widely recognized, the emergence of VITT resulted in regulatory actions by the Center for Disease Control and Prevention (CDC) and the Food and Drug Administration (FDA) in 2021.

Conversely, the thromboembolic side effects of mRNA COVID-19 vaccines (Pfizer (New York, NY, USA); Moderna (Cambridge, MA, USA)) have been rarely reported, with only a few case reports published within medical literature [18–23]. The underlying pathogenesis and clinical characteristic of VTE after mRNA COVID-19 vaccines has not been well explored when compared with VITT induced by virus vector COVID-19 vaccines. In addition, the relationship between VTE, COVID-19 vaccination, and OCP use in women of reproductive age is not well understood. Therefore, we have reported a rare case of CVST in a female on OCPs after an mRNA Pfizer COVID vaccination.

2. Case

A 32-year-old female with a history of depression and acne was presented to the Emergency Department (ED) with concern for stroke. She received her second Pfizer mRNA COVID-19 vaccination 16 days prior to admission and started oral combined contraceptives (OCPs) approximately 4 months prior. The patient does not have a personal or family history of atypical headaches, hypercoagulation disorders/thrombosis or autoimmune disease. She does not use tobacco products. Medications prior to admission included norgestimate-ethinyl estradioL (TRINESSA, 28,) 0.18/0.215/0.25 mg-35 mcg (28) Tablet, Sulfacetamide Sodium 10 % Cleanser, and Dapsone (ACZONE) 5 % topical gel. The patient was brought to the ED by her mother when she fell at home and was unable to talk or ambulate. She presented with aphasia, right hemiplegia, and collapse, subsequently resulting in a stroke alert upon arrival. Three days prior to presentation, the patient began to develop new onset headaches with no other associated symptoms. She was seen at an urgent care twice, where she was diagnosed with a migraine and prescribed sumatriptan and ibuprofen. The patient opted to stay with her parents due to the increasing severity of headaches.

Upon arrival to the ED, the patient's vitals were blood pressure of 114/80 mmHg with a MAP of 93 mmHg, P 78 bpm, oxygen saturation of 100% on room air, axillary temperature of 96.9 °F (36.1 °C) and weight of 67.1 kg. The patient was awake and alert but unable to answer orientation questions secondary to expressive aphasia. She was able to follow most commands, however, she struggled with complex commands. Neurological physical exam findings were significant for expressive aphasia, left superior hemianopsia, right facial droop, 3/5 left shoulder strength (Motor strength scale 1 to 5: 0 = no muscle contraction; 1 = flicker or trace of contraction is seen; 2 = active movement in the same plane, not against gravity; 3 = active movement against gravity but not resistance; 4 = active movement against gravity with some resistance; 5 = active movement against gravity with full resistance), 1/5 right shoulder strength, flaccid paralysis of her right upper extremity and bilateral lower extremities. Deep tendon reflexes were all 2/4 except for 3 s at the right brachioradialis and bilateral knees. Upgoing Babinski reflex was noted on the right side but not the left side. Sensation was decreased on the right upper extremity compared with the left; bilateral lower extremities sensations were intact.

The patient proceeded with the stroke workup. CT of the head showed relative hyper density of the superior sagittal, left transverse, and straight sinuses suggesting dural venous sinus thrombosis. No evidence of parenchymal or extra-axial hemorrhage were noted. CT angiogram of the head and neck revealed occlusion of the superior sagittal sinus, left transverse and sigmoid sinuses extending into the internal jugular vein, straight sinus, left internal cerebral vein. Nonocclusive thrombus involves the vein of Galen; right transverse sinus with normal contrast opacification of the right sigmoid sinus. There was no evidence of arterial stenosis, occlusion, or aneurysm in the head. Bilateral carotid systems and vertebral arteries were all enhanced normally. Extravascular findings were unremarkable. Her initial NIH Stroke Score (NIHSS) was 19. In the absence of other inciting injuries or underlying medical comorbidities, cerebral venous sinus thrombosis secondary to contraceptive use, COVID vaccinations, underlying autoimmune process, and occult malignancy was suspected. The patient was started with a high-dose heparin drip to prevent thrombus extension and inpatient seizure precautions with close neurologic monitoring. The patient was then transferred to a larger hospital for further workup and neurocritical management.

Additional labs showed Complete Blood Count (CBC) within acceptable limits, Basic Metabolic Panel (BMP) significant with glucose of 142 mg/dL, normal cardiac troponin level, and a negative urine drug screen. Urinalysis showed a small amount of blood but no evidence of infection. Genetic hypercoagulable labs, including antinuclear antibody, antineutrophil cytoplasmic antibodies, anti-cardiolipin, anti-Beta-2-glycoprotein, Factor V Leiden, and a lupus anticoagulant assay, were also unremarkable. Several hypercoagulable tests including antithrombin, protein C, and protein S were deferred, as results would have been confounded by the acute thrombotic event. Of note, the patient had abnormal findings on the lipid panel consisting of high cholesterol, triglyceride, and VLDL, and a low HDL level. Ultrasound Venous Doppler of the bilateral lower extremities showed no deep vein thrombosis. MRI brain/MRV (Magnetic Resonance Imaging (MRI) is a technique that uses magnetic fields and computer-generated radio waves to create images of organs and tissues in your body. Magnetic Resonance Venography (MRV) uses magnetic resonance technology and intravenous contrast dye to visualize the veins. Diffusion-Weighted Imaging (DWI) is a form of MRI that uses the diffusion of water molecules to generate images) with and without contrast confirmed acute venous infarct in the left subcortical frontal and parietal lobes as well as the left splenium of the corpus callosum. Thrombosis of the superior sagittal sinus, cortical veins, straight sinus, left internal cerebral vein, vein of Galen and the bilateral transverse sinuses, as well as the left sigmoid sinus, were also confirmed. A small hemorrhagic focus in the left occipital lobe was noted and was likely venous hemorrhages (Figures 1 and 2). The final diagnosis was diffuse cerebral venous sinus thrombosis likely related to OCP use with possible contribution by recent COVID vaccination.

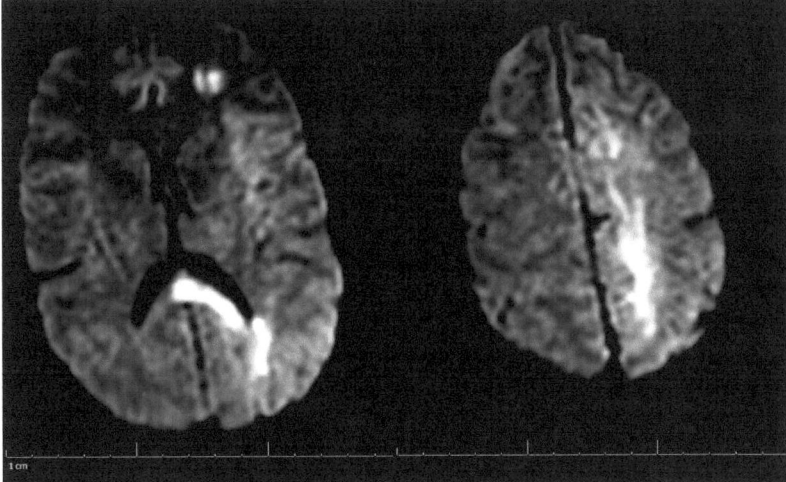

Figure 1. MRI of the Brain without contrast (DWI) (Magnetic Resonance Imaging (MRI) is a technique that uses magnetic fields and computer generated radio waves to create images of organs and tissues in your body. Magnetic Resonance Venography (MRV) uses magnetic resonance technology and intravenous contrast dye to visualize the veins. Diffusion-Weighted Imaging (DWI) is a form of MRI that uses the diffusion of water molecules to generate images).

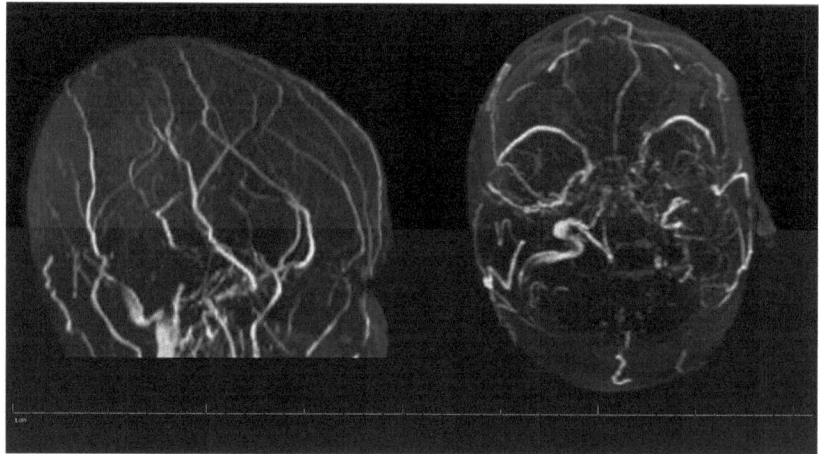

Figure 2. MRV of the Head during Hospital Admission.

On hospital day two, the patient remained more aphasic than would be expected by her imaging results. A 24-h video electroencephalogram (EEG) was ordered to rule out nonconvulsive seizure activity secondary to CVST. The EEG did not show seizure activity but did show a high burden of abnormal epileptiform discharges, and levetiracetam (Keppra) 1000 mg twice daily was started for seizure prophylaxis. By hospital day three, the patient has significantly improved in motor strength, speech, and activity. NIHSS at this time was three. She was discontinued on the heparin drip and started on rivaroxaban (Xarelto), for long-term thrombus stabilization and prophylaxis against future clotting events, and atorvastatin (Lipitor) 40 mg. Her peripherally inserted central catheter (PICC) line, foley catheter, and intravenous fluids were also discontinued and she was transferred to a stepdown unit. She continued to improve clinically and was discharged on hospital day six to acute rehabilitation remaining on current medications.

On her outpatient neurology clinic follow-up six weeks later, the patient was doing very well and largely back to her baseline. She still endorsed mild headaches about every other day and was using acetaminophen (Tylenol) for pain relief. The patient had been progressing well from attending regular physical therapy, occupational therapy, and speech therapy. Due to no seizure-like events, Keppra was to be weaned off to 500 mg every two weeks. Decreased Tylenol use was also suggested to avoid a rebound phenomenon. She was medically cleared to return to work and driving. Her three-month post-hospitalization MRV of the head showed stable left occipital intraparenchymal hemorrhage concerns for venous hemorrhage; partial thrombosis of the left transverse sinus improved in appearance compared with the previous examination three months ago; unremarkable appearance to the superior sagittal sinus, internal cerebral veins, inferior sagittal sinus, right transverse sinus, right and left sigmoid sinuses and internal jugular veins (Figure 3). A lipid panel showed improvement from inpatient levels. At the following telemedicine visit five months later, the patient reported only residual right hand weakness associated with reduced hand grip, but no further headaches. She discontinued Keppra at her last visit and has tolerated it well. Based on her most recent MRV, lipid panel, and clinical improvement, Xarelto and Lipitor were discontinued. The patient was advised to continue to follow a healthy diet and exercise to keep cholesterol under control, and avoid estrogen-containing birth control. There are no limitations on her activities from a neurological perspective. Another follow-up was scheduled in six months to ensure there are no new concerns, however, the patient did not show for this visit.

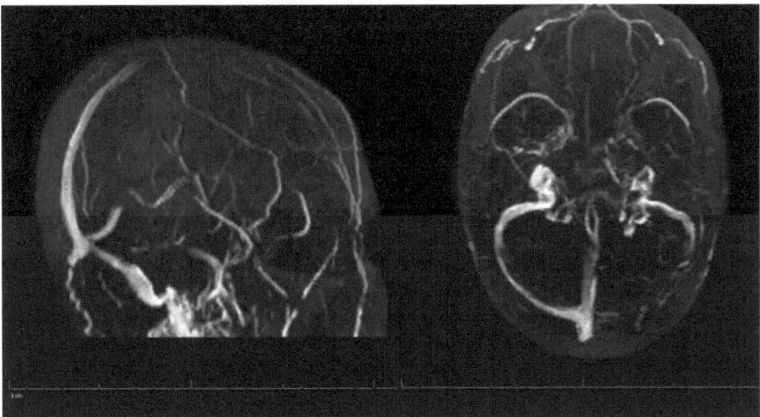

Figure 3. MRV of the Head on 3-Months Post-Hospitalization.

3. Discussion

According to our literature review, this is the first published case report of CVST following recent completion of the Pfizer mRNA COVID-19 vaccination series alongside oral combined contraceptives in a reproductive age female in the United States. Dias and colleagues also reported a similar phenomenon in Portugal in a 47 year old female, though the length of time the patient had been on OCPs is unclear [19]. Globally, it appears the reporting rate of unexpected cerebral venous thrombosis for post COVID-19 mRNA vaccinations is 0.9% for mRNA-1273 (Moderna) and 0.4% for BNT1626b2 mRNA (Pfizer) [20]. Of note, this data may be challenging to assess due to differing databases. Park and colleagues analyzed the pharmacovigilance database from the World Health Organization and found 756 (0.07%) cases of cerebral venous thrombosis events out of 1,154,023 sampled mRNA COVID19 vaccines (620 (0.05% for Moderna, and 136 (0.01%) for Pfizer) [24]. In Singapore, as of 31 May 2021, 4,047,651 million doses of the mRNA vaccine had been delivered with three possible COVID-19 vaccine associated cerebral venous thrombosis events [20]. Finally, one recent systematic review found 11 cases of CVST that occurred following mRNA vaccinations [25]. Thus, as the data continues to evolve, the importance of quick recognition of cerebral venous thrombosis events is critical for patient outcomes.

The pathophysiology of mRNA vaccine-induced VTE remains unclear, but some have proposed it may be due to endothelial dysfunction [20,21]. More specifically, the disruption of the blood-brain barrier may allow the spike glycoprotein to directly cause platelet aggregation, promote IL-6 inflammatory response, and activation of the alternative complement pathway [20,21]. This is in contrast to the proposed VITT mediated reaction which is due to PF4-reactive antibodies [16]. The mechanism behind endothelial dysregulation supports why OCPs, and other risk factors including hematologic disease or autoimmune disease, may increase the risk of a hypercoagulable state post-COVID19 mRNA vaccination. More specifically, OCPs affect blood clotting by increasing plasma fibrinogen, the activity of coagulation factors, and platelet activity while decreasing antithrombin III [26]. Thus, when combined with mRNA vaccines, a hypercoagulable state could potentially lead to obstruction of the cerebral sinuses when a thrombus does not resolve. It is important to consider that the COVID-19 infection has also been demonstrated to cause a hypercoagulable state and is responsible for a number of CVST's [27–29]. The risk of a COVID-19 infection itself may be more likely to cause CVST in comparison to the mRNA vaccines [30]. More specifically, Taquet and colleges found the incidence of cerebral venous thrombosis two weeks after a COVID-19 diagnosis to be 42.8 million people (95% CI 28.5–64.2), which was significantly higher than in a matched cohort of people who received an mRNA vaccine (RR = 6.33, 95% CI 1.87–21.40, $p = 0.00014$) [30]. Another study analyzed over 200 different hospitals and found the incidence of CVST in COVID-19 hospitalized patients to be 231 per 100,000 person years (95% CI, 152.1–350.8) [31]. The mechanism appears to be similarly mediated through endothelial damage caused by viral protein binding to the ACE-2 receptor, resulting in endothelial damage promoting a hypercoagulable state [27].

It is very possible that this patient's stroke was provoked by her recent COVID-19 vaccine, however, it is difficult to definitively prove. While we believe that the risk of coagulopathy provoked by mRNA vaccines should be further investigated, we do recognize that this presentation could be coincidental and not directly associated with the mRNA vaccination. CVST accounts for roughly 0.5–0.7% of all strokes and is commonly seen in younger populations [32]. It is more common in females than males, and a multitude of risk factors exist including genetic thrombophilia, infectious etiologies, and trauma [33]. In our patient, the CVST could have been due to OCPs alone, or there may be an underlying hematologic disorder that was not identified upon initial testing. Therefore, the patient would benefit from seeing a hematologist for further workups of genetic hypercoagulable conditions, including antithrombin, protein C, protein S, heparin induced thrombocytopenia antibodies, and specific coagulation factor activity levels.

In sum, the literature on COVID-19 vaccination and COVID-19 infections is challenging to report. Large data sets and the continually evolving COVID-19 pandemic make it difficult to draw specific conclusions. However, it is important for clinicians to consider that COVID-19 or mRNA vaccinations may predispose patients with risk factors for hypercoagulable states to CVSTs.

4. Conclusions

This case report shows one rare instance of CVST in a patient who received her second dose of the mRNA vaccination and was recently put on OCPs. This is not to deter the usage of mRNA vaccination as demonstrated by an increased risk for CVST for patients who are infected with COVID-19. However, other risk factors, such as OCPs that result in a hypercoagulable state, may increase the risk for CVST in patients who receive the mRNA vaccination. Clinicians should consider COVID-19 vaccine-induced CVST in patients recently vaccinated. Early diagnosis and treatment may ultimately improve health outcomes.

Author Contributions: Conceptualization, T.C.F. and S.P.F.; investigation, T.C.F., G.V.B. and S.P.F.; writing—original draft preparation, T.C.F., T.W., M.M.G. and G.V.B.; writing—review and editing, T.C.F., T.W., M.M.G. and G.V.B. and S.P.F.; visualization, S.P.F.; supervision, S.P.F.; project administration, S.P.F. All authors have read and agreed to the published version of the manuscript.

Funding: This research was funded in part by an unrestricted grant from the Wright State University Department of Pharmacology and Toxicology.

Institutional Review Board Statement: Ethical review and approval were waived for this study as study sample is less than 3 patients and patient is de-identified.

Informed Consent Statement: Written informed consent has been obtained from the patient to publish this paper.

Data Availability Statement: Not applicable.

Acknowledgments: The authors appreciate helpful suggestions by Jeffrey B. Travers, Wright State University.

Conflicts of Interest: The authors declare no conflict of interest.

References

1. Idiculla, P.S.; Gurala, D.; Palanisamy, M.; Vijayakumar, R.; Dhandapani, S.; Nagarajan, E. Cerebral Venous Thrombosis: A Comprehensive Review. *Eur. Neurol.* **2020**, *83*, 369–379. [CrossRef] [PubMed]
2. Saposnik, G.; Barinagarrementeria, F.; Brown, R.D.; Bushnell, C.D.; Cucchiara, B.; Cushman, M.; DeVeber, G.; Ferro, J.; Tsai, F.Y. Diagnosis and management of cerebral venous thrombosis: A statement for healthcare professionals from the American Heart Association/American Stroke Association. *Stroke* **2011**, *42*, 1158–1192. [CrossRef]
3. Bousser, M.-G.; Ferro, J.M. Cerebral venous thrombosis: An update. *Lancet Neurol.* **2007**, *6*, 162–170. [CrossRef]

4. Ferro, J.M.; Canhão, P.; Stam, J.; Bousser, M.G.; Barinagarrementeria, F.; ISCVT Investigators. Prognosis of Cerebral Vein and Dural Sinus Thrombosis: Results of the International Study on Cerebral Vein and Dural Sinus Thrombosis (ISCVT). *Stroke* **2004**, *35*, 664–670. [CrossRef]
5. Ferro, J.M.; Canhão, P.; de Sousa, D.A. Cerebral venous thrombosis. *Presse Méd.* **2016**, *45*, e429–e450. [CrossRef]
6. Van Vlijmen, E.F.W.; Wiewel-Verschueren, S.; Monster, T.B.M.; Meijer, K. Combined oral contraceptives, thrombophilia and the risk of venous thromboembolism: A systematic review and meta-analysis. *J. Thromb. Haemost.* **2016**, *14*, 1393–1403. [CrossRef] [PubMed]
7. Amoozegar, F.; Ronksley, P.E.; Sauve, R.; Menon, B.K. Hormonal Contraceptives and Cerebral Venous Thrombosis Risk: A Systematic Review and Meta-Analysis. *Front. Neurol.* **2015**, *6*, 7. [CrossRef] [PubMed]
8. Lidegaard, Ø.; Løkkegaard, E.; Svendsen, A.L.; Agger, C. Hormonal contraception and risk of venous thromboembolism: National follow-up study. *BMJ* **2009**, *339*, b2890. [CrossRef]
9. De Bastos, M.; Stegeman, B.H.; Rosendaal, F.R.; Vlieg, A.V.H.; Helmerhorst, F.M.; Stijnen, T.; Dekkers, O.M. Combined oral contraceptives: Venous thrombosis. *Cochrane Database Syst. Rev.* **2014**, CD010813. [CrossRef] [PubMed]
10. Dentali, F.; Crowther, M.; Ageno, W. Thrombophilic abnormalities, oral contraceptives, and risk of cerebral vein thrombosis: A meta-analysis. *Blood* **2006**, *107*, 2766–2773. [CrossRef]
11. Porfidia, A.; Valeriani, E.; Pola, R.; Porreca, E.; Rutjes, A.W.; Di Nisio, M. Venous thromboembolism in patients with COVID-19: Systematic review and meta-analysis. *Thromb. Res.* **2020**, *196*, 67–74. [CrossRef]
12. Spratt, D.I.; Buchsbaum, R.J. COVID-19 and Hypercoagulability: Potential Impact on Management with Oral Contraceptives, Estrogen Therapy and Pregnancy. *Endocrinology* **2020**, *161*, bqaa121. [CrossRef] [PubMed]
13. Scully, M.; Singh, D.; Lown, R.; Poles, A.; Solomon, T.; Levi, M.; Goldblatt, D.; Kotoucek, P.; Thomas, W.; Lester, W. Pathologic Antibodies to Platelet Factor 4 after ChAdOx1 nCoV-19 Vaccination. *N. Engl. J. Med.* **2021**, *384*, 2202–2211. [CrossRef]
14. Schultz, N.H.; Sørvoll, I.H.; Michelsen, A.E.; Munthe, L.A.; Lund-Johansen, F.; Ahlen, M.T.; Wiedmann, M.; Aamodt, A.-H.; Skattør, T.H.; Tjønnfjord, G.E.; et al. Thrombosis and Thrombocytopenia after ChAdOx1 nCoV-19 Vaccination. *N. Engl. J. Med.* **2021**, *384*, 2124–2130. [CrossRef] [PubMed]
15. Muir, K.-L.; Kallam, A.; Koepsell, S.A.; Gundabolu, K. Thrombotic Thrombocytopenia after Ad26.COV2.S Vaccination. *N. Engl. J. Med.* **2021**, *384*, 1964–1965. [CrossRef] [PubMed]
16. Greinacher, A.; Thiele, T.; Warkentin, T.E.; Weisser, K.; Kyrle, P.A.; Eichinger, S. Thrombotic Thrombocytopenia after ChAdOx1 nCov-19 Vaccination. *N. Engl. J. Med.* **2021**, *384*, 2092–2101. [CrossRef]
17. See, I.; Su, J.R.; Lale, A.; Woo, E.J.; Guh, A.Y.; Shimabukuro, T.T.; Streiff, M.B.; Rao, A.K.; Wheeler, A.P.; Beavers, S.F.; et al. US Case Reports of Cerebral Venous Sinus Thrombosis with Thrombocytopenia after Ad26.COV2.S Vaccination, March 2 to April 21, 2021. *JAMA* **2021**, *325*, 2448–2456. [CrossRef]
18. Zakaria, Z.; Sapiai, N.A.; Ghani, A.R.I. Cerebral venous sinus thrombosis 2 weeks after the first dose of mRNA SARS-CoV-2 vaccine. *Acta Neurochir.* **2021**, *163*, 2359–2362. [CrossRef]
19. Dias, L.; Soares-Dos-Reis, R.; Meira, J.; Ferrão, D.; Soares, P.R.; Pastor, A.; Gama, G.; Fonseca, L.; Fagundes, V.; Carvalho, M. Cerebral Venous Thrombosis after BNT162b2 mRNA SARS-CoV-2 Vaccine. *J. Stroke Cerebrovasc. Dis.* **2021**, *30*, 105906. [CrossRef] [PubMed]
20. Fan, B.E.; Shen, J.Y.; Lim, X.R.; Tu, T.M.; Chang, C.C.R.; Khin, H.S.W.; Koh, J.S.; Rao, J.P.; Lau, S.L.; Tan, G.B.; et al. Cerebral venous thrombosis post BNT162b2 mRNA SARS-CoV-2 vaccination: A black swan event. *Am. J. Hematol.* **2021**, *96*, E357–E361. [CrossRef]
21. YYamaguchi, Y.; Kimihira, L.; Nagasawa, H.; Seo, K.; Wada, M. Cerebral Venous Sinus Thrombosis after BNT162b2 mRNA COVID-19 Vaccination. *Cureus* **2021**, *13*, e18775. [CrossRef]
22. Syed, K.; Chaudhary, H.; Donato, A. Central Venous Sinus Thrombosis with Subarachnoid Hemorrhage Following an mRNA COVID-19 Vaccination: Are These Reports Merely Co-Incidental? *Am. J. Case Rep.* **2021**, *22*, e933397. [CrossRef] [PubMed]
23. Nakagawa, I.; Okamoto, A.; Kotsugi, M.; Yokoyama, S.; Yamada, S.; Nakase, H. Endovascular mechanical thrombectomy for cerebral venous sinus thrombosis after mRNA-based SIRS-CoV-2 vaccination. *Interdiscip. Neurosurg.* **2022**, *30*, 101644. [CrossRef]
24. Park, J.; Park, M.-S.; Kim, H.J.; Song, T.-J. Association of Cerebral Venous Thrombosis with mRNA COVID-19 Vaccines: A Disproportionality Analysis of the World Health Organization Pharmacovigilance Database. *Vaccines* **2022**, *10*, 799. [CrossRef]
25. Jaiswal, V.; Nepal, G.; Dijamco, P.; Ishak, A.; Dagar, M.; Sarfraz, Z.; Shama, N.; Sarfraz, A.; Lnu, K.; Mitra, S.; et al. Cerebral Venous Sinus Thrombosis Following COVID-19 Vaccination: A Systematic Review. *J. Prim. Care Community Heal.* **2022**, *13*, 21501319221074450. [CrossRef]
26. Bonnar, J. Coagulation effects of oral contraception. *Am. J. Obstet. Gynecol.* **1987**, *157*, 1042–1048. [CrossRef]
27. Dakay, K.; Cooper, J.; Bloomfield, J.; Overby, P.; Mayer, S.A.; Nuoman, R.; Sahni, R.; Gulko, E.; Kaur, G.; Santarelli, J.; et al. Cerebral Venous Sinus Thrombosis in COVID-19 Infection: A Case Series and Review of The Literature. *J. Stroke Cerebrovasc. Dis.* **2020**, *30*, 105434. [CrossRef]
28. Ahmad, S.A.; Kakamad, F.H.; Mohamad, H.S.; Salih, B.K.; Mohammed, S.H.; Abdulla, B.A.; Salih, A.M. Post COVID-19 cerebral venous sinus thrombosis; a case report. *Ann. Med. Surg.* **2021**, *72*, 103031. [CrossRef] [PubMed]
29. Anipindi, M.; Scott, A.; Joyce, L.; Wali, S.; Morginstin, M. Case Report: Cerebral Venous Sinus Thrombosis and COVID-19 Infection. *Front. Med.* **2021**, *8*, 741594. [CrossRef] [PubMed]

30. Taquet, M.; Husain, M.; Geddes, J.R.; Luciano, S.; Harrison, P.J. Cerebral venous thrombosis and portal vein thrombosis: A retrospective cohort study of 537,913 COVID-19 cases. *Eclinicalmedicine* **2021**, *39*, 101061. [CrossRef]
31. McCullough-Hicks, M.E.; Halterman, D.J.; Anderson, D.; Cohen, K.; Lakshminarayan, K. High Incidence and Unique Features of Cerebral Venous Sinus Thrombosis in Hospitalized Patients with COVID-19 Infection. *Stroke* **2022**, *53*, e407–e410. [CrossRef] [PubMed]
32. Stam, J. Thrombosis of the Cerebral Veins and Sinuses. *N. Engl. J. Med.* **2005**, *352*, 1791–1798. [CrossRef] [PubMed]
33. Payne, A.B.; Adamski, A.; Abe, K.; Reyes, N.L.; Richardson, L.C.; Hooper, W.C.; Schieve, L.A. Epidemiology of cerebral venous sinus thrombosis and cerebral venous sinus thrombosis with thrombocytopenia in the United States, 2018 and 2019. *Res. Pract. Thromb. Haemost.* **2022**, *6*, e12682. [CrossRef] [PubMed]

Disclaimer/Publisher's Note: The statements, opinions and data contained in all publications are solely those of the individual author(s) and contributor(s) and not of MDPI and/or the editor(s). MDPI and/or the editor(s) disclaim responsibility for any injury to people or property resulting from any ideas, methods, instructions or products referred to in the content.

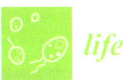

Article

Challenges in Cerebral Venous Thrombosis Management—Case Reports and Short Literature Review

Florentina Cristina Pleșa [1,2], Alina Jijie [1], Gabriela Simona Toma [3], Aurelian Emilian Ranetti [1,4,*], Aida Mihaela Manole [1], Ruxandra Rotaru [1], Ionuț Caloianu [1], Daniela Anghel [5,6] and Octaviana Adriana Dulămea [7,8]

1. Department of Neurology, "Dr. Carol Davila" Central Military Emergency University Hospital, 134 Calea Plevnei, 010242 Bucharest, Romania
2. Department of Preclinical Disciplines, "Titu Maiorescu" University, 031593 Bucharest, Romania
3. Department of Radiology, "Dr. Carol Davila" Central Military Emergency University Hospital, 010242 Bucharest, Romania
4. Department of Endocrinology, "Dr. Carol Davila" Central Military Emergency University Hospital, 010242 Bucharest, Romania
5. Department of Medico-Surgical and Prophylactic Disciplines, Faculty of Medicine, "Titu Maiorescu" University, 031593 Bucharest, Romania
6. Department of Internal Medicine, Central Military Emergency University Hospital, 010242 Bucharest, Romania
7. Neurology Department, Fundeni Clinical Institute, 022328 Bucharest, Romania
8. Neurology Department, Carol Davila University of Medicine and Pharmacy, 050474 Bucharest, Romania
* Correspondence: ranetti@gmail.com

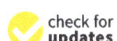

Citation: Pleșa, F.C.; Jijie, A.; Toma, G.S.; Ranetti, A.E.; Manole, A.M.; Rotaru, R.; Caloianu, I.; Anghel, D.; Dulămea, O.A. Challenges in Cerebral Venous Thrombosis Management—Case Reports and Short Literature Review. *Life* **2023**, *13*, 334. https://doi.org/10.3390/life13020334

Academic Editor: Jessica Mandrioli

Received: 25 November 2022
Revised: 7 January 2023
Accepted: 23 January 2023
Published: 26 January 2023

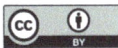

Copyright: © 2023 by the authors. Licensee MDPI, Basel, Switzerland. This article is an open access article distributed under the terms and conditions of the Creative Commons Attribution (CC BY) license (https:// creativecommons.org/licenses/by/ 4.0/).

Abstract: Cerebral venous thrombosis (CVT) is a rare type of stroke, with a complex clinical presentation that can make it a diagnostic challenge for the swift initiation of anticoagulation. When a hemorrhagic transformation is added, therapeutic management becomes even more complex. We describe a series of four cases, aged between 23 and 37 years old, with cerebral venous thrombosis. They were admitted to our clinic between 2014 and 2022. All cases presented significant challenges in either diagnostic, therapeutic or etiologic evaluation, at different stages of the disease. Late complications such as epilepsy or depression and other behavioral disorders represent long-term sequelae for the patient. Therefore, through its late complications, CVT is not only an acute disease but a chronic disorder with long-term follow-up requirements. The first case of the series is of a postpartum woman with focal neurological deficit caused by CVT with hemorrhagic transformation that presented multiple thrombotic complications and severe depression. The second case is of a man with extensive cerebral thrombosis who developed bilateral papillary edema under therapeutic anticoagulation treatment. The third case is of a woman with bilateral cavernous sinus thrombosis who later developed depressive disorder and focal seizures. The fourth case is of a pregnant woman in the first trimester presenting with a steep decline in consciousness level secondary to deep cerebral vein thrombosis requiring intensive care and subsequently developing a memory disorder. For a long period of time, due to being underdiagnosed, few things were known about CVT. Nowadays, we have all the tools to diagnose, treat, and follow up cases of CVT.

Keywords: cerebral venous thrombosis; pregnancy; seizure; postpartum; hemorrhage; depression

1. Introduction

Cerebral vein and dural sinus thrombosis (CVT) is one of the least frequent types of strokes, although it represents one of the most important causes of stroke in young adults, with an average age of 37 years old [1,2].

Epidemiologically, CVT has an annual incidence of 1.16 to 2.02 cases per 100,000 and is more frequent in females than males, with a ratio of 3:1 [2] due to the association with the use of oral contraceptives, pregnancy, and postpartum period. There are other prothrombotic factors involved such as thrombophilia, malignancy, and localized or systemic infections.

Thrombosis of the veins or venous sinuses, through the alteration of the blood–brain barrier and the reduction in CSF absorption, causes an increase in intracranial pressure (ICP). In 26% of patients, this can be the only manifestation of the onset of the disease, misguiding the diagnosis [2]. Sometimes the symptoms are complex and non-specific and further complicate the diagnosis which can be established using cerebral CT venography or MRI venography with contrast if MRI imaging is rapidly available [3].

The most common locations are at the level of the superficial venous sinuses and, frequently, several sinuses are involved. The treatment of acute CVT is primarily aimed at stopping the progression of the thrombus, restoring venous blood flow, and preventing thrombotic relapses.

With its myriad of clinical manifestations and challenging imaging diagnosis, CVT requires careful management, particularly in the treatment strategy. Overall, CVT has a favorable prognosis. However, it may sometimes be complicated by various, yet rare, coexistent pathologies such as focal deficits or altered state of consciousness and, in the long term, epileptic seizures or mental disorders [4].

In this article, we present four different cases that represented a diagnostic and therapeutic challenge in terms of symptoms, etiology, evolution, and complications.

2. Results

2.1. Case Presentation 1

A 23-year-old obese woman developed right-arm paresthesia followed by ipsilateral arm and leg weakness, as well as right-sided hemi-face paresthesia 4 days post-partum (cesarean delivery), complicated by pulmonary thromboembolism and deep vein thrombosis in the acute phase, long-term sequelae of moderate depression, and one severe episode of major depression, with an autolytic attempt 2 years later.

Regarding the pregnancy, she was a primigravida, with no miscarriages (spontaneous or medical) and no history of oral contraception use or smoking. The pregnancy had not been complicated, and the delivery by cesarean section was due to prolonged labor; subsequently, the mother and child took 4 days of antibiotics because of meconium contaminating the amniotic fluid. Her medical and family history were unremarkable.

Four days later, she was transferred to our clinic due to the development of neurological symptoms. The neurological exam showed a conscious and cooperative patient with no signs of meningeal irritation or right lateral homonymous hemianopsia and no other cranial nerve involvement, with right hemiparesis of 3/5 brachial on the Medical Research Council Scale (MRC) and 4/5 MRC crural, as well as hyperesthesia, brisk deep tendon reflexes, and a positive Babinski sign, all on the right side.

She underwent an unenhanced cerebral CT that revealed a parietal hypodensity with hemorrhagic transformation. (Figure 1).

Routine bloodwork at admission revealed a hypochromic microcytic anemia (iron deficiency) and an inflammatory syndrome (associating fever); microbiological examination of vaginal secretions came back positive for *Klebsiella pneumoniae* and *Escherichia coli*.

Therefore, she was started on antibiotics and supportive treatment. Throughout the course of the investigations, the patient was clinically stable.

The imaging aspect and the clinical picture of the patient made a positive diagnosis difficult. Due to her age, we had to look for the more common etiologies of stroke in a young patient. She underwent transthoracic and transesophageal echocardiography, in search of a patent foramen ovale or endocarditis, taking into account the recent history of infection. Both suspected diagnoses were disproven. We also looked for a collagen vascular disease (such as systemic lupus erythematous, antiphospholipid syndrome, ANCA-associated vasculitis, and large-vessel vasculitis), syphilis, and atrial fibrillation (24-h Holter monitor), but none of them came back positive. No arterial dissection or stenosis/occlusion was found at the cervical Doppler ultrasound and a tumor pathology or arteriovenous malformation was discussed; all these etiologies were later disproved.

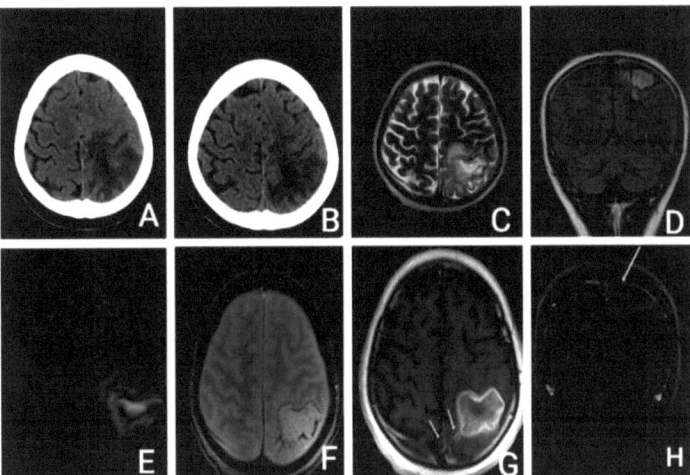

Figure 1. (**A**,**B**)—Unenhanced CT axial: (**A**)—acute parietal stroke with hemorrhagic transformation; (**B**)—9 days apart—Unenhanced head CT axial: subacute parietal stroke with hemorrhage resorption. (**C**–**H**): Brain MRI with and without contrast enhancement: (**C**)—T2 axial, (**D**)—FLAIR coronal, (**E**)—DWI axial, (**F**)—T2* hemo axial, (**G**)—T1 axial after i.v. contrast, (**H**)—T1 coronal after i.v. contrast. Ischemic area with hemorrhage transformation, hemosiderinic deposits mostly in periphery, central restricted diffusion and peripheral enhancement, filling defects of the sagittal venous sinus and of a cortical vein towards the affected left parietal area. CT—computer tomography; T1—weighed image; T2 weighted image; FLAIR—fluid attenuated inversion recovery; DWI—diffusion weighted imaging; T2* hemo—T2 weighted sequence.

The head CT scan, performed 9 days after admission, showed that the hemorrhage was in a resorptive stage. The diagnosis of CVT was then considered and contrast-enhanced cerebral MRI confirmed sagittal venous sinus thrombosis.

In the meantime, the patient started complaining of left ilioinguinal and lower leg pain with minimal left-leg swelling. She underwent lower-limb Doppler ultrasonography which revealed left ilio–femoral–popliteal thrombosis. She was then immediately transferred to the cardiovascular intensive care unit and was started on continuous i.v. heparin and close neurologic monitoring was initiated. Considering that she also had a progressive thrombocytosis, from 321 k/μL to 619 k/μL (with the lab reference values 140–440 k/μL) and iron deficiency, the risk–benefit balance was in favor of anticoagulation.

After six days under heparin treatment with therapeutic dose, she started to complain of interscapular pain and dyspnea with slight oxygen desaturation (SpO$_2$ 94%). She immediately underwent a chest–abdomen–pelvis contrast-enhanced CT that revealed moderate pulmonary embolism and a left inferior vena cava thrombosis (Figure 2). Having a high risk of cerebral bleeding and extensive deep vein thrombosis, the placement of a filter on the inferior vena cava was considered.

She was hospitalized for 40 days and discharged with a positive clinical and paraclinical outcome, with an improvement in motor deficits to 4/5 MRC right hemiparesis, and long-term acenocoumarol anticoagulation with target INR between 2 and 3.

The thrombophilia test, partially performed one year after the acute event, revealed positive results: antithrombin III deficit, low activated protein C resistance, and hyperhomocysteinemia, thus making her a candidate for chronic anticoagulation.

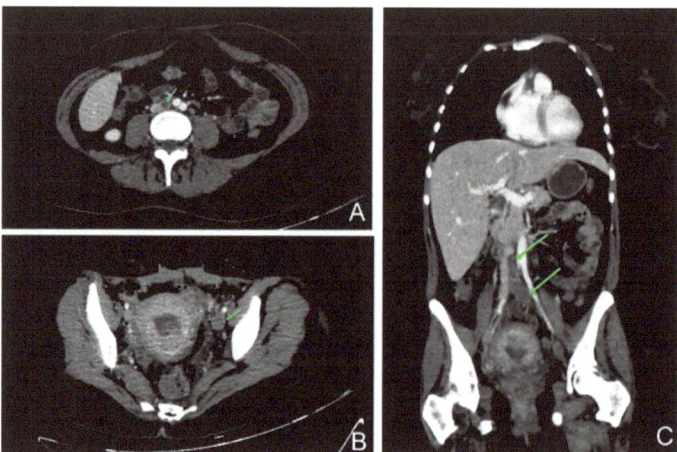

Figure 2. Contrast-enhanced thorax abdominal and pelvis CT: (**A**)—axial abdominal CT shows thrombus in inferior vena cava; (**B**)—axial pelvis CT reveals the extension of the thrombus in the left external iliac vein; (**C**)—coronal CT encompasses the length of the thrombus.

Close monitoring was performed after discharge, clinically, biologically, and radiologically. Three months after the CVT, she had completely recovered all her motor functions with the use of neurorehabilitation therapy. However, she developed symptoms of depression, for which she started receiving antidepressant medication. The brain MRI (Figure 3) showed the lesion as being chronic with the hemorrhage partially resolved at three months, with an aspect of organizing hematoma.

Three years later, she underwent another brain MRI (Figure 3) that showed a chronic ischemic left parietal lesion with partial peripheral gliosis and peripheral hemosiderin deposits.

However, her depression advanced to moderate, having had one severe episode. Following this event, she was closely managed psychiatrically with antidepressant treatment and psychotherapy. The depression was kept under control, with no further major or moderate episodes.

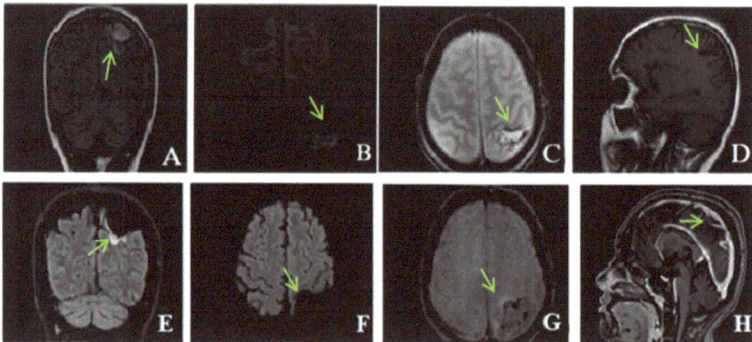

Figure 3. (**A–D**): Unenhanced brain MRI (at 3 months): (**A**)—Fluid attenuated inversion recovery (FLAIR) coronal, (**B**)—Diffusion-weighted imaging (DWI) axial, (**C**)—T2* hemo axial, (**D**)—T1 sagittal: Chronic ischemic left parietal lesion with hemorrhagic transformation partially resolved. E-H: Unenhanced and enhanced brain MRI (at six years): (**E**)—FLAIR coronal, (**F**)—DWI axial, (**G**)—T2* hemo axial, (**H**)—T1 sagittal after i.v. contrast administration: Chronic ischemic left parietal lesion with slightly peripheral gliosis, without restricted diffusion and minimal hemosiderin peripheral deposits, without filling defect of the veins and venous sinuses.

A follow-up brain MRI at six years showed the chronic lesion with no filling defect of cerebral veins and sinuses.

We also performed complete thrombophilia tests, including Factor V G1691A (Leiden), Factor V H1299R (R2), MTHFR C677T, MTHFR A1298C, Factor XIII V34L, PAI-1 4G/4G, Factor II G20210A and Endothelial Protein C Receptor (EPCR) A1/A2 coupled with serology for: Ac anti-cardiolipin IgG and IgM, Ac anti-Beta2 glycoprotein 1, Ac-anti phospholipid IgG and IgM, lupus anticoagulant, homocysteine, and protein C and S activity. The results came back positive for Factor V Leiden heterozygous and PAI-1 homozygous, having thrombophilia with a medium-to-high risk, with the subsequent need for chronic anticoagulation. She is still under acenocumarol therapy at the indication of the hematologist. She is no longer in need of antidepressants, while still attending her weekly psychotherapy.

2.2. Case Presentation 2

A 37-year-old overweight male patient with no past medical history presented with severe diffuse headache that started several days prior. The headache was refractory to usual analgesic medicine and got progressively worse. His wife recalled an episode of disorientation and slurred speech disturbance that lasted for a short period of time and stopped spontaneously. Upon arrival, vital signs were normal. The objective neurological examination was unremarkable.

In what concerns the laboratory blood testing, inflammatory markers had increased values. The ECG showed bradycardia at the beginning, with normalization afterward.

Native head CT performed at admission (Figure 4) showed increased dimensions of sinuses, and hyperdense content in the superior longitudinal sagittal sinus, the right sinus, and, contiguously, the inferior longitudinal sinus as well as in the right transverse sinus and partially the right sigmoid sinus. Additionally, a hyperdense appearance of the cerebellar tentorium raised the suspicion of a subarachnoid hemorrhage. The hypoattenuating brain tissue is suggestive of diffuse cerebral edema.

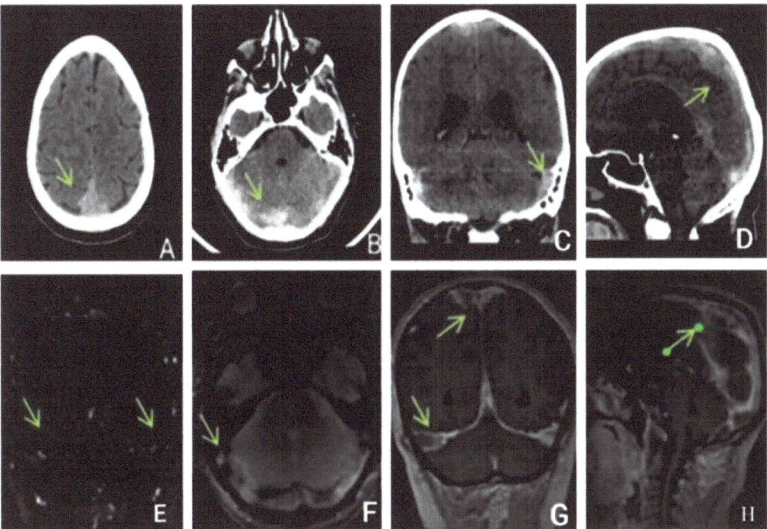

Figure 4. Unenhanced CT: (**A**,**B**)—axial, (**C**)—coronal, (**D**)—sagittal exhibits hyperdensity of the venous sinuses (sagittal superior and inferior, right sinus, transverse and sigmoid sinuses). (**E**–**H**) MRI, (**E**)—TOF (time of fligt angiography) venous coronal; (**F**)—T2*hemo axial, (**G**)—T1 coronal after i.v. contrast, (**H**)—T1 sagittal after i.v. contrast, expressed extensive thrombosis of all veins.

Blood samples were collected and tested for thrombophilia: lupus anticoagulant, antithrombin III levels, factor V Leiden levels and protein C and S levels did not have significant values. Afterwards, the anticoagulant treatment with unfractionated heparin in continuous perfusion was started.

Further investigations highlighted increased homocysteine levels (17,1 µmol/l—with normal range < 10 µmol/L) and normal Vitamin B12 values (195 pg/mL, normal range: 187–883 pg/mL) for which the hematological consultation recommended anticoagulant treatment in combination with vitB12 and folic acid.

Two days after admission, the patient underwent a contrast-enhanced brain MRI that showed extensive venous thrombosis at the level of the sagittal, transverse, and right sigmoid sinus with an increase in vascular caliber, absence of flow, and post-contrast filling defect. The association of fine bilateral high parietal subarachnoid hemorrhagic suffusions was also present, without constituted superficial parenchymal lesions. Inflammatory MRI signal changes at the level of the mastoids, frontal sinuses, and the ethmoidal cellular system were noticed, in keeping with pansinusitis.

The oral anticoagulant treatment was started with acenocoumarol, with a target INR range between 2 and 3. Clinically, the patient was stationary, without new complaints or neurological signs. Another brain MRI was performed after 9 days. Compared to the previous examination, this was showing a slightly improved appearance, with the corresponding thrombi at the level of the superior sagittal sinus being reduced.

With a favorable clinical evolution and stable desired INR, the patient was deemed medically fit for discharge after 20 days. Long-term acenocumarol treatment was prescribed and follow-up imaging and hematologic review at three months were booked.

Ten days after the discharge, he presented again to the emergency department with headache, dizziness, visual acuity disorders, and diplopia. Upon admission, an ophthalmological examination was performed, revealing bilateral papilledema. INR was within therapeutic limits (INR = 2.66). Given the symptomatology, a new angio-MRI was performed that showed improvement in thrombosis compared to the previous examination.

After three days of associated antiedematous treatment, the patient was discharged again with no further complaints.

The fluctuating symptomatology under anticoagulant treatment, in the context of an extensive cerebral venous thrombosis, in a patient with hyperhomocysteinemia recommends the continuation of the anticoagulant with clinical and imaging re-evaluation at one year.

At the one-year follow-up, the tests for thrombophilia were normal except for the maintenance of homocysteine at elevated values.

MRI reassessment was also performed which revealed T2 and FLAIR hypersignal, but no DWI signal of the right subcortical frontal structures—a spot of ischemic gliosis. Furthermore, parietal FLAIR and flow void signal of the transverse sinuses was present in keeping with chronic thrombosis.

2.3. Case Presentation 3

A 36-year-old, overweight, female patient with medically controlled hypertension as the sole known cardiovascular risk factor came to the emergency department for intense headaches at the level of the right hemicranium, predominantly fronto-orbital, associated with dizziness. The symptoms were refractory to treatment and started three days before presentation. After the debut, the headache significantly progressed in severity, being also accompanied by dizziness, diplopia, mild photophobia, nausea, and inconstant paresthesia in the right limbs, along with a hypertensive spike. The neurological examination identified right external rectus muscle paralysis, mild palpebral edema, and redness at the level of the eyeballs, predominantly on the right side, alongside dysarthria. The patient complained of diplopia on frontal and bilateral horizontal gaze. Otherwise, the exam was unremarkable, without fever. The contrast CT Head performed was found to be normal.

The ophthalmological examination showed no signs of papilledema. On the same day, a lumbar puncture was performed, with unremarkable results.

A brain MRI (Figure 5) showed flow asymmetry at the level of the cavernous sinuses, left more than right, coupled with fluid accumulation in the left mastoid cells, whilst cerebral parenchyma had morphology and signals within normal limits, thus establishing the diagnosis of bilateral (left > right) cavernous sinus thrombosis. The patient was started on continuous heparin infusion followed by treatment with acenocoumarol.

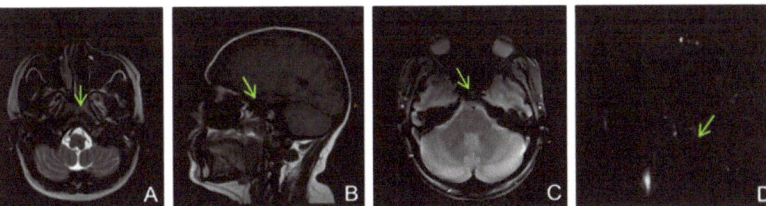

Figure 5. Non-enhanced MRI (at onset): ((**A**)—T2 axial, (**B**)—T1 sagittal, (**C**)—T2* axial, (**D**)—venous TOF coronal) shows unremarkable parenchyma and absence of flow in cavernous sinuses on TOF imagesFive months later, the patient came back to our clinic complaining of paroxysmal episodes of altered state of consciousness with language disorders such as verbal barrage followed by disorientation. An EEG was performed, showing a low-voltage background path, weakly modulated in spindles in the left derivations, reactive when opening the eyes, and rare isolated degraded peak-wave complexes, thus concluding that the patient was experiencing focal onset impaired awareness seizures; she was then started on antiepileptic treatment with oxcarbazepine 300 mg twice daily. She also was psychiatrically examined due to emotional lability confirming the diagnosis of depression and allowing antidepressant treatment to be started.

The six-month follow-up MRI identified persistent left maxillary sinusitis and cavernous sinus asymmetry but with an improved flow in the left one. Additionally, after 2 weeks of subcutaneous low-weight heparin, the panel for thrombophilia was requested and a protein C and S deficit was found, with the other tests (lupus anticoagulant, antithrombin III, factor V Leiden, IgM and IgG antiphospholipid antibodies, IgM and IgG anti-cardiolipin antibodies, IgM and IgG anti beta-2 glycoprotein I, p-ANCA, and c-ANCA) being within normal values. Thus, thrombophilia was diagnosed and the indication of lifelong anticoagulation established.

The patient continues to present a depressive disorder that improves under treatment and rare paroxysmal seizures with intermittent speech impairment. She was noted to be otherwise stable, with no further neurological sings.

2.4. Case Presentation 4

A 24-year-old woman in the seventh week of pregnancy was brought to the emergency department for a confusional syndrome onset in the morning of presentation.

As per her obstetrical history, she was a primigravida, with no miscarriages (spontaneous or medical) and no history of oral contraception use or smoking. Her medical history was unremarkable. Her sister had a full-term pregnancy, without complications and a spontaneous miscarriage in first trimester.

The patient presented an intense headache four days prior to the current admission, followed by dizziness and fatigue, for which she was investigated in an obstetrics–gynecology department and received symptomatic treatment.

She was admitted to our hospital with a heart rate of 98 bpm, in sinus rhythm, with a blood pressure of 180/100 mmHg, an oxygen saturation (SpO$_2$) of 99%, and a temperature of 36.9 Celsius.

The neurological exam showed a confused patient, with whom it was hard to cooperate. She was able to execute simple orders and had no signs of meningeal irritation, no cranial-nerve involvement, a bilateral Babinski sign, and was apparently without motor deficits.

Routine bloodwork at admission revealed slightly increased inflammation markers, without other abnormalities.

We decided to have an emergency MRI, but considering that the patient was pregnant, contrast was not used.

MRI showed (Figure 6) changes evoking venous thrombosis of left transverse and sigmoid sinuses, straight sinus, vein of Galen, internal cerebral and basal veins with extensive venous infarcts at the level of bilateral basal ganglia and a left temporo-occipital subcortical area.

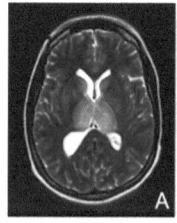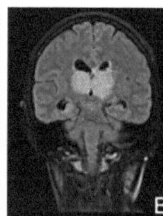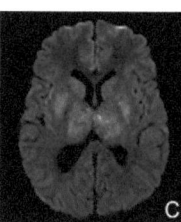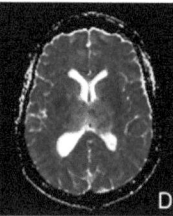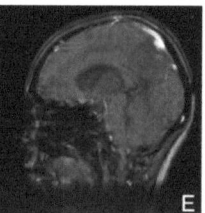

Figure 6. MRI without contrast enhancement ((**A**)—T2 axial, (**B**)—FLAIR coronal, (**C**)—DWI axial, (**D**)—ADC axial, (**E**)—venous TOF sagittal) shows hyperintensities of the thalamic nuclei on T2, FLAIR and DWI, with areas of restricted diffusion included and no flow in Galen's vein, internal cerebral veins, straight sinus, and inferior sagittal sinus.

She was admitted to the intensive care unit for continuous monitoring and started receiving anticoagulant and supportive treatment represented by continuous intravenous unfractionated heparin with flow adapted to the APTT value, isotonic fluids, vitamin therapy, physical therapy, pneumatic compression, and empiric antiviral therapy until encephalitis was excluded.

On the first day after admission, the patient's clinical condition deteriorated. She became febrile, presented episodes of drowsiness alternating with spontaneous wakefulness and psychomotor agitation, involuntary hyperextension movements at the thoracic level, bilateral grasping, and plantar clonus bilaterally, and she was only reacting to nociceptive stimuli. The ophthalmological examination ruled out papilledema. A lumbar puncture was performed, and the result was negative for bacteria and viruses. The thrombophilia profile tests were requested and were found to be positive for: homozygous V H129 R mutation, heterozygous PAI1 4G/5G, and homozygous MTHFR A 1289C mutation.

In the following days, the patient's condition continued to worsen. She did not respond to nociceptive stimuli, spontaneously mobilized her limbs, and had involuntary movements of the jaw. Considering the unfavorable and unpredictable evolution, in agreement with the family, we decided to perform therapeutic abortion. A new brain CT was performed (Figure 7).

Subsequently, with a decreasing Glasgow Coma Scale down to 5 points, the patient needed to be intubated and mechanically ventilated.

After a few days, her condition improved, leading to the patient's extubation. Then, she was transferred back to the neurology department.

In the meantime, the intravenous heparin therapy was switched to oral anticoagulant therapy—acenocoumarol. Prior to this, brain imaging was repeated and revealed minimal hemorrhagic transformation, but due to the patient's agitated state during the MRI, we could not achieve enhanced sequences.

Neurological evolution was slowly favorable. Clinical examination before hospital discharge showed a conscious and cooperative patient, without motor and sensory deficits, with memory impairment.

During hospitalization, the patient could not be cognitively evaluated because she was not always cooperative and had trouble focusing. Later, at the re-evaluation after 2 months, the MMSE and MOCA tests were performed, with a score of 29 and 25 points, respectively, which showed the persistence of a slight cognitive impairment.

Even if the pregnancy was in the first trimester, the association with coagulation disorders led to an increased risk of cerebrovascular phenomena.

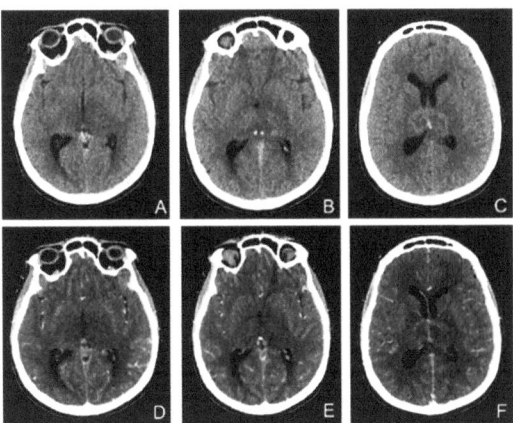

Figure 7. CT without contrast (**A–C**) and with (**D–F**) contrast enhancement shows hyperdensities in the Galen vein and internal cerebral veins with nonhomogeneous thalamic nuclei. After contrast enhancement, there was a slight enhancement in the veins and hypoperfusion of the thalamic nuclei.

3. Discussion

There are several risk factors, transient or permanent, that may increase the likelihood of developing cerebral venous thrombosis. Thrombophilia due to antithrombin III or protein C and S deficiency, mutation of factor V Leiden, or hyperhomocysteinemia are permanent risk factors. They are frequently "to blame" in young patients with cerebral venous thrombosis. They can also be incriminated in other situations, such as the ongoing pregnancy or other thrombotic complications such as deep vein thrombosis or pulmonary thromboembolisms. In these cases, and especially if no other associated risk factors are found, it is necessary to perform the thrombophilia genetic profile. It should be noted that mutations in the PAI-1 gene and protein Z are not considered a risk factor for cerebral venous thrombosis [2].

Air pollution is now identified as an independent risk factor for many diseases, including the neurological ones. Air pollution is held responsible for 30% of stroke cases in developing countries [5]. New studies are required to establish the relationship between this new risk factor and CVT.

In our cases, the thrombophilia state was identified through antithrombin III deficiency, respectively, protein C and S deficiency, while two patients had hyperhomocysteinemia. In the case of the pregnant patient, the homozygous mutation V H129 R, the heterozygous PAI-1 4G/5G, and the homozygous mutation MTHFR A 1289C were identified. The latter, being frequently present in the general population, only in association with other prothrombotic factors (especially hyperhomocysteinemia) can be considered of increased risk for CVT. Hyperhomocysteinemia is known to be harmful to endothelial cells and has atherosclerotic and prothrombotic effects. It has been correlated with higher cardiovascular mortality and stroke [6].

There are acquired prothrombotic conditions, such as the use of oral contraceptives, smoking, estrogen receptor modulators, pregnancy and puerperium, infections, malignancy, obesity or head trauma [2]. It is also common for the underlying etiology or risk factors not to be identified (37% of older adults), in which case, CVT is considered cryptogenic [2]. In the largest cohort study on CVT (624 patient), the risk factors for an unfavorable outcome were identified and included: male sex, age over 37 years, coma or mental status disorder, intracranial hemorrhage at onset, thrombosis of the deep cerebral venous system, infection of the central nervous system, and malignances [7].

It is necessary to state that women during puerperium are more susceptible to hypercoagulability conditions related to this period: pregnancy, caesarean section, massive bleeding, thrombocytosis, fluctuation of intracranial pressure during labor, and pre-eclampsia [8]. During pregnancy, the equilibrium state between the fibrinolytic and hemostatic systems changes in favor of the prothrombotic status to prevent major bleeding during pregnancy and delivery [9]. Thrombocytosis is caused by anemia associated with pregnancy and childbirth, which can cause thrombosis [10], several articles have shown a link between CVT and iron deficiency, with anemia playing a consistent role in the development of CVT [11].

Cesarean delivery increases the risk of venous thromboembolism by three times compared with vaginal delivery [12]. During pregnancy, the women develop resistance to protein C, in addition to losing it through surgery [13].

In the first case of the postpartum female, the onset and evolution of CVT were determined by the postpartum prothrombotic condition, aggravated by caesarean section. The complex profile of thrombophilia genetic status, along with the burden of temporary risk factors (anemia, genital infection, obesity, and limitation of mobilization) influenced the response to treatment and the appearance of multiple thrombotic complications.

The infectious state was present in most of the cases exposed, with localized infections being more frequent in our analysis: two cases with an infection in the field of otorhinolaryngology and the postpartum patient having a genital infection. The literature maintains the association with generalized infections as more common in the etiology of CVT. Infectious causes are responsible for only 6–12% of cerebral venous thromboses, with systemic infections being a more frequent cause than local infections (more commonly of the sinuses and mastoid, just as those encountered in our cases) [7].

The onset is frequently associated with signs of cranial hypertension (HIC): variable headaches (intense from the beginning or progressively worse); focal neurological signs or an altered state of consciousness, the latter appearing in up to 61.5% of patients, according to a study from 2007 [14]; and other signs and symptoms such as epileptic seizures (30–40%), papilledema (30–60%), focal motor deficits (30–50%), aphasia (15–20%), mental status disorder (15–25%), coma (5–15%), and movement disorders (rare) [15].

Three patients presented intense and persistent headaches; two of them complained of visual acuity disorder and the patient in the first case had focal onset symptoms similar to a stroke. The initial symptomatology of the pregnant patient (case 4) was with headaches, followed by the alteration of the state of consciousness. This raised the suspicion of cerebral thrombosis, being quickly diagnosed using the angio-MRI. In pregnant patients, the signs and symptoms of thrombosis are generally attributed to their status, as in the case of our patient, and can often cause a delay in the diagnosis and treatment.

MRI with venous TOF sequence is preferred; contrast enhancement is to be avoided in pregnant women with suspected CVT [16]. MRI angiography is superior to CT venography which has low sensitivity for cortical veins. Brain CT is the first intention investigation in which indirect signs such as the chord sign, the dense triangle sign, and the empty delta sign can be observed, and can associate hemorrhagic lesions, focal hypodensities or cerebral edema. In 30% of cases, the CT without enhancement can appear normal [17], as it was in one of the cases presented by us. DSA (digital subtraction angiography) has the highest diagnostic accuracy and is recommended when the basic techniques do not elucidate the diagnosis or when a dural fistula is suspected [3]. The ESO guidelines suggest MRI venography or CT venography to confirm the diagnosis of CVT.

Hemorrhagic transformation can complicate both an arterial stroke and a CVT stroke. In CVT, hemorrhages appeared as a result of increased intracranial pressure due to impaired venous return or the use of heparin used to treat CVT. These hemorrhagic stigmas can also be observed later on the SWI sequence of a brain MRI, with the sequelae of brain parenchyma lesions with hemorrhagic stigma being observed in two of our patients. An imaging feature related to non-hemorrhagic venous infarcts can appear on the follow-up CT, while some of the non-hemorrhagic lesions may disappear, a phenomenon known as "disappearing infarcts" [2].

The presence of the hemorrhagic lesions from the onset, in the first case, delayed the initiation of anticoagulant treatment in the therapeutic dose, putting in balance the risks and benefits, until the diagnosis was established. The association of deep venous thrombosis together with cerebral hemorrhage raised problems regarding the anticoagulant regimen, which could be counterbalanced by the enlarging cerebral hematoma.

Regarding the location of the thrombosis, it is specified to preferentially affect the large sinuses or the confluence of sinuses [7]. The most common locations of CVT occurrence according to the International Study on Cerebral Vein and Dural Sinus Thrombosis (ISCVT) are listed as: transverse sinus (86%), superior sagittal sinus (62%), straight sinus (18%), cortical veins (17%), jugular veins (12%), and vein of Galen and internal brain veins (11%) [14]. In general, there is an association between several sinuses or venous structures, an aspect also observed in our analysis. A study from 2019 mentions the involvement of multiple venous sinuses in 76% of cases, with left heart attacks being twice as frequent as right ones (36% versus 18%) [18]. In the vast majority of people, the cerebral veins on the right side are dominant; hence, an obstruction of the right transverse sinus will have a greater clinical impact [3].

The same reviews mention hemorrhagic transformation in 17.3% of CVT cases and 3.8% in intraparenchymal hemorrhage. Extensive vascular damage as well as the presence of bleeding worsens the prognosis through the severity of intracranial hypertension and the increased risk of complications.

The main objective of the treatment of cerebral venous thrombosis is to stop the progression of the thrombotic phenomenon with the restoration of the flow in the venous system and the prevention of recurrences. For this purpose, the anticoagulant treatment options differ and one can choose between continuous unfractionated heparin (UFH) or subcutaneous low-molecular-weight heparin (Enoxaparin) twice a day [19]. UFH requires dose adjustments based on APTT, this being short-lived, and the effect can be reversed with protamine sulfate. Meanwhile, the effect of Enoxaparin can be reversed only partially, and in a patient with severe renal failure, it is contra-indicated. Thus, the European Stroke Association Guideline recommends the use of enoxaparin instead of UFH, excluding situations in which the patient has renal failure or is likely to require neurosurgical intervention in the near future, or if the patient is pregnant or in the postpartum period [20].

The issue of using new oral anticoagulants for chronic post-CVT anticoagulation is still being studied [20]. The RE-SPECT CVT trial compared the risks and benefits of using warfarin and dabigatran and found both to be safe and without the recurrence of thromboembolic events [21]. A similar result was also obtained in a comparative study of rivaroxaban versus warfarin published in 2020 [22] after which there is no different significant efficiency and safety. A 2022 meta-analysis mentions that the use of direct-acting oral anticoagulants (DOAC) in CVT is as effective and safe as using vitamin K antagonists, with a better recanalization rate in favor of DOAC, but requires prospective randomized studies for confirmation [23]. In addition, due to their targeted effect in the coagulation cascade, compared to Warfarin, they also have the advantage of a much lower risk of hemorrhagic complications. These observations were mentioned in comparative studies performed on patients with symptomatic deep vein thrombosis [24]. Without imposing dietary restrictions, with a reduced number of drug interactions, a constant therapeutic concentration, and no need for periodic monitoring as required by vitamin K antagonists, DOAC gives them multiple advantages and, through that, increases the compliance as well. In addition, the existence of a specific medication to reverse the effect of DOACs increases their safety even in the event of acute complications such as hemorrhage, emergency surgeries, or ischemic stroke in a therapeutic window [25]. New clinical trials are needed to analyze their benefits and risks in cerebral venous thrombosis, thus contributing to the development of the next guidelines.

However, the European Stroke Association Guideline, published before the results of these studies, does not recommend the use of oral anticoagulants (thrombin or factor Xa inhibitors) for the prevention or treatment of the acute phase of CVT (ESO 2017). The use of a vitamin K antagonist is recommended for 3 to 12 months after acute CVT [19].

Regarding hemorrhagic complications of CVT, nowadays, the same guideline recommends the initiation of anticoagulant treatment in the therapeutic dose, regardless of the presence of bleeding, with close clinical and paraclinical monitoring [20].

We noticed that although the patients were under effective anticoagulant treatment, three of them presented clinical fluctuations, different thrombosis ages, and extracerebral thrombotic events. A possible explanation is the summation of thrombophilia risk factors (possibly in association with homocysteine increase) in addition to an inflammatory response to an infectious background that could lead to neurologic fluctuations.

The first episode of CVT with transient risk factors requires ACO treatment for three to six months (six to twelve months if cryptogenic). The presence of properly diagnosed thrombophilia (at a distance from temporary conditions that can change the real values) requires permanent anticoagulant treatment.

In the case of a patient with permanent risk factors (genetic thrombophilia), the oral anticoagulation treatment is administered continuously. Case number four is on a two-month course of anticoagulant treatment and was to return in three months for a new clinical imaging and thrombophilia reassessment to decide the indication of anticoagulants.

The vast majority of patients require anticoagulant treatment for a minimum of 3 to a maximum of 12 months, but in the four cases presented, three of them required chronic anticoagulant treatment due to the type of thrombophilia and the risk associated with it [15].

The following studies, as well as the following guide regarding CVT, should offer recommendations regarding the possibility of using the new oral anticoagulants, taking into account the aspect identified in the three cases (the need for permanent anticoagulation).

Additionally, future studies/guides should take into account the conclusions of the study led by Mrs. Aguiar de Sousa et al. (2020), namely the fact that venous recanalization begins in the first 8 days and that the age of the patient must also be taken into account, so as to reduce the hemorrhagic risks associated with anticoagulant therapy [26]. Pathogenic therapy is combined with symptomatic and risk factor therapy, which imposes the long-term therapy of CVT. It should be noted that anticonvulsant therapy should not be recommended as a preventive measure and if it is necessary, it is recommended to choose a medication that does not interfere with the anticoagulant medication. These patients will be clinically and paraclinical monitored under anticonvulsant treatment for a minimum of one year [27].

Complications are relatively rare and can be grouped into acute or chronic. Acute complications are venous infarction and/or hemorrhage, subarachnoid hemorrhage, pulmonary thromboembolism, motor or language deficits, rapid progressive deterioration of mental status or coma, or in cavernous sinus involvement, Korsakoff-like amnestic syndrome with confabulation, bilateral temporal lobe infarction, inadequate antidiuretic hormone secretion, and blindness. Hemorrhagic complications were present in two of the patients, alongside the rapid alteration of the state of consciousness in case 4: that of the pregnant woman who required the rapid intervention of intensive care.

The most common chronic complications are arterio-venous fistulas, epilepsy, and psychiatric complications (cognitive impairments, depression, and anxiety) [4,28].

Neurological deficits, such as paresis or slurred speech, can also persist if the venous damage has also caused damage to the brain parenchyma, which deprives these functions.

Regarding the long-term complications of cerebral venous thrombosis, we also draw attention to the fact that depression can be a chronic complication of CVT [4] and various other behavioral disorders can occur, depending on the site, resulting in a significant burden for the patient and their family if not treated and closely monitored. Although in most cases neurological recovery after cerebral thrombosis is very good, depression and anxiety occur frequently between 1/3 and 2/3 of the cases [29].

Post-stroke depression, an emotional incontinence, is strongly influenced by lesion location, probably associated with the chemical neuroanatomy related to the frontal/temporal lobe–basal ganglia–ventral brainstem circuitry. Michaela C et al. reported that hyperhomocysteinemia is correlated with an increased risk of clinical depression. Depression is the most prevalent psychiatric complication among stroke survivors. Post-stroke depression is correlated with reduced motor function and poorer outcome [30].

Abulia, executive deficits, and amnesia may result from thrombosis of the deep venous system, causing bilateral thalamic infarcts. Recovery is variable, but memory deficits, behavioral problems, or executive deficits may persist [31]. Regarding case four, we noticed behavioral disorders such as quickly abandoning a just-started activity and lack of patience. Patients should be encouraged to return to previous occupations and hobbies.

In case one, the patient with the hemorrhagic left parietal lesion, the depression after CVT was severe without finding a correlation between the affected brain aria and its specific syndrome. We mention that the patient had no previous depression. A study on depression and its relation to lesion location after stroke reported an association between lesions on the right hemisphere, particularly the anterior region and depression [31]. Another 2010 study of six patients with depression and suicide attempts after stroke found that five of them had moderate neurological deficits; moreover, in five cases, lesions were identified at the temporo-parietal cortex level, with dominance slightly on the left side (three versus two), but without statistical significance. There was no evidence of hemorrhagic transformation in any of the cases [32].

The patient with a longer evolution of CVT at the level of the cavernous sinuses developed depression and later focal convulsions.

One in ten patients may have late seizures after a CVT [33]. According to the International Epilepsy League, we can diagnose epilepsy after one unprovoked seizure if there are specific conditions that imply a 60% or higher risk of developing subsequent epilepsy, which was the case in our third patient, who presented not only interictal discharge on their EEG, but also a favorable factor—CVT [34].

In the last case reported with the dominant acute symptomatology of the altered state of consciousness and memory disorders, we observed an improvement in cognitive deficits at the evaluation after 2 months. A psychological assessment of each type of cognitive function will bring us additional data in the future. The long-term follow-up of this patient should particularly take notice of focusing difficulties and behavioral impairment.

We thought it important to draw attention to depression as a potentially life-threatening complication of CVT. The identification of additional risk factors and the rigorous neuropsychiatric monitoring of these patients are essential in the ad vitam prognosis.

Further investigations studying the pathophysiological correlations between cerebral venous thrombosis lesions and psychiatric complications could lead to their prevention and appropriate management.

The prognosis of patients with CVT is generally favorable and depends on the speed of diagnosis and treatment. Complete clinical recovery is achieved in approximately 75% of cases, but there is also the risk of residual neurological deficit or death (15%) [7].

The CVT-GS grading scale can be used to calculate outcome prediction after a CVT (Table 1). In our cases, the score was as follows: case 1–5 points, moderate CVT with a 30-day mortality rate of 9.9%; case 2–2 points, mild CV with a 30-day mortality rate of 0.4%; case 3–0 points, mild CVT with a 30-day mortality rate of 0.4%; and case 4–11 points, severe CVT with 30-day mortality of 61.4% [35].

Negative prognostic factors are represented by intracranial hemorrhage, male sex, CVT outside of pregnancy, puerperium, or the use of oral contraceptives, and were present in three of our patients. In the literature, it is mentioned that in 85% of cases, they have at least one risk factor present [36,37].

The risk of recurrence of any other thrombotic event after a CVT is approximately 6.5%, and most recurrences appear in the first year [38] after the thrombotic event. Men tend to have a worse recovery compared to women: 81% of women will have a full recovery, while men only 71% of them. Severe and mild thrombophilia are the most important relapse risk factors (four times higher). Mild thrombophilia is considered to be one of the following: heterozygous factor V Leiden and prothrombin G20210A mutation, while protein C, S and antithrombin III deficiencies, antiphospholipid antibodies, and homozygous factor V Leiden are considered to be a severe form of thrombophilia [29]. The risk of recurrence was also increased in patients who stopped anticoagulant treatment early [39].

Table 1. CVT-GCS Scale—Risk of mortality at 30 days calculated for each case presented.

CVT-GS Scale	Case 1	Case 2	Case 3	Case 4
Parenchymal lesion > 6cm—3pt	3	0	0	3
Bilateral Babinski sign—3pt	0	0	0	3
Male sex—2pt	0	2	0	0
Parenchymal hemorrhage—2pt	2	0	0	2
Level of consciousness - Coma 3pt - Stupor 2pt - Alert 0pt	0	0	0	3
TOTAL	5	2	0	11
30-day case fatality	9.9%	0.4%	0.4%	61.4%

The 2017 ESO guideline does not recommend screening for thrombophilia in order to prevent recurrences or improve the prognosis; yet, in patients with a high probability of having thrombophilia, it can be considered. This category includes a patient's high pre-test probability to suffer from a severe form of it, young age at the onset of CVT, no other risk factors, and personal or family history of a form of venous thrombosis.

Based on the available evidence, CVT is not a contraindication for future pregnancies, but if a prothrombotic condition or a previous thrombotic event exists, antithrombotic prophylaxis is necessary during pregnancy and in the puerperium period.

4. Conclusions

The association of multiple risk factors in the case of cerebral venous thrombosis determines a negative prognosis and unexpected late complications. The presence of bleeding at the onset makes it difficult to establish a quick diagnosis and the therapeutic decision balances risk–benefit, requiring close monitoring. An anticoagulant treatment, even in the therapeutic dose, may not offer safe protection for the development or occurrence of other thrombotic complications. The recurrences and severity of CVT encountered in real life can determine new directions of study regarding the identification of additional risk factors involved as well as conditions that determine the choice of a certain type of anticoagulant. The successful management of CVT depends on the rapidity of the etiological diagnosis and the promptness of the therapy in the acute phase, coupled with the careful monitoring of the patient to prevent or intervene immediately in case of acute or chronic complications. Epilepsy, depression, or cognitive impairment are complications in the evolution of patients requiring close monitoring to prevent unpredictable behavior.

Author Contributions: Conceptualization, F.C.P. and D.A.; methodology, F.C.P.; software, I.C.; validation, F.C.P., I.C., A.E.R. and O.A.D.; formal analysis, F.C.P., A.E.R. and D.A.; investigation, F.C.P., R.R. and D.A.; resources, F.C.P., A.J. and G.S.T.; data curation, F.C.P., G.S.T. and D.A.; writing—original draft preparation, F.C.P., A.J., A.M.M. and D.A.; writing—review and editing, A.J., A.E.R., R.R. and O.A.D.; visualization, I.C and O.A.D.; supervision, F.C.P. and O.A.D.; project administration, G.S.T.; funding acquisition, A.M.M. All authors have read and agreed to the published version of the manuscript.

Funding: This research received no external funding.

Institutional Review Board Statement: The study was conducted according to the guidelines of the Declaration of Helsinki and approved by the Ethics Commission of "Dr. Carol Davila" Central Military Emergency University Hospital Nr 544/16.09.2022.

Informed Consent Statement: Informed consent was obtained from all subjects involved in the study.

Data Availability Statement: Third-party data restrictions apply to the availability of these data. The data were obtained from "Dr. Carol Davila" Central Military Emergency University Hospital Bucharest and are available from the authors with the permission of the Institutional Ethics Committee of Clinical Studies of the "Dr. Carol Davila" Central Military Emergency University Hospital Bucharest.

Conflicts of Interest: The authors declare no conflict of interest.

References

1. Ulivi, L.; Squitieri, M.; Cohen, H.; Cowley, P.; Werring, D.J. Cerebral venous thrombosis: A practical guide. *Pract. Neurol.* **2020**, *20*, 356–367. [CrossRef] [PubMed]
2. Ferro, J.C.P. *Cerebral Venous Thrombosis: Etiology, Clinical Features, and Diagnosis*; Post, T.W., Ed.; UpToDate; UpToDate Inc.: Waltham, MA, USA, 2022; Available online: https://www.uptodate.com/contents/cerebral-venous-thrombosis-etiology-clinical-features-and-diagnosis (accessed on 2 October 2022).
3. Jianu, D.C.; Jianu, S.N.; Dan, T.F.; Munteanu, G.; Copil, A.; Birdac, C.D.; Motoc, A.G.M.; Axelerad, A.D.; Petrica, L.; Arnautu, S.F.; et al. An Integrated Approach on the Diagnosis of Cerebral Veins and Dural Sinuses Thrombosis (a Narrative Review). *Life* **2022**, *12*, 717. [CrossRef] [PubMed]
4. Siddiqui, F.M.; Kamal, A.K. Complications associated with cerebral venous thrombosis. *J. Pak. Med. Assoc.* **2006**, *56*, 547–551.
5. Sîrbu, C.A.; Stefan, I.; Dumitru, R.; Mitrica, M.; Manole, A.M.; Vasile, T.M.; Stefani, C.; Ranetti, A.E. Air Pollution and Its Devastating Effects on the Central Nervous System. *Healthcare* **2022**, *10*, 1170. [CrossRef]
6. Anghel, D.; Sîrbu, C.A.; Hoinoiu, E.-M.; Petrache, O.-G.; Pleşa, C.-F.; Negru, M.M.; Ioniţă-Radu, F. Influence of anti-TNF therapy and homocysteine level on carotid intima-media thickness in rheumatoid arthritis patients. *Exp. Ther. Med.* **2022**, *23*, 59. [CrossRef] [PubMed]
7. Ferro, J.M.; Canhão, P.; Stam, J.; Bousser, M.G.; Barinagarrementeria, F.; ISCVT Investigators. Prognosis of cerebral vein and dural sinus thrombosis: Results of the International Study on Cerebral Vein and Dural Sinus Thrombosis (ISCVT). *Stroke* **2004**, *35*, 664–670. [CrossRef]
8. Florea, A.A.; Sirbu, C.A.; Ghinescu, M.C.; Plesa, C.F.; Sirbu, A.M.; Mitrica, M.; Ionita-Radu, F. SARS-CoV-2, multiple sclerosis, and focal deficit in a postpartum woman: A case report. *Exp. Ther. Med.* **2022**, *21*, 92. [CrossRef]
9. Ferro, J.M.; Coutinho, J.M.; Dentali, F.; Kobayashi, A.; Alasheev, A.; Canhão, P.; Karpov, D.; Nagel, S.; Posthuma, L.; Roriz, J.M.; et al. Safety and Efficacy of Dabigatran Etexilate vs. Dose-Adjusted Warfarin in Patients With Cerebral Venous Thrombosis: A Randomized Clinical Trial. *JAMA Neurol.* **2019**, *76*, 1457–1465. [CrossRef]
10. Coutinho, J.M.; Zuurbier, S.M.; Gaartman, A.E.; Dikstaal, A.A.; Stam, J.; Middeldorp, S.; Cannegieter, S.C. Association Between Anemia and Cerebral Venous Thrombosis: Case-Control Study. *Stroke* **2015**, *46*, 2735–2740. [CrossRef]
11. Ezeh, E.; Katabi, A.; Khawaja, I. Iron Deficiency Anemia as a Rare Risk Factor for Recurrent Pulmonary Embolism and Deep Vein Thrombosis. *Cureus* **2021**, *13*, e13721. [CrossRef]
12. Blondon, M.; Skeith, L. Preventing Postpartum Venous Thromboembolism in 2022: A Narrative Review. *Front. Cardiovasc. Med.* **2022**, *9*, 886416. [CrossRef] [PubMed]
13. Walker, M.C.; Garner, P.R.; Keely, E.J.; Rock, G.A.; Reis, M.D. Changes in activated protein C resistance during normal pregnancy. *Am. J. Obstet. Gynecol.* **1997**, *177*, 162–169. [CrossRef] [PubMed]
14. Bousser, M.-G.; Ferro, J.M. Cerebral venous thrombosis: An update. *Lancet Neurol.* **2007**, *6*, 162–170. [CrossRef] [PubMed]
15. Silvis, S.M.; de Sousa, D.A.; Ferro, J.M.; Coutinho, J.M. Cerebral venous thrombosis. *Nat. Rev. Neurol.* **2017**, *13*, 555–565. [CrossRef] [PubMed]
16. American College of Obstetricians and Gynecologists. Committee Opinion No. 723: Guidelines for Diagnostic Imaging during Pregnancy and Lactation. *Obstet. Gynecol.* **2017**, *130*, e210–e216. [CrossRef]
17. Chiras, J.; Bousser, M.G.; Meder, J.-F.; Koussa, A.; Bories, J. CT in cerebral thrombophlebitis. *Neuroradiology* **1985**, *27*, 145–154. [CrossRef]
18. Saroja, A.O.; Thorat, N.N.; Naik, K.R. Depression and quality of life after cerebral venous sinus thrombosis. *Ann. Indian Acad. Neurol.* **2019**, *23*, 487–490. [CrossRef]
19. Ferro, J.C.P. *Cerebral Venous Thrombosis: Treatment and Prognosis*; Post, T.W., Ed.; UpToDate; UpToDate Inc.: Waltham, MA, USA, 2022; Available online: https://www.uptodate.com/contents/cerebral-venous-thrombosis-treatment-and-prognosis (accessed on 2 October 2022).

20. Ferro, J.M.; Bousser, M.-G.; Canhão, P.; Coutinho, J.M.; Crassard, I.; Dentali, F.; di Minno, M.; Maino, A.; Martinelli, I.; Masuhr, F.; et al. European Stroke Organization guideline for the diagnosis and treatment of cerebral venous thrombosis—Endorsed by the European Academy of Neurology. *Eur. Stroke J.* **2017**, *2*, 195–221. [CrossRef]
21. Bajko, Z.; Motatainu, A.; Stoian, A.; Barcutean, L.; Andone, S.; Maier, S.; Drăghici, I.-A.; Balasa, R. Postpartum Cerebral Venous Thrombosis—A Single-Center Experience. *Brain Sci.* **2021**, *11*, 327. [CrossRef]
22. Maqsood, M.; Khan, M.I.H.; Yameen, M.; Ahmed, K.A.; Hussain, N.; Hussain, S. Use of oral rivaroxaban in cerebral venous thrombosis. *J. Drug Assess.* **2020**, *10*, 1–6. [CrossRef] [PubMed]
23. Nepal, G.; Kharel, S.; Bhagat, R.; Shing, Y.K.; Coghlan, M.A.; Poudyal, P.; Ojha, R.; Shrestha, G.S. Safety and efficacy of Direct Oral Anticoagulants in cerebral venous thrombosis: A meta-analysis. *Acta Neurol. Scand.* **2022**, *145*, 10–23. [CrossRef] [PubMed]
24. Hokusai-VTE Investigators; Büller, H.R.; Décousus, H.; Grosso, M.A.; Mercuri, M.; Middeldorp, S.; Prins, M.H.; Raskob, G.E.; Schellong, S.M.; Schwocho, L.; et al. Edoxaban versus warfarin for the treatment of symptomatic venous thromboembolism. *NEJM* **2013**, *369*, 1406–1415.
25. Pleșa, C.F.; Nicolae, C.; Sirbu, C.A.; Nemeș, R.O.X.A.N.A.; Păunescu, A.L.I.N.A.; Țânțu, M.M. Use of anticoagulants in cerebral vascular pathology. *Farmacia* **2019**, *67*, 27–33. [CrossRef]
26. De Sousa, D.A.; Neto, L.L.; Arauz, A.; Sousa, A.L.; Gabriel, D.; Correia, M.A.; Gil-Gouveia, R.; Penas, S.; Dias, M.C.; Carvalho, M.; et al. Early Recanalization in Patients With Cerebral Venous Thrombosis Treated With Anticoagulation. *Stroke* **2020**, *51*, 1174–1181. [CrossRef] [PubMed]
27. Lewis, S.L. CONTINUUM: Lifelong Learning in Neurology. 22 - Volume 28 – Issue 2. *Epilepsy* **2022**, *28*, 228–229. [CrossRef]
28. Ferro, J.M.; Aguiar de Sousa, D. Cerebral Venous Thrombosis: An Update. *Curr. Neurol. Neurosci. Rep.* **2019**, *19*, 74. [CrossRef]
29. Ferro, J.M.; Canhão, P. Complications of Cerebral Vein and Sinus Thrombosis. *Handb. Cereb. Venous Thromb.* **2008**, *23*, 161–171.
30. Lindén, T.; Blomstrand, C.; Skoog, I. Depressive disorders after 20 months in elderly stroke patients: A case-control study. *Stroke* **2007**, *38*, 1860–1863. [CrossRef]
31. MacHale, S.M.; O'Rourke, S.J.; Wardlaw, J.M.; Dennis, M.S. Depression and its relation to lesion location after stroke. *J. Neurol. Neurosurg. Psychiatry* **1998**, *64*, 371–374. [CrossRef]
32. Katayama, M.; Naritomi, H.; Oomura, M.; Nukata, M.; Yamamoto, S.; Araki, K.; Kato, H.; Kinoshita, M.; Ito, T.; Shimode, A.; et al. Case reports of unexpected suicides in patients within six months after stroke. *Kobe J. Med. Sci.* **2011**, *56*, E184–E194.
33. van Kammen, M.S.; Lindgren, E.; Silvis, S.M.; Hiltunen, S.; Heldner, M.R.; Serrano, F.; Zelano, J.; Zuurbier, S.M.; Mansour, M.; de Sousa, D.A.; et al. Late seizures in cerebral venous thrombosis. *Neurology* **2020**, *95*, e1716–e1723. [CrossRef] [PubMed]
34. Fisher, R.S.; Acevedo, C.; Arzimanoglou, A.; Bogacz, A.; Cross, J.H.; Elger, C.E.; Engel, J., Jr.; Forsgren, L.; French, J.A.; Glynn, M.; et al. ILAE Official Report: A practical clinical definition of epilepsy. *Epilepsia* **2014**, *55*, 475–482. [CrossRef] [PubMed]
35. Barboza, M.A.; Chiquete, E.; Arauz, A.; Merlos-Benitez, M.; Quiroz-Compeán, A.; Barinagarrementería, F.; Cantú-Brito, C. A Practical Score for Prediction of Outcome After Cerebral Venous Thrombosis. *Front. Neurol.* **2018**, *9*, 882. [CrossRef] [PubMed]
36. Martinelli, I.; Bucciarelli, P.; Passamonti, S.M.; Battaglioli, T.; Previtali, E.; Mannucci, P.M. Long-Term Evaluation of the Risk of Recurrence After Cerebral Sinus-Venous Thrombosis. *Circulation* **2010**, *121*, 2740–2746. [CrossRef]
37. Miranda, B.; Ferro, J.M.; Canhão, P.; Stam, J.; Bousser, M.G.; Barinagarrementeria, F.; Scoditti, U. ISCVT Investigators Venous thromboembolic events after cerebral vein thrombosis. *Stroke* **2010**, *41*, 1901–1906. [CrossRef]
38. Gosk-Bierska, I.; Wysokinski, W.; Brown, R.D., Jr.; Karnicki, K.; Grill, D.; Wiste, H.; Wysokinska, E.; McBane, R.D., II. Cerebral venous sinus thrombosis: Incidence of venous thrombosis recurrence and survival. *Neurology* **2006**, *67*, 814–819. [CrossRef]
39. Saposnik, G.; Barinagarrementeria, F.; Brown, R.D., Jr.; Bushnell, C.D.; Cucchiara, B.; Cushman, M.; deVeber, G.; Ferro, J.M.; Tsai, F.Y.; American Heart Association Stroke Council and the Council on Epidemiology and Prevention. Diagnosis and management of cerebral venous thrombosis: A statement for healthcare professionals from the American Heart Association/American Stroke Association. *Stroke* **2011**, *42*, 1158–1192. [CrossRef] [PubMed]

Disclaimer/Publisher's Note: The statements, opinions and data contained in all publications are solely those of the individual author(s) and contributor(s) and not of MDPI and/or the editor(s). MDPI and/or the editor(s) disclaim responsibility for any injury to people or property resulting from any ideas, methods, instructions or products referred to in the content.

MDPI AG
Grosspeteranlage 5
4052 Basel
Switzerland
Tel.: +41 61 683 77 34

Life Editorial Office
E-mail: life@mdpi.com
www.mdpi.com/journal/life

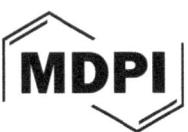

Disclaimer/Publisher's Note: The title and front matter of this reprint are at the discretion of the Guest Editors. The publisher is not responsible for their content or any associated concerns. The statements, opinions and data contained in all individual articles are solely those of the individual Editors and contributors and not of MDPI. MDPI disclaims responsibility for any injury to people or property resulting from any ideas, methods, instructions or products referred to in the content.

www.ingramcontent.com/pod-product-compliance
Lightning Source LLC
LaVergne TN
LVHW072357090526
838202LV00019B/2565